Population Health:

Management, Policy, and Technology

First Edition

EXECUTIVE EDITORS

Robert J. Esterhay | LaQuandra S. Nesbitt
James H. Taylor | H.J. Bohn, Jr.

FOREWORD BY
David B. Nash

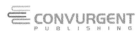
CONVURGENT
PUBLISHING

D0920806

Praise for Population Health: Management, Policy, and Technology

This book provides a refreshing and long overdue link among technology, management and policy – the critical components of leadership required to improve population health – and applies these to the most pressing health challenges we face in aging, chronic illness, mental health and health systems reform. Brilliant!

Donna J. Petersen, ScD, MHS, CPH
Interim Senior Vice President, USF Health
Dean, College of Public Health
Professor of Global Health
University of South Florida, Tampa, Florida

The book takes a comprehensive approach to addressing how best to tackle the increasingly diverse landscape affecting the health of communities, and presents examples that readers from multiple sectors would do well to read and incorporate into their thinking since reconnecting public health knowledge and practice and care delivery isn't the no-brainer it should be.

Pierre N.D. Vigilance, MD, MPH
Associate Dean for Public Health Practice, Milken Institute School of Public Health
The George Washington University, Washington, DC
Former Director District of Columbia Department of Health
Former Director Baltimore County Health Department
Former Assistant Commissioner Baltimore City Health Department

To my knowledge, no other work examines the topic of population health with this level of detail, rigor, and clarity. This book comes at just the right time, as we recognize the urgency of shifting our thinking from patient-centered to "citizen-centered" policies to improve the health of communities. This book will prove invaluable to anyone undertaking this work.

Steven H. Woolf, MD, MPH
Director, VCU Center on Society and Health
Professor, Department of Family Medicine and Population Health
Virginia Commonwealth University School of Medicine
Richmond, Virginia

Praise for Population Health (cont.)

This book is for those cross-sector leaders needed to build the bridge between health and health care. It addresses some of the major challenges to improving the health of individuals and communities. Spot on.

Stephen M. Shortell, PhD, MPH, MBA
Blue Cross of California Distinguished Professor of Health policy and Management
Dean Emeritus, School of Public Health
Professor of Organizational Behavior, Haas School of Business
UC-Berkeley

This timely volume provides a marvelous opportunity for health professionals and the public to understand the evolving issues at the intersection of health policy, management, and the increasingly important and enabling role of information technology. An anthology by top leaders in these areas, the volume serves both as an authoritative textbook and as a key reference for stakeholders in the health arena – that is, for all of us!

Edward H. Shortliffe, MD, PhD, MACP, FACMI
Professor of Biomedical Informatics
College of Health Solutions, Arizona State University
Phoenix, Arizona

This textbook embraces the point that health has to be seen in the context of the broader issues of social determinants, which are the major forces that shape the health outcomes of people and communities. Collaboration of individuals and teams in community settings, rethinking policies, and using information technologies are all valuable in order to achieve health for all. This textbook makes an outstanding contribution to help us better understand population health.

Adewale Troutman, MD, MPH, MA, CPH
Professor and Director of Public Health Practice and Leadership
University of South Florida, Tampa, Florida
Past President of the American Public Health Association
Former Director, Louisville Metro, Department of Public Health and Wellness

Praise for Population Health (cont.)

By highlighting the importance of collaboration for addressing today's population health challenges, this book makes an important new contribution to our understanding of how to solve complex health problems. Using a rich set of case examples, the book shows how structured collaborations – value alliances – among multiple organizations are central to achieving the goals of 21st century population health improvement.".

Rich McKeown
Co-author of *Finding Allies, Building Alliances* with Mike Leavitt, founder and chairman of Leavitt Partners and former Secretary of Health and Human Services and former governor of Utah
President, CEO and co-founder of Leavitt Partners
Former Chief of Staff, Department of Health and Human Services

ISBN-13: 978-0-9834824-9-9
ISBN-10: 0983482497

Convurgent Publishing, LLC
4445 Corporation Lane, Suite #227
Virginia Beach, VA 23462
Phone: (877) 254-9794; Fax: (757) 213-6801
Web Site: www.convurgent.com
E-mail: info@convurgent.com

Special Orders.

Bulk Quantity Sales.
Special discounts are available on quantity purchases. Please contact sales@convurgent.com.

Library of Congress Control Number: 2014940075

Bibliographic data:

Population Health: Management, Policy, and Technology, first edition / Robert J. Esterhay, LaQuandra S. Nesbitt, James H. Taylor, H.J. Bohn, Jr.

p. cm.

1. Population health. 2. Network transitions. 3. Health policy. 4. Health information technology. 5. Mental and behavioral health. 6. Complexity science. 7. Chronic disease. 8. Public health. 9. Social determinants of health.

ISBN: 978-0-9834824-9-9

Credits
Copy Editing: Rebecca J. Frey, PhD (rebeccafrey@snet.net)
Corresponding Editor: H.J. Bohn, Jr. (jb@km4i.com)

EDITORIAL TEAM

Robert J. Esterhay, MD, is the chair of the Department for Health Management and Systems Sciences in the School of Public Health and Information Sciences at the University of Louisville.

LaQuandra S. Nesbitt, MD, MPH, is a board-certified family physician and director of the Louisville Metro Department of Public Health and Wellness in Louisville, Ky.

James H. Taylor, DMan, MBA, MHA, served as president of the University of Louisville Hospital from August 1996 through February 2013. He assumed the role of special advisor to the Executive Vice President for Health Affairs at the University of Louisville and as CEO of University Medical Center in March 2013.

H.J. Bohn, Jr., MBA, is a published author, book designer, and corresponding editor on contemporary healthcare issues, and principal of KMI Communications, LLC.

FOREWORD: David B. Nash, MD, MBA, founding dean of the Jefferson School of Population Health of Thomas Jefferson University in Philadelphia, Pa. Nash is also the editor-in-chief of *Population Health Management* and is the Doris N. Grandon Professor of Health Policy in the Jefferson School of Population Health.

ACKNOWLEDGMENTS

A journey to produce a new academic and health industry textbook that took over 21 months from start to finish brought together the efforts of a coordinating executive editorial team and a group of authors from the health care, public health, and academic communities in Louisville, Kentucky, along with several authors from outside the Louisville area.

The hard work and unwavering commitment to producing rigorously researched chapters by this group of faculty members, industry professionals, and policy makers will be useful to readers in academia and in the public and private sectors for years to come. The executive editorial team extends its sincerest gratitude and appreciation for their efforts and contributions.

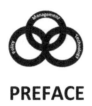

PREFACE

"Action without vision is only passing time, vision without action is merely day dreaming, but vision with action can change the world."

Nelson Mandela
Former President of South Africa
1918–2013

Public health and health care have become increasingly population-focused in the twenty-first century. Some might argue it's about time. Initiatives to improve the health of communities today require a new way of thinking, acting, and leading across a multisectoral landscape. My introduction to public or population health took root in the community psychology movement of the 1960s and 1970s—systems change or research-based social change. Those who seek to impact population health today are compelled to put effective and integrated health-related, social, and economic policies in place, as they will affect the opportunities of current and future generations to live healthier lives. Further, population health is becoming synonymous with global health. Addressing the health of communities and nations at both the individual and population levels requires improving the information and communications infrastructure to support health care, behavioral health, and wellness services throughout each community's population health ecosystem. This book seeks to marry a vision for the future with a desire to stimulate action. Will this book change the world? Likely not. But it is the authors' intent that, if exposed to the right leaders, it can contribute to enough of a shared vision and common calls to action to make measured progress possible.

Such landmark federal policy reforms as the 2009 American Recovery and Reinvestment Act and the 2010 Patient Protection and Affordable Care Act, enacted in recent years, have established new programs and initiatives to improve the health and wellness of individuals and families; and have provided the tools and infrastructure for caregivers to help tackle the challenges faced by the health system in the United States. Yet simple global comparisons paint a picture of a U.S. health delivery system still struggling to produce competitive population health parameters.

About This Book

Population Health: Management, Policy, and Technology, first edition is a 14-chapter anthology that dives into many issues confronting today's stakeholders (i.e., consumers, patients and their families, care providers, clinicians, health care workers, public health workers, community leaders, academics, policy researchers, and technologists) in each community's healthcare and public health network.

Population health issues are addressed in the context of systemic challenges, enabling transitions with new information and communication technologies, and the ways in which leadership, policy, and innovation are affecting the quality of the nation's health and wellness.

The launch of the Medicare Shared Savings Program in 2011 introduced the Three-Part Aim, which focused on "better care for individuals, better health for populations, and lower growth in expenditures" per the Centers for Medicare and Medicaid Services Summary Final Rule Provisions for Accountable Care Organizations. To achieve these aims, the U.S. healthcare and public health systems are enabled through collaborative community leadership bridging multisectoral industries. This book emphasizes the importance of a Health in All Policies (HiAP) approach to comprehensive community health and wellbeing improvement strategies.

The chapters of this book cover the following topics:

- *Chapter 1. Introduction to Population Health*

- *Chapter 2. Network Leadership: Improving Population Health through Networks of People and Organizations*

- *Chapter 3. Population Health Impact Assessment and Policy Development*

- *Chapter 4. Understanding the Numbers: The New Demographic Realities and the Future of Population Health*

- *Chapter 5. Envisioning an Expanded Model of Population Health*

- *Chapter 6. Changing the Context: Promoting Wellness through Systems and Policy Change*

- *Chapter 7. Chronic Disease in the United States: Progress and Today's Challenges*

- *Chapter 8. Mental and Behavioral Health Services: The Need for Renewed Focus*

- *Chapter 9. Developments in Population Health for an Aging Population*

- *Chapter 10. Building a Bridge to Nowhere: A Case Study of a State-run Health Information Exchange*

- *Chapter 11. Using Terminology Standards to Count the Healthy and Sick*

- *Chapter 12. Advancing the Use of Personal Health Data: Information for Population Health*

- *Chapter 13. "Big Data", Analytics, and Population Health*

- *Chapter 14. The Future of Population Health: Moving Forward with Networks, Policies, and Innovation*

Three central themes are addressed throughout the book: network leadership; the implications of Health in All Policies; and data-driven technological innovations. The first chapter establishes these themes, while subsequent chapters target specific features of the overall system.

Moving Forward with Population Health

As an endorsement both of the academic rigor in this new book and testament to its value to the student, practitioner, and policy making communities, the intent of *Population Health* is that it should serve as a new literary compilation by a diverse group of authors and executive editors which transcends the boundaries of the health and healthcare, social sciences, technology, and policy domains. Models, illustrations, and theories are provided throughout the book to stimulate critical thinking around the evolving complexities in population health management.

Additional information can be found at www.population-health.info.

Continued refinement of our approaches, tools, and abilities to improve population health management in the United States is essential. The executive editors and group of authors hope that *Population Health* serves as a guide for insights, references, and ideas to spawn awareness, education, creative thinking, and new policy initiatives for the nation to work toward and support population health initiatives. Strategy and action can change the world.

As dean of the University of Louisville School of Public Health and Information Sciences, I encourage you to make intensive use and application of the extensive work provided in the following chapters.

June 2014

Craig H. Blakely, PhD
Dean
University of Louisville
School of Public Health and Information Sciences

Table of Contents

Chapter 12. Advancing the Use of Personal Health Data: Information for Population Health 402

Chapter 13. "Big Data", Analytics, and Population Health 436

Chapter Contributors

CHAPTER 1

Robert J. Esterhay, MD
Associate Professor and Chair,
Department of Health Management and
Systems Sciences,
School of Public Health and Information
Sciences
University of Louisville

H.J. Bohn, Jr., MBA
Principal
KMI Communications, LLC

CHAPTER 2

Judah Thornewill, PhD
Founder and CEO, GroupPlus, LLC
Assistant Professor (adjunct), School of
Public Health and Information Sciences,
University of Louisville

Robert J. Esterhay, MD
Associate Professor and Chair,
Department of Health Management and
Systems Sciences,
School of Public Health and Information
Sciences
University of Louisville

CHAPTER 3

Susan Olson Allen, PhD
Assistant Professor, School of Public
Health and Information Sciences,
University of Louisville

Raymond Austin, PhD
Assistant Professor, School of Public
Health and Information Sciences,
University of Louisville

CHAPTER 4

Ron Crouch, MA, MSSW, MBA
Director of Research and Statistics,
Kentucky Education and Workforce
Development Cabinet

CHAPTER 5

Robert William Prasaad Steiner, MD,
MPH, PhD
Professor, School of Public Health and
Information Sciences,
University of Louisville

Barry Wainscott, MD, MPH, ABPM
Assistant Professor, School of Public
Health and Information Sciences,
University of Louisville

CHAPTER 6

Sara E. Walsh, PhD, MPH
Assistant Professor of Health
Administration School of Health
Sciences,
Eastern Michigan University

LaQuandra S. Nesbitt, MD, MPH
Director of Louisville Metro Department
of Public Health and Wellness

CHAPTER 7

Renee Vannucci Girdler, MD, FAAFP
Associate Professor and Vice Chair,
Department of Family and Geriatric
Medicine,
University of Louisville

James G. O'Brien, MD, FRCPI
Margaret Dorward Smock Endowed
Chair in Geriatrics, Director of the
Institute for Sustaining Health and
Optimal Aging,
University of Louisville

CHAPTER 8

Catherine Batscha, DNP, PMHCNS-BC, PMHNP-BC,
Assistant Professor, School of Nursing
University of Louisville

Scott Hedges, MD
Senior Vice President for Medical
Services, Seven Counties Services, Inc.

Anthony Zipple, Sc.D, MBA
CEO
Seven Counties Services, Inc.

Sandra Wilkniss, PhD
Former Senior Health Policy Legislative
Assistant to U.S. Senator Jeff Bingaman

CHAPTER 9

William Altman, JD, MA
Senior Vice President of Strategy and
Public Policy
Kindred Healthcare, Inc.

Marc Rothman, MD
Chief Medical Officer and Senior Vice
President for the Nursing Center
Division
Kindred Healthcare, Inc.

John P. Reinhart, CPA, MBA, CNA
Founder and CEO, International Center
for Long Term Care Innovation
(InnovateLTC)

Kathleen Smith, MBA, MPH, Manager,
Government Affairs and Public Policy,
Kindred Healthcare, Inc.

CHAPTER 10

John H. Tobin, DMan, MPH
Retired CEO,
Waterbury Hospital, Waterbury,
Connecticut

James H. Taylor, DMan, MBA, MHA
Special Advisor to the Executive Vice
President for Health Affairs,
University of Louisville

CHAPTER 11

Mark Samuel Tuttle, AB, BE, FACMI
Board of Directors
Apelon

Stephanie Suzanne Lipow, MLIS,
Senior Biomedical Informatics Analyst
Medical Sciences and Computing, Inc.

CHAPTER 12

William Yasnoff, MD, PhD, FACMI
Managing Partner, National Health
Information Infrastructure Advisors,
CEO of Health Record Banking Alliance

CHAPTER 13

Bert B. Little, PHD
Associate Vice President for Academic
Research, Professor of Computer
Science and Mathematics
Tarleton State University

CHAPTER 14

Richard Wilson, DHSc
Professor and Chair, Department of
Health Promotion and Behavioral
Sciences, School of Public Health and
Information Sciences
University of Louisville

LaQuandra S. Nesbitt, MD, MPH
Director of Louisville Metro Department
of Public Health and Wellness

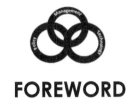

FOREWORD

by

David B. Nash, MD, MBA
Dean, School of Population Health
Thomas Jefferson University

Population Health: Management, Policy, and Technology

by Robert J. Esterhay, et al.

What exactly is population health? This is not an inconsequential question! It is especially important as I am the dean of the only School of Population Health in the country—namely, the Jefferson School of Population Health on the campus of Thomas Jefferson University in Philadelphia.

Esterhay and colleagues have essentially provided the Rosetta Stone of population health. They have successfully linked the work of Donald Berwick and the Three-Part Aim (also called the Triple Aim) of the Centers for Medicare and Medicaid Services with the national goals embedded in *Healthy People 2020* and the core requirements of the Affordable Care Act. They have done this in a thoughtful and comprehensive textbook that will undoubtedly be widely read.

The Three-Part Aim calls for better care for individuals; better health for populations; and a lower growth in per capita expenditure. These important objectives, largely attributed to Donald Berwick and other key national leaders, have never gained real political traction after Berwick left the Center for Medicare and Medicaid Services. Here comes Esterhay and his team, eager to reconnect the worthy goals of the Three-Part Aim to a critically important national initiative like *Healthy People 2020*. The core of *Healthy People 2020* includes such laudable goals, for example, as longer lives, free of preventable disease, disability, injury, and premature death.

Savvy readers, however, recognize that the Institute of Medicine noted in its January 2013 report, titled *U.S. Health in International Perspective: Shorter Lives and Poorer Health*, that our country faces a major challenge. How will we reconcile the Three-Part Aim, *Healthy People 2020*, and the Affordable Care Act when our top national leaders believe that our children are at risk of having shorter lives than their parents for the first time since the close of World War II? We ought to be taking to the streets demanding more from our leaders.

Esterhay and his team have divided the book according to three basic concepts, focusing on network leadership, health in all policies, and technological innovation. The first is an uphill battle, as clearly leadership in our healthcare system is our core challenge. Second, health in all policies conjures up for me such key questions as what's for lunch in your hospital cafeteria? Are you still serving French fries and oily pizza? And as for technological innovation, well, just take a look at what children do every day to harness technology; we will need to learn from them how to make innovations in health care in the next decade.

Esterhay and his colleagues also have great political courage in tackling unpopular and often controversial areas. I was particularly taken by Chapter 8 on Mental and Behavioral Health Services, as so little of merit has been written about the way in which these services will be tucked into health reform. Similarly, Chapter 10 admits that health information exchanges, especially those at the state level, have been largely failures and have not produced the kinds of results that the country deserves. This failure is especially disturbing in light of the nearly $19 billion that was pumped into the health information technology industry at the height of the recession in 2007 and 2008.

This book will serve as a great platform for the future. Not only is it the Rosetta Stone translating our current situation, but I believe Esterhay and colleagues have also given us a kind of roadmap. The roadmap will enable us to interpret the impact of poverty in our country as it remains one of the most important predictors of health and wellness. We're going to need new kinds of measures of accountability for accountable care organizations. These measures might be very difficult for the healthcare system to tackle—such as the number of families on public assistance and the number of persons suffering bankruptcy due to unpaid medical bills. Will provider organizations take greater responsibility for these largely social determinants of health care? The National Quality Forum believes that that's exactly what provider groups will confront under reform. Enter Esterhay again, as this book might help organizations to navigate these new "potholes" that appear on the road toward true reform.

Finally, I believe that this book should be in every graduate school program—in medicine, public health, nursing, and pharmacy. It is time for all trainees across the professional spectrum to understand the core tenets of *Population Health*. The appendix will also be very helpful, especially to newcomers to our field because the glossary and test questions are excellent!

Kudos to Esterhay and his team in producing a highly readable and politically courageous textbook that I am confident will have a positive impact on our nascent field of population health. Our School of Population Health salutes Esterhay and his team of executive editors and authors!

Chapter 1. Introduction to Population Health

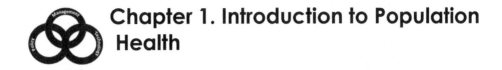

Robert J. Esterhay, MD

H.J. Bohn, Jr., MBA

"THE MAINTENANCE of the public's health allows—some would say demands—concern with almost every aspect of life."[1]

Paul Starr, Professor of Sociology and
Public Affairs, Princeton University

Chapter 1 Learning Objectives

- Obtain an understanding of the comprehensive meaning of population health.

- Understand at a high level the importance of network leadership, Health in All Policies, and technological innovation in relation to population health.

- Be able to articulate the role of leaders in population health.

- Define four elements or components of the total population health ecosystem.

- State the factors that contribute to the United States' health disadvantage as noted in the IOM's 2013 report on U.S. health.

How do we lead and effect change to improve the health and wellness of our communities?

Ask a thousand people and you get a myriad of answers. In order to effectively change the behaviors that contribute to the health and wellness of society, a nation must first recognize the need for and then chart a course to a future of comprehensive betterment for all in the society. In recent years the healthcare[*] and public health sectors have seen a shift toward a focus on population health issues, surveillance, and management from the perspective of policy setting, new initiatives, and measurement of progress or lack thereof in some cases. There can, however, be differing perspectives on the application and meaning of the phrase "population health" when viewed from the medical, sociological, and public health perspectives. The views and perspectives applied will influence the direction and type of challenges identified for a given population and the needs of those included in any given population. During the past decade, health reforms in the United States have moved toward more coordinated, integrated, and comprehensive health and wellness initiatives for the population of each community, state, and the nation as a whole;[2] however, it is an iterative process in which great progress has been made but many challenges lie ahead. In fact, from a global perspective the United States lags behind several comparable nations in prevalence of heart disease; obesity and diabetes; drug and alcohol-related mortalities; and disabilities among the elderly. These points were emphasized in the 2013 Institute of Medicine (IOM) report, *U.S. Health in International Perspective: Shorter Lives, Poorer Health*, which went on to state that the United States is at a disadvantage with peer nations due in part to a large number of health determinants that include but are not limited to:[3]

- Patterns of food consumption shaped by environmental issues;

- Social inequalities, unemployment, and lack of health insurance;

- High-stress environments leading to a higher prevalence of substance abuse, illness, violence, and criminal activity; and

- Greater firearms availability in the United States compared to peer nations.

Each community in the United States and other nations, and its stakeholders set priorities that shape decisions which in turnaffect the health and wellness of its population.

Addressing such dilemmas as these issues, which affect the larger society and the stakeholders in the ecosystem of each community, can lead to innovations (e.g., health information technologies, processes, and constructs)

---

[*] For the purpose of this book, *healthcare* (one word) is used when referring to the health system (e.g., the U.S. healthcare system; the healthcare and public health sector, etc.) and *health care* (two words) is used when referring to care provided as a service.

and potential solutions that improve people's health and wellness, and provide opportunities for the population of each community to overcome its sociological challenges. At the center of the collective ecosystem are those stakeholders who strive to improve the community, its systems, and its processes for the benefit of their own and future generations. A network transformation has been ongoing for decades across the healthcare, wellness, and public health sectors. The technology renaissance continues to drive and support this transformation. Cultures are merging, new standards are being established, and communications are improving through adoption of advanced health information technologies. These are only a few of the components contributing to the status of population health that will be discussed throughout this book.

Enhancing the Meaning of Population Health

Defining a population is a critical step in establishing the health status of any group in question, whether the focus is a community, region, nation, or the entire globe. So how should we define the population? For the purpose of this text, a population can be defined as the people within a given geographic region and stratified on the basis of their demographics or statistical characteristics. From a demographic perspective, there are the physical, behavioral and mental, gender, age, and economic characteristics, to name a few. As noted by Scheck McAlearney in 2003, population health is multidimensional.[4] These dimensions can be viewed on the basis of how we live; where we live; and to some extent on the constraints of the environment that surrounds a given population. One means of viewing a population is typically done with the aid of population pyramids. These graphic illustrations serve as tools that show the distribution of a given population based on a selected demographic. Figure 1-1 provides an example from the U.S. Census Bureau of the 2013 age distribution of males and females in the United States.

Figure 1-1. Population Pyramid: U.S. Age Distribution[5]

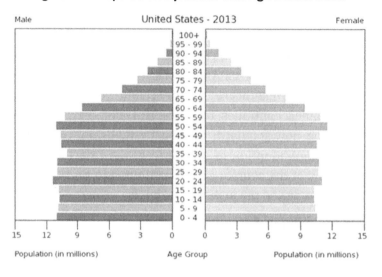

This figure is a representative illustration of a population distribution and is based on estimated data from the U.S. Census Bureau. Given the impact of the Baby Boomer segment of the population in the United States, one can envision the shift that will occur in a pyramid based on a similar scale in future years. Chapter 4 on Quantitative Perspectives will provide additional insights with other population pyramids.

There are numerous determinants of the health of a population. In the World Health Organization's 2008 report, *Closing the Gap in a Generation: Health Equity through Action on the Social Determinants of Health*, a key element of improving population health must address social and economic policies for both urban and rural communities.[6] The urban-versus-rural community dimension for a population is significant in light of the inequality that may exist in resources made available to people in these different types of communities. This inequality holds true for the United States and globally for both developed and underdeveloped nations. Considering the number of potential determinants, another dynamic to consider in understanding population health is how we derive the cumulative measurement of the health of a population.

Here the question must be asked: does the aggregation of individual health (the micro perspective) necessarily provide a meaningful assessment of a community, region, nation, or global population's health (the macro perspective)? In a 2005 article in the *Journal of Epidemiology and Community Health*, Reidpath addressed this issue, noting that "Wealth, sex, race, environment, behavior, culture, etc., all influence health outcomes," and went on to establish that the distribution of these determinants can be more a matter of equity than of health for the population.[7] If this is the case, then the argument that the sum of the parts does not always equal the aggregate of the population holds true, and deeper analysis of health determinants is needed to assess any given population's health. Today, capabilities with predictive, descriptive, and optimization analytics integrated with electronic health records (EHRs), health information exchanges, and community health data banks have greatly advanced the opportunities for researchers and practitioners in accountable care organizations and other clinical practices to "use sophisticated data mining to identify care practices that result in better outcomes, such as reduced readmissions."[8] These capabilities can also produce insights on population-level trends and relationships between health determinants and outcomes that may be nonlinear or appear dissociated on the surface, but have underlying relationships and correlations that provide evidence to support future clinical decision making. The scope of the determinants making up a population's composite health, however, is broader than what is available in these health record resources. So the full meaning of the "total" health of the population should account for other determinants, as will be described throughout the chapters in this book.

A definition of population health is essential and is recognized as a relatively new term in the industry. Table 1-1 provides several definitions of population health.

Table 1-1. Definitions of and Perspectives on Population Health

Year	Authors/Report/Article	Definition
1995	(Frank) *Canadian Journal of Public Health* article[9]	"A broad population health perspective requires us to examine with a critical eye, the conditions of life and work that damage the health of our communities. . . ."
2002	(Raphael and Bryant) *Health Promotion International* article.[10]	". . . processes by which system-level variables influence the health of populations."
2003	(Kindig and Stoddart) *American Journal of Public Health* article[11]	". . . the health outcomes of a group of individuals, including the distribution of such outcomes within the group". . . population health also includes patterns of health determinants, policies and interventions that connect the two.
2008	Minnesota eHealth Initiative	". . . an approach to health that aims to improve the health of an entire population. . .

Year	Authors/Report/Article	Definition
	white paper[12]	addressing a broad range of factors that impact health on a population level, such as environment, social structure, resource distribution and the relative minor impact that medicine and healthcare have on improving health overall."
2010	*Public Health 101*, a Jones and Bartlett Learning book[13]	"The concept of population health can be seen as a comprehensive way of thinking about the modern scope of public health."
2012	(Jacobson and Teutsch) Report commissioned by the Institute of Medicine[14]	". . . a cohesive, integrated, and comprehensive approach to health considering the distribution of health outcomes in a population, the health determinants that influence the distribution of care, and the policies and interventions that impact and are impacted by the determinants."

John Frank's perspective on population health emerged from the work of the Canadian Institute for Advanced Research (CIAR) as Canada's movement toward nationalized medicine occurred in the 1990s. Kindig and Stoddart's definition is from a well-known seminal work done in 2003 on defining population health; while the 2012 report by Dawn Marie Jacobson, MD, MPH, and Steve Teutsch, MD, MPH, emphasized the need for the industry to change its favored vocabulary of "population health" to "total population health." The need for health systems to evaluate outcomes and distinguish between subpopulations in identifying needs and solutions from a multisectoral stakeholder approach becomes increasingly important for such twenty-first-century care delivery models as accountable care organizations (ACOs), clinically integrated networks (CINs), and patient-centered medical homes (PCMHs).

From a healthcare perspective, the Medicare Payment Advisory Commission (MedPAC) stated in their June 2012 report to Congress, *Medicare and the Health Care Delivery System*, that they stratified their beneficiary population as rural, urban, under-65, dual-eligible, and high-risk, based on the needs of beneficiaries within each segment.[15] This report is an example of a breakdown of the sector of the population that the Centers for Medicare and Medicaid Services (CMS) seek to provide financing for their medical, wellness, and behavioral health care across our nation (addressed further in Chapter 9). This is only one example of a population segment, but indicative of the driving need to focus on care for the nation as a whole, and the ongoing redesign of the care delivery system around integrated, accountable, and patient-centric care processes—that is, care that is accountable to the individual consumer and the various segments of the population we all serve.

Given these different ways of dissecting the population, Figure 1-2 proposes a model for the population health ecosystem.

Figure 1-2. Population Health Ecosystem[16]

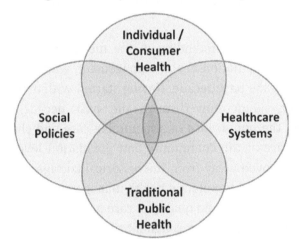

Population health models differ in light of differing causal relationships, interactions among factors, and distinctions between individual and population health.[17] Figure 1-2 identifies four ellipses in the population health ecosystem model.

First is the individual/consumer health ellipse. Throughout the past decade consumers have become increasingly engaged in the management of their health and health care.[18] During this time consumers have assumed more responsibility for their health plans; expanded their use of personal health records (PHRs); and increased their adoption of mobile health technologies and social media.[19] Second is the healthcare systems ellipse. The IOM's 2001 report titled *Crossing the Quality Chasm: A New Health System for the 21st Century* highlighted the challenges to and the importance of redesigning healthcare organizations.[20] Since that time, hospitals, physician practices, and other health services organizations have engaged vigorously in more process improvement, adoption of health information technology (health IT), and establishing new structures focused on refining accountability for outcomes and performance. Third is the traditional public health ellipse. Funded through a complex stream of local, state, federal, and private sources that vary from one community to another based on community need and health determinant factors, traditional public health services have usually served as safety-net health services focused on preventive care and care of at-risk populations. While accounting for a small percentage of total health care spending, evidence has shown these services reduce mortality rates.[21] Fourth is the social policies ellipse. This final ellipse represents social health determinants and the importance of Health in All Policies (HiAP) at the federal, state, and local levels that can affect an individual's quality of life in the communities in which he or she is born, lives, and works.

With a foundational understanding of the meaning of population health, comes the concept of population health management, which is a relatively new focus in healthcare in the past decade. Having started with managed care in the 1990s and gaining momentum through the past decade, the healthcare industry's focus on the importance of accountable care and clinical integration to provide better care at the community and population levels has increased significantly. It has moved away from the historical cottage industry structure. In fact, McAlearney defined population health management in 2003 as "a variety of approaches to foster health and quality of care improvements."[22] This concept has gained significant momentum throughout the decade and is being echoed by health IT vendors, consulting firms, legislators, medical researchers, practicing physicians, and caregiver teams as one of the keys to solving some of the United States' daunting challenges in the quality and cost of medical care.

Complexity: Its Effect on a Nation's Health and Wellness

The four overlapping ellipses of the population health ecosystem model as illustrated in Figure 1-2 are considered the major parts of the complexity of the nation's health infrastructure. Complexity science invokes the concepts of chaos theory, self-organization, principal-agent theory (from the perspective of the role of incentives in healthcare), feedback loops, dynamic nonlinear behavior systems, and ultimately the forming of a network of systems within an ecosystem resulting in complex adaptive systems. In a 2011 article in *Emerging Themes in Epidemiology*, Jayasinghe notes,

> Complexity science would view population health outcomes in the context of an 'open' system . . . the patterns of population health outcomes are an emergent property of the system.[23]

This notion of an open system is indicative of the nonlinearity of complex adaptive systems and the involvement of independent intelligent agents, as has been the case in healthcare throughout history. On the other hand, the formation of ACOs, integrated care delivery models, and increased standardization in healthcare systems and practices carries the potential to diminish free and open actions within the system over time. Health information technologies, while accompanied by some unintended adverse consequences noted throughout the past decade,[24,25] are believed to improve the efficiency, effectiveness, and integration of health care delivery services, but they also increase the complexity of managing the technologies themselves. Therefore, with the adoption of such new health information technologies as EHRs and health information exchanges (HIEs), there exist tremendous opportunities to affect the health and wellness of the stakeholders in each community, but multiple health care and public health interventions must accompany the implementation of these new technologies at the same time. How community members interact and effectively engage the resources available in a care delivery system for medical, mental or behavioral health, or public health needs, can raise or lower the quality of life achieved in these communities.

The subtitle of this work, *Population Health: Management, Policy, and Technology, first edition*, lists three areas of influence that play an active role in the strategic guidance and achievement of total population health across all dimensions.

So where is the interplay of these levers? And how do they influence the determination of outcomes, whether health-, economically, or socially oriented?

Figure 1-3 is adapted from Paul Plsek's Appendix B in the IOM's 2001 report, *Crossing the Quality Chasm: A New Health System for the 21st Century*.[26] Plsek attributes the original model to Ralph Stacey's 1996 work on complexity theory to explain the importance of understanding how organizations operate as complex adaptive systems—an advance beyond historically mechanical process-oriented thinking. Stacey later went on to change his perspective on organizational complexity to one focused on patterns of relationships.[27] In fact the underlying complexity of many social processes could be characterized as generally ignored, underappreciated, and insufficiently studied—something that should be explored further for the benefit of all stakeholders throughout the population health ecosystem. The terms *complexity* and *complicated* have often been used interchangeably. To understand the perspective taken throughout this book, the reader should regard *complexity* as the nonlinear dynamics of people, organizations, and networks throughout an ecosystem, while understanding *complicated* as referring to the multifaceted difficult-to-comprehend aspect of any given situation and its associated people, processes, and technologies.

The certainty-versus-agreement model has been used widely across industries as one contingency theory approach for managers to understand the implications of various actions and how they may affect their organizations. Our rendition of Figure 1-3 illustrates the concept of three spheres of influence to help steer organizations and stakeholders toward achieving agreement and certainty about outcomes in navigating the zone of complexity between total planning and control over outcomes and the realm of chaos characterized by a low degree of certainty over outcomes.

Figure 1-3. Population Health: Spheres of Influence to Manage Complexity[26]

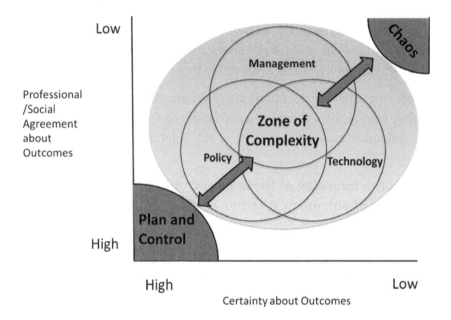

Management initiatives tend to provide vision and goals, and to focus on solution development, while policy initiatives provide structure and frameworks that allow management initiatives to operate. The third sphere, technology, involves advanced tools and technical innovations that enable the accomplishment of management initiatives to meet the objectives of certain regulatory frameworks. A case in point is the CMS legislation for the Medicare Shared Savings Program issued in April 2011.[28] This new program (focused around shared savings strategies and risk sharing) is being implemented as a new mechanism for CMS with provider and hospital organizations across the United States, with over 250 Medicare ACOs established as of early 2013.[29] The guiding federal policy requires the adoption and use of enabling health IT; establishing an underlying clinical integration program and physician leadership; and reporting on clinical quality measures to evaluate and drive accountability for improvement of population-level clinical health.[30] Navigating the zone of complexity can require dealing with known and unknown factors that precipitate a need for "stability-focused interventions, enactment tools, pattern management, and perspective filtering" as part of a dynamic sense-making process to develop optimal solutions to contemporary challenges.[31] As Stacey's own perspective on complex adaptive systems changed over the years, those with an interest in this element of organizational dynamics and complexity science should consult Chapter 10 by Tobin and Taylor for further discussion of this topic.

Role of Leaders in Solving Population Health Challenges

As the nation moves forward in the twenty-first century, collaborative community leadership with an underlying transformative and adaptive approach is a key to addressing the challenges that lie ahead. Empowerment and engagement of stakeholders helps facilitate the overcoming of systemic barriers. In order to transform communities and improve the United States' health status among peer countries, we must engage and develop collaborative leaders from all sectors of each community (e.g., government, law enforcement, public health, medical, technology and trade, religion, nonprofit) to address such community-based challenges as "workforce development, improving access to care, reducing disparities, and improving data" as demonstrated through the Public Health Leadership Institute program.[32] System disorganization and lack of accountability are two challenges that clinical integration programs and ACOs are positioned to address under collaborative physician leadership with a focus on achieving better health for populations. As new organizational capacity emerges through collaboration and multisectoral partnerships, common goals can be established with action plans that target meeting the needs of all stakeholders across the ecosystem.[33] The question should be asked here as well as in the concluding chapter:

How will leaders not only balance the risks and rewards of transformational and innovative change, but also accomplish this task in the face of accelerating or exponential change?

Leaders of every generation face challenges; however, in the early twenty-first century there is an added dynamic, as noted by Terrell and Bohn in 2012:

> . . . adoption of new technologies and process of information exchange are accelerating the pace of change in the delivery of health services, promising the possibility of a true renaissance in the way we live and work. . . [34]

Along with this acceleration in the pace of change, a number of challenges affect specific subpopulations. Some areas to be addressed throughout this book include mental and behavioral health; chronic conditions; the health network transition; the complexities and challenges posed by health IT; the aging of the general United States population; and the need for continued innovation. Leadership is required to address all these issues, along with recognizing the importance of the consumerist movement that has also contributed significantly to the quality of health care and public health initiatives throughout the past decade.[35] As consumers have gained access to their health information, they have become more active partners in decision making and understanding their options. At the same time, this access to personal health information has also created new challenges for physicians and care provider teams in resolving misunderstandings with or misinterpretations by patients.

Mental and behavioral health challenges in the United States have surged to the forefront of American society in light of such critical issues as firearms violence associated with mentally ill patients; privacy protections for mental and behavioral health records; help needed by many American veterans with combat-related posttraumatic stress disorder (PTSD); and abuse of illegal subtances across demographic sectors—among many other issues. Is it not a worthy priority for societal and population health to address these issues? It is; and a paradigm shift is needed, followed by deep corrective action at local, state, and federal levels that will require strong collaborative leadership to alter the current path. Relevant issues that will be addressed later in Chapter 8 include but are not limited to:

- Historical reductions in funding that have resulted in the defunding of psychiatric services;[36]

- The need for integration of mental and behavioral health services with primary care services and the potential for coordination with PCMH models;[37,38] and

- New strategies to support members of the U.S. armed forces as well as veterans and their families in dealing with the emotional effects of combat and extended military deployments.[39,40]

These challenges and others that have evolved over the last three decades, along with identifying potential solutions at the community level for mitigating risk and serving as a positive contribution to the health of various subpopulations, will be identified and addressed. A multitude of issues exist where effective collaborative leaders can make a difference in the health of their communities in the twenty-first century.

Central Themes

Three central themes are addressed throughout the following chapters. Figure 1-4 identifies these themes as interlocking.

Figure 1-4. Central Themes

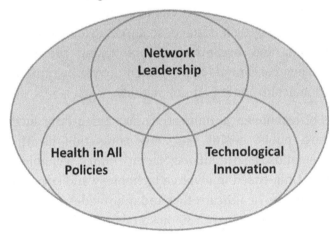

Each of these themes is uniquely important in relation to the functioning of the population health ecosystem; and each author will address them in different degrees within their chapters. First is network leadership. A network transition is under way and symbolizes the transformation occurring throughout the healthcare system—"a transition to a world in which change is primarily influenced by networks."[41] Good leadership is essential to ensure that sound health decision making occurs both for individuals and the population, along with strong administrative decision making to propel organizations and networks forward to provide the services and products needed to benefit everyone. Second is Health in All Policies. Improving the health, wellness, and eradication of disease in any population is influenced by many factors—economic, sociological, financial, and medical—and the policies that govern a population's lives have far-reaching ramifications at the community, state, and national levels. As Blumenthal and Cortese noted in a 2009 *Huffington Post* article, Health in All Policies is an approach to re-engineering all policies (e.g., federal, state, and local) that influence the health of the population served.[42] It is not a new concept but one that requires strong coordination to be effective. It can be summarized as follows:

> Health in All Policies refers to a simple fact: areas other than health services have the greatest impact on people's health. Our health depends more on what kind of work we have, where we live, what food is available to buy and so on. Health in all Policies provides a concrete roadway to strengthen population health promotion.[43]

Third is technological innovation. Information and communication technologies (ICTs) have been a driving force over the last two decades across all organizational types throughout the population health ecosystem. As new innovations have been diffused, consumers and patients have been empowered; caregiver teams and physicians have acquired evidence of the quality and outcomes achieved; and organizations are taking the incremental steps necessary to achieve continuous improvement across the multiple dimensions of total population health and its subpopulations.

Thousands of technological innovations are being introduced each year in the medical care, public health, and now population health domains. One example of population health management (PHM) technology comes from Health Catalyst, a Utah-based innovative technology and services provider with roots in Intermountain Healthcare that today provides data warehousing and analytic solutions to more than 135 hospitals and 1,700 clinics focused on quality improvement, population health, and ACO initiatives.

Community Care Physicians Deliver Effective Population Health Management with Clinical Analytics

Health Catalyst Case Study

A healthcare system in the western United States has established an infrastructure that enables its clinics to manage the health of its patient populations more effectively. These clinics needed the ability to:

- Promote preventive care;
- Identify and engage patients with multiple chronic diseases to help them

**Community Care Physicians Deliver Effective Population Health
Management with Clinical Analytics
Health Catalyst Case Study**

achieve optimal care;

- Measure regulatory and performance results against national benchmarks;
- Free RN navigator and RN nurse care coordinator time that was spent cobbling together reports; and
- Effectively compare providers and clinics across the system

The Challenge: Manual Reporting Processes

The health system knew that moving to population health management would require significant analytics capabilities—particularly the ability to aggregate, analyze, and report data. Without an analytics platform in place to handle this heavy lifting, clinic staff members were spending valuable time piecing together reports from the available data. This process left little to no time for analysis, and took staff away from more important work. For example:

- RN care coordinators were tasked with scanning through data from the electronic medical record (EMR) delivered to them in the form of large Excel files or static PDF reports. They would use these data to cobble together reports on which to base decisions for managing their populations. They then spent valuable time putting together graphical representations of the data in an attempt to engage other providers with the data.

- The patient navigator, tasked with helping patients overcome barriers to care, didn't have an analytics platform in place to identify the patients who required outreach. She had to spend 50–60 percent of her time conducting chart reviews to identify these patients.

The Solution: An Enterprise Data Warehouse and Clinical Analytics

To create an analytics foundation, the health system implemented a healthcare enterprise data warehouse (EDW), which aggregates data from the EMR, financial systems, patient satisfaction systems, and others to create an enterprise-wide, consistent view of all health system data. On top of this EDW platform, the system deployed clinical analytics designed to enable PHM processes.

Community Care Physicians Deliver Effective Population Health Management with Clinical Analytics
Health Catalyst Case Study

Results

Aggregated data from sources across the continuum

The health system has currently aggregated data from inpatient sources and the ambulatory EMR. Users now have the infrastructure in place to gather data from an unlimited number of sources, including pharmacies, long-term care facilities, HIEs, and health record banks.

Integrated near-real-time reporting of regulatory and performance measures

The PHM initiative has given clinicians access to near-real-time reporting of more than 20 regulatory and performance measures. These measures include such social determinant factors as tobacco cessation and preventive measurements: screenings, immunizations, etc.; and disease management.

Seventy-five percent reduction in reporting and chart abstraction time

The patient navigator estimates that the analytics infrastructure enables her to perform reporting and chart reviews 75 percent faster. She is able to identify patients for care coordinator outreach more rapidly.

Graphic visuals that encourage provider engagement and free RN resources

The analytics platform saves RN patient care coordinators an estimated 25–30 percent of their time per clinic. They spend less time creating reports, and can quickly communicate progress and results to the clinics' providers and management. By showing performance information in graphic formats, they are better able to engage the clinics' providers in effecting improved results.

Timely patient outreach for overdue treatment and upcoming reminders

The analytics infrastructure delivers a summarized community follow-up view that has enabled the clinics to generate near-real-time lists of patients who aren't compliant with recommended evidence-based care guidelines. Clinicians are now able to reach out to patients in a timely manner.

Such innovative technology solutions as this and others, introduced by both global technology developers and entrepreneurial firms alike, will help meet the health information needs of community leaders, healthcare providers, and policy makers seeking to improve the health of the populations they serve.

Regulatory Reforms

There has been intense debate about the cost and effectiveness of U.S. healthcare reforms, starting with the elements of the 2009 American Recovery and Reinvestment Act (ARRA) and continuing with the 2010 Patient Protection and Affordable Care Act (ACA). The nation had been in need of reforming how its citizens pay for, deliver, and evaluate the cost and quality of health care in the United States for several years. Health IT has and will continue to play a significant role in the reshaping of communications, health records management, and emerging analytics capabilities as the CMS Meaningful Use of EHRs continues to work toward a nationwide health information network.[43] These capabilities will support improvements in the ways in which care is delivered, altering the structure of care delivery with the establishment of ACOs, clinical integration programs, and the network of safety-net care delivery organizations throughout the country in urban and rural areas.

In addition, the private payer health insurance industry has been in turmoil in preparation for significant change with the introduction of health insurance exchanges across the country. Stemming from the ACA, the new health insurance exchanges began operations on January 1, 2014, serving as a new market for small businesses and consumers to evaluate and purchase private health plans.[44] Exchanges are being established at the state level; however, nineteen (19) states have elected to opt out and allow the federal government to establish insurance exchanges for them.[45] While a major part of this new mandate in the healthcare industry overhaul resulting from ARRA and the ACA, it is a totally new concept for small businesses and consumers to purchase private insurance plans online. Other major changes from the regulatory reforms affecting the private insurance industry that have a significant impact on various segments of the U.S. population have included:[46]

- Establishment of new consumer assistance programs for help with the private insurance market and system;

- Controls on health plan premiums (enforcement of a medical loss ratio of 85% for large employer plans and 80% for small employers and individual plans) and premium increases;

- Expansion of Medicaid population coverage; and

- Prohibited denial of coverage based on preexisting conditions.

Many issues related to these health reforms will be discussed throughout the following chapters given the importance of these landmark reform laws.

Legal Perspectives on Public and Population Health

An additional and final critical dimension that underlies the challenges for resolving these complex issues is the underlying constitutional authority passed down to public health officials from federal to state and local levels. In the Institute of Medicine's 2003 report titled *The Future of the Public's Health in the 21st Century*, the authors identified one of the systemic challenges facing the nation:

> The governmental public health infrastructure is built on a legal foundation replete with obsolete and inconsistent laws and regulations, and a great deal of public health law is not coordinated among states and territories.[47]

This statement made over a decade ago was emblematic of the state of public health and the need for improvement and new legislation at the federal level. Improved coordination is still a challenge today due to variation across states in policy and technology; however, standards and capabilities are improving and progress is being made.

Definitions of population health and the broad intention of solving the social determinants of health dilemmas faced by our nation and each respective community have been touched on throughout this opening chapter. There is, however, a bottleneck. The police powers conveyed to public health officials of each state by the U.S. Constitution predominantly empower and fund them to:[48]

- Regulate individuals to stop or reduce the transmission of communicable disease; and

- Regulate professions and businesses through licensure and the maintenance of safe and healthy conditions.

While other challenges certainly exist, when one considers the ramifications of the social determinants of health, there are constraints on what can be feasibly and realistically accomplished by public health officials versus the responsibilities that the general public and private sector should accept in order to improve the health of the population.

From a sociological point of view, achieving greater health for the population can be said to be everyone's responsibility; but from the legal perspective there are only certain powers bestowed upon states, and ". . . state constitutions and statutes impart the authority for local governments to influence health."[49] Over the last two centuries many improvements have been made, due in part to legal mandates for public health initiatives. A few of these improvements include:[50]

- Responses to natural disasters;

- Vaccination programs;

- Workplace safety measures;

- Better control of communicable diseases; and

- Fluoridation of drinking water.

The legal boundaries of what can be done and what is funded by the federal government to improve population health provide a narrow context and guidelines for public health responsibilities assumed by the government. The laws, statutes, and regulations in effect have led to the present U.S. public health infrastructure. In a 2012 article in the *American Journal of Public Health*, the authors state that a key objective should be "to understand law's contribution to community health . . . the association between legal structures and population health indicators."[51]

Each local government will have different socioeconomic variables to deal with in efforts to improve the health of the population it serves. However, such twenty-first-century health policies as the ACA have and will continue to have significant effects as springboards for new community-level health initiatives that provide better funding for the development of public health assets within their constitutional authority. The ACA provided the legislative authorization of funding to support testing of such various delivery system innovations as ACOs, interdisciplinary community health teams, and community transformation programs. As an additional example, Section 4002 of the ACA established the Prevention and Public Health Fund, which provided $500 million in 2010 to support public health programs in communities across the country, and authorized funding to increase to $2 bilion annually for 2015 and beyond.[52]

Such policy changes as these do not change the constitutional police powers of a state or local public health department, but they do provide needed infrastructural funding that has been lacking for years in communities across the country. Such initiatives as the Prevention and Public Health Fund serve as new legal mandates that help bolster community-level assets to improve population health over multiyear periods.

Further discussion and research is warranted for future editions of this work in terms of the legal authority that determines who should be responsible; who is presently responsible; and what actions can and should be taken to improve the health of a population in any specific community given twenty-first-century societal changes in the United States. In addition, there are other issues related to the legal perspective of population health the will require further treatment in the future. Some of these issues include: (1) the use of health policy to create economic incentives as social levers to influence healthy behaviors; (2) gaps in services needed by specific populations and the identification of those responsible for closing those gaps; and (3) the continued tension between the need to balance restraints on individual liberties that have the potential to affect the health of the greater community against the needs of the full population and the need to protect the public's heath.[53]

Policy Implications and Conclusion

One of the key themes in this book is the importance of Health in All Policies (HiAP). In 2013 a joint report was issued by the American Public Health Association and the Public Health Institute titled *Health in all Policies: A Guide for State and Local Governments*. This report identified five critical elements of HiAP: (1) promoting health equity and sustainability; (2) supporting intersectoral collaboration; (3) benefiting multiple partners; (4) engaging stakeholders; and (5) creating structural or procedural change.[55] The authors of the report recommend focusing on these elements to help ensure that a comprehensive health perspective is taken in all key government decisions.

To build on the premise of the need to collaborate, organizations throughout the population health ecosystem can improve policy making and oversight of outcomes by engaging more multisectoral partnerships in their communities. As noted by Woulfe and colleagues in 2010, this approach leads to

> . . . shifting the focus from individuals and organizations to networks, rules, social norms, and/or laws to affect health behaviors and outcomes that recognize the connection between health and social institutions, surroundings, and social relationships.[56]

Multisectoral partnerships are also contributing to the management of complexity through shared and distributed responsibility across industry participants. One example is the Office of the National Coordinator for Health Information Technology (ONC-HIT) and its federal advisory committees that draw their membership from organizations across the healthcare ecosystem:

technology vendors, government agencies, nonprofits, integrated delivery networks, private insurance payers, and others. This type of engagement with stakeholders leads to greater opportunities for examiming industry challenges and reaching effective solutions for the good of the public through a balance of federal policy setting and industry innovations.

A number of issues have been addressed throughout this chapter as an introduction. An additional distinction to keep in mind throughout this book is that between *health care* and *healthcare*. *Health care* is defined as provider actions taken in the provision of medical, public health, or behavioral health services; *healthcare* refers to an organizational system(s) that delivers these services. The following chapters are intended to provide a significant contribution to current thinking on population health, on management, policy, and technological issues. As Krieger noted in her 2012 *Milbank Quarterly* article, "Who and What Is a 'Population'? Historical Debates, Current Controversies, and Implications for Understanding 'Population Health' and Rectifying Health Inequities," "critical population-based thinking" will be essential in the future for understanding evidence, defining new principles, and recognizing the dynamics in relationships among members within a given population.[57]

The remainder of this book is divided into three sections, each with four chapters, followed by a concluding chapter. Each section was overseen by a member of the executive editor team who provided strategic guidance to the authors on the chapters in their section. *Section I. Population Health in a Complex World* (Executive Editor, Robert J. Esterhay, MD) is focused on issues related to the ongoing transformation of health networks; ways to assess the causes of health problems across the total population; statistical analyses; and an examination of the differences between and the need for growing integration of traditional public health and medical care models into population health models. *Section II. Critical Business Aspects of Health and Wellness of a Nation* (Executive Editor, LaQuandra S. Nesbitt, MD, MPH) covers core issues involving chronic conditions; wellness strategies; the importance of mental and behavioral health issues, and the aging of the population with the upward movement of the Baby Boomers on the population pyramid. *Section III. Health Technologies: Enablers of Change* (Executive Editor, James H. Taylor, DMan, MBA, MHA) addresses several important issues in the growth of health information technology and the complexities faced by stakeholder executives working to improve the quality of health and healthcare for individuals and the populations they serve.

Communities and nations can change; we can improve the environment to make better opportunities for generations to come.

"…Healthy People *reminds us about the importance of prevention. It reminds us about the importance of the gift of health and it gives us new directions to reach for the future.*"

> Opening remark, presentation on *Healthy People 2020*,
> September 10, 2012
> Howard K. Koh, MD, MPH, Assistant Secretary for Health
> U.S. Department of Health and Human Services

ACKNOWLEDGMENTS

The authors would like to thank Leslie Hough Falk, RN, PMP, CIPP, and Greg Miller from Health Catalyst for their case study contribution to Chapter 1.

In addition, special thanks are owed to John Chenault, Associate Professor and librarian of the Kornhauser Health Sciences Library at the University of Louisville, for his mentoring and teaching on citation management issues, along with periodic reviews of the book manuscript that proved to be invaluable to our team in the compilation and editing process.

CHAPTER 1 DISCUSSION QUESTIONS

Discussion questions are provided for team building or class exercises. Answers to all questions are provided in Appendix C.

Question Number	Question
1	What is population health—a concept, field of study, or a new discipline of management?
2	What are the three central themes that will appear throughout the following chapters in this book?
3	What are the four ellipses in the figure depicting the total population health ecosystem?
4	What are some of the factors that contribute to the United States' health disadvantage, as noted in the Institute of Medicine's 2013 report?
5	In general, what are the police powers granted to local public health officials through the U.S. Constitution?

CHAPTER 1 SUMMARY

- Multiple definitions of population health have been proposed over the past two decades.

- The social determinants of health are of growing importance on a global scale in the twenty-first century. These factors are often not within the direct ability of public health departments to address but are a definite society-level concern that affects the health of populations.

- Three central themes were enumerated that will be covered throughout the book: network leadership; health in all policies; and technological innovation.

- Collaborative community leadership will be essential to resolving the complex challenges in population health. The ability to manage the dynamics of such matrixed organizations as ACOs, clinically integrated networks, and other types of health care delivery structures is critical to improving measures of individual and community-level health.

- The Patient Protection and Affordable Care Act of 2010 (ACA) while controversial, is bringing sweeping changes with new programs that will affect how we access, pay for, and assess the quality of health care services in the United States.

- The chapter discussed three levers used to manage complexity in healthcare: management, policy, and technology. The U.S. healthcare system is a complex adaptive system that operates with numerous independent intelligent agents.

- Community public health departments and officials possess constitutional authority to enact health-related initiatives to protect individuals from transmission of communicable diseases; to regulate individuals and businesses for licensure; and to ensure safe and healthy workplaces.

CHAPTER 1 REFERENCES

1. Starr P. The boundaries of public health. In: *The social transformation of American medicine*. New York, N.Y.: HarperCollins Publishers; 1982:180-197.

2. Department of Health and Human Services. HHS announces the nation's new health promotion and disease prevention agenda. *HHS News*. December 2, 2010. http://www.healthypeople.gov/2020/about/DefaultPressRelease.pdf. Accessed June 10, 2014.

3. National Research Council and Institute of Medicine. Summary. Woolf SH, Laudan AE, trans. *U.S. health in international perspective: shorter lives, poorer health*. Washington, D.C.: National Academies Press; 2013:1-11.

4. McAlearney AS. Introduction. *Population health management: strategies to improve outcomes*. Chicago, Ill.: Health Administration Press; 2003:3-10.

5. US Census Bureau. Population pyramid of the U.S. population distribution by age for 2013. http://www.census.gov/population/international/data/idb/region.php?N=%2 0Results%20&T=12&A=separate&RT=0&Y=2013&R=-1&C=US. Accessed February 3, 2013.

6. Commission on Social Determinants of Health. Health equity through action on the social determinants of health. Geneva, Switzerland: World Health Organization;2008.

7. Reidpath DD. Population health. More than the sum of the parts? *J Epidemiol Community Health*. 2005;59(10):877-880.

8. Bradley P. Predictive analytics can support the ACO model. *Healthc Financ Manage*. 2012;66(4).

9. Frank JW. Why "population health"? *Can J Public Health*. 1995;86(3):162-164.

10. Raphael D, Bryant T. The limitations of population health as a model for a new public health. *Health Promot Int*. 2002;17(2):189-199.

11. Kindig D, Stoddart G. What is population health? *Am J Public Health*. 2003;93(3):380-383.

12. Minnesota e-Health Initiative. Population Health and Health Information Technology Framework of the Minnesota e-Health Initiative Population Health Workgroup Minnesota Department of Health; 2008.

13. Riegelman R. Public health: the population health approach. In: *Public health 101: healthy people—healthy populations*. Sudbury, Mass.: Jones & Bartlett Learning; 2010:3-15.

14. Jacobson DM, Teutsch S. *An environmental scan of integrated approaches for defining and measuring total population health by the clinical care system, the government public health system and stakeholder organizations*. Los Angeles, Calif.: Public Health Institute and County of Los Angeles Public Health Department; 2012.

15.   Medicare Payment Advisory Commission. *Report to Congress: Medicare and the health care delivery system*. Washington, D.C.: Medicare Payment Advisory Commission; 2012.

16.   Riegelman R. Figure 1-1. The full spectrum of population health. *Public Health 101: healthy people—healthy populations*. Sudbury, Mass.: Jones & Bartlett Learning; 2010:8.

17.   Friedman DJ, Starfield B. Models of population health: their value for US public health practice and research. *Am J Public Health*. 2003;93(3):366-369.

18.   Robinson JC, Ginsburg PB. Consumer-driven health care: promise and performance. *Health Aff (Millwood)*. 2009;28(2):w272-281.

19.   Konschak CB, Jarrell LP. *Consumer-centric healthcare: opportunities and challenges for providers*. Chicago, Ill.: Health Administration Press; 2011.

20.   Institute of Medicine, Committee on Quality of Health Care in America. Building organizational supports for change. In: *Crossing the quality chasm: a new health system for the 21st century*. Washington, D.C.: National Academies Press; 2001:111-144.

21.   Mays GP, Smith SA. Evidence links increases in public health spending to declines in preventable deaths. *Health Aff (Millwood)*. 2011;30(8):1585-1593.

22.   McAlearney AS. Integrating population health management concepts and strategies. In: *Population health management: strategies to improve outcomes*. Chicago, Ill.: Health Administration Press; 2003:175-189.

23.   Jayasinghe S. Conceptualising population health: from mechanistic thinking to complexity science. *Emerg Themes Epidemiol*. 2011;8(1):2.

24.   Campbell EM, Sittig DF, Ash JS, Guappone KP, Dykstra RH. Types of unintended consequences related to computerized provider order entry. *J Am Med Inform Assoc*. 2006;13(5):547-556.

25.   Ash JS, Sittig DF, Poon EG, Guappone K, Campbell E, Dykstra RH. The extent and importance of unintended consequences related to computerized provider order entry. *J Am Med Inform Assoc*. 2007;14(4):415-423.

26.   Plsek P. Institute of Medicine, Committee on Quality of Health Care in America. Appendix B: Redesigning health care with insights from the science of complex adaptive systems. In: *Crossing the quality chasm: a new health system for the 21st century*. Washington, D.C.: National Academies Press; 2001:312-317.

27.   Stacey R. *Tools and techniques of leadership and management: meeting the challenge of complexity*. New York, N.Y.: Routledge; 2012.

28.   Centers for Medicare and Medicaid Services. I.(C) Overview and intent of Medicare Shared Savings Program. *Federal Register*. April 7, 2011;76(67).

29.   Department of Health and Human Services. More doctors, hospitals partner to coordinate care for people with Medicare. [press release]. HHS Press Office; January 10, 2013.

30. Flareau BF, Yale K, Bohn JM, Konschak C. Chapter 1. History and Case for Action. In: Frey RJ, ed. *Clinical integration: a roadmap to accountable care.* 2nd ed. Virginia Beach, Va.: Convurgent Publishing; 2011:25-26.

31. Kurtz CF, Snowden DJ. The new dynamics of strategy: sense-making in a complex and complicated world. *IBM Systems Journal.* 2003;42(3):462-483.

32. Umble K, Steffen D, Porter J, et al. The National Public Health Leadership Institute: evaluation of a team-based approach to developing collaborative public health leaders. *Am J Public Health.* 2005;95(4):641-644.

33. Corrigan J, McNeill D. Building organizational capacity: a cornerstone of health system reform. *Health Aff (Millwood).* 2009;28(2):w205-215.

34. Terrell GE, Bohn JM. Pace of change accelerates. In: *MD 2.0: Physician leadership for the information age: from hero to Duyukdv.* Tampa, Fla.: American College of Physician Executives; 2012:91-105.

35. Cohen SB, Grote KD, Pietraszek WE, Laflamme F. Increasing consumerism in healthcare through intelligent information technology. *Am J Manag Care.* 2010;16(12 Suppl HIT):SP37-43.

36. Applebaum PS. The "quiet crisis" in mental health services. *Health Aff (Millwood).* 2003;23(5):110-116.

37. Agency for Healthcare Research and Quality. Experts call for integrating mental health into primary care. *Research Activities.* Rockville, Md.: Agency for Healthcare Research and Quality;2012.

38. Hogan MF, Sederer LI, Smith TE, Nossel IR. Making room for mental health in the medical home. *Prev Chronic Dis.* Nov 2010;7(6):A132.

39. Bonner L. Community mental health services for young adults challenged. *News Observer.* December 22, 2012. http://www.newsobserver.com/2012/12/22/2561984/community-mental-health-services.html. Accessed June 24, 2013.

40. Obama B. Executive Order—Improving access to mental health services for veterans, service members, and military families. Washington, D.C.: Office of the Press Secretary;2012.

41. Reinhart JP, Esterhay R. The new horizon—a network transition to individual and population health. In: Spooner B, Reese B, Konschak C, eds. *Accountable care: bridging the health information technology divide.* 1st ed. Virginia Beach, Va.: Convurgent Publishing; 2012:380-421.

42. Blumenthal S, Cortese D. Health in All Policies. *Huffington Post.* July 31, 2009. http://huffingtonpost.com/susan-blumenthal/health-in-all-policies_b_249003.html. Accessed June 13, 2014.

43. Fajuri SP. Health in All Policies: The emperor's old clothes. 2011; http://www.healthypolicies.com/2011/08/health-in-all-policies-the-emperor%E2%80%99s-old-clothes/. Accessed July 18, 2013.

44. US Department of Health and Human Services. American Recovery and Reinvestment Act. Title IV: Medicare and Medicaid Health Information Technology; Miscellaneous Medicare Provisions. Sec. 4101. Incentives for

Elegible Professionals. (a) Incentive Payments. *Public Law 111-5*. Washington, D.C.: US Department of Health and Human Services; February 17, 2009.

45. Herman B. HHS publishes final rule on PPACA's health insurance exchanges. *Becker's Hospital Review*. March 12, 2012. http://www.beckershospitalreview.com/finance/hhs-publishes-final-rule-on-ppacas-health-insurance-exchanges.html. Accessed January 20, 2014. Accessed June 5, 2014.

46. Alonso-Zaldivar R. State insurance exchanges approved by White House. *Huffington Post*. January 3, 2013. http://www.huffingtonpost.com/2013/01/03/state-insurance-exchanges_n_2404173.html. Accessed June 13, 2014.

47. US Department of Health and Human Services. Key features of the Affordable Care Act by year. http://www.hhs.gov/healthcare/facts/timeline/timeline-text.html. Accessed July 18, 2013.

48. Institute of Medicine, Committee on Assuring the Health of the Public in the 21st Century. Assuring America's Health. In: *The future of the public's health in the 21st century*. Washington, D.C.: National Academies Press; 2003:26.

49. Gostin LO, Thompson EF, Grad FP. The law and the public's health: the foundations. In: Goodman RA, Hoffman RE, Lopez W, Matthews GW, Rothstein MA, Foster KL, eds. *Law in public health practice*. 2nd ed. New York, N.Y.: Oxford University Press; 2007:37-42.

50. Turnock BJ. Law, government and public health. In: Riegelman R, ed. *Essentials of public health*. Sudbury, Mass.: Jones and Barlett Publishers; 2007:75.

51. Novick LF, Morrow C.B. Defining public health: historical and contemporary developments. In: Novick LF, Morrow CB, Mays GP, eds. *Public health administration: principles for population-based management*. Second ed. Sudbury, Mass.: Jones and Bartlett Publishers, Inc.; 2008:14.

52. Costich JF, Patton DJ. Local legal infrastructure and population health. *Am J Public Health*. Oct 2012;102(10):1936-1941.

53. H.R. 3590. Patient Protection and Affordable Care Act. Sec. 4002. Prevention and Public Health Fund; 2010.

54. Rothstein MA. Guest editorial: the future of public health ethics. *Am J of Public Health*. 2012;102(1):9.

55. Rudolph L, Caplan J, Ben-Moshe K, Dillon L. The five key elements of Health in All Policies. *Health in all policies. a guide for state and local governments*. Washington, D.C., and Oakland, Calif.: American Public Health Association and Public Health Institute; 2013.

56. Woulfe J, Oliver TR, Zahner SJ, Siemering KQ. Multisector partnerships in population health improvement. *Prev Chronic Dis*. 2010;7(6):A119.

57. Krieger N. Who and what is a "p opulation"? historical debates, current controversies, and implications for understanding "population health" and rectifying health inequities. *Milbank Q.* 2012;90(4):634-681.

SECTION I. Population Health in a Complex World

Executive Editor,

Robert J. Esterhay, MD

Section I Overview

Population Health in a Complex World
(Network Leadership)

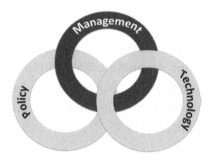

The dynamics of improving the health of a community in this second decade of the twenty-first century are vast and ever-increasing. However, as Dean Nash noted in the foreword, Dean Blakely mentioned in the preface, and the authors of Chapter 1 pointed out, health reforms here in the United States (U.S.) and abroad are moving stakeholders in health and wellness to think upstream about a more efficient, effective, integrated, and well-coordinated population health ecosystem.

Chapters 2 through 5, which comprise Section I of this book, address several management topics that include network leadership and systems dynamics; health impact assessments and their value to community transformation and policy setting; statistical analysis of U.S. and global trends in light of population health improvement needs; and a perspective on the importance of the social determinants of health as a different way to think about population health for the next decade of the twenty-first century.

A few key points from the chapters that follow in this section:

Chapter 2 discusses today's increasingly interconnected world, with collaboration among and between many different groups and organizations becoming increasingly important. Moreover, collaboration is required to address most population health challenges in the categories of infectious, chronic, and social diseases. There are many opportunities for network leadership in population health. Opportunities include *Healthy People 2020* service areas, Health in All Policies (HiAP) initiatives, population health research networks, clinically integrated networks, and community health management systems.

Chapter 3 focuses on health impact assessments (HIAs) as useful tools to aid community and policy decision makers in identifying challenges related to health determinants. HIAs can also improve a community's understanding of health risks or effects that may arise from implementation of new policies, programs, or projects. The HIA approach provides a potentially useful means of developing and evaluating policies related to managing population health.

Chapter 4 points out that the United States as well as the rest of the world is experiencing a demographic revolution. The nation is becoming more diverse and its citizens are living longer. All of us need to understand these realities. The longevity revolution changes all the rules; it will require us to rethink issues like education, work, retirement, and the like.

Chapter 5 offers an understanding of the inherent differences between the traditional medical care model and the public or population health model. The global perspective of the social-cultural-ecological construct and the evolving need for adoption and incorporation of this model into contemporary thinking on population health is presented. A model for managing population health is introduced that includes a medical care model which is not driven by measures of disease or illness, but rather by measures for community health which depend on societal measures to a greater extent.

The health of our nation is everyone's responsibility; however, those who study and work in the fields of health care and public health serve on the front lines of community service to help deliver care and improve the health of the population they serve. The Department of Health and Human Services' *Healthy People 2020* program illustrates the comprehensive perspective used to evaluate the health of the country and its citizens.

As readers study the content of the following chapters, they should keep one thing in mind: population health is a community good and one that we can all strive to improve for the hopes and health of the next generation.

Robert J. Esterhay, MD
Department Chair,
University of Louisville School of Public Health and Information Sciences

Chapter 2. Network Leadership: Improving Population Health Through Networks of People and Organizations

Judah Thornewill, PhD

Robert J. Esterhay, MD

"Collaboration among allies is more than a cooperative attitude—it is a skill you can improve when you understand how to organize and manage the various participants in an alliance or network. The ability to get things done with collaborative networks is the next evolution in human productivity. Those who develop these skills will prosper in the next quarter-century. Those who don't will fall behind."[1]

Mike Leavitt
Former Governor of Utah and U.S. Secretary for DHHS,
and
Rich McKeown
Former Chief of Staff, DHHS

Chapter 2 Learning Objectives

- Why is collaboration important to achieving the goals of twenty-first century population health?
- What is network leadership and why does it matter?
- What is a network?
- What are collaborative networks?
- What are some other terms used to describe collaborative networks?
- What are the three steering mechanisms leaders use to effect change?
- What are the strengths and limitations of each of these mechanisms?
- What are some ways in which network leaders measure and manage trust?
- What are some emerging opportunities for network leadership?

Introduction

Starting in 2003, we (Judah Thornewill and Bob Esterhay at the University of Louisville's School of Public Health and Information Sciences) started conducting research at the intersection of population health, information sciences, and organizational sciences. Our interest was to better understand factors influencing the success of new kinds of *collaborative networks*, broadly defined as two or more entities collaborating to achieve a shared goal. We were also interested in how collaborative networks might be influenced by the use of new kinds of information and communications technology (ICT), including the Internet, cloud-based computing, and social media.

This focus led us to participate in several real-world participatory action research initiatives between 2003 and 2012 in areas including community and state health information exchanges; biosurveillance; and infectious disease tracking networks. In addition, we became familiar with an emerging academic literature on collaborative networks in such areas as network sciences, inter-organizational networks, and inter-organizational systems. In 2012, as a way to share what we were learning with our students, we also developed and taught a graduate-level course titled *Network Leadership: How to Lead and Succeed in a World of Networks*.

In this chapter, we will share some of the insights we have gained in the last decade about the increasingly important role of network leadership—that is, the leadership of collaborative networks—in achieving population health goals in the twenty-first century. What we share is part of a rapidly developing area of research and practice with evolving terminology and findings. The key finding, however, is empirically well established: the growth of many new kinds of collaborative networks, in which people and organizations collaborate to achieve shared goals, is occurring worldwide in many different industries. The growing impact of these new kinds of collaborations recently led Yochai Benkler of Harvard Law School to document the emergence of a twenty-first century transformed by "the wealth of networks."[2] Other academics postulate that inter-organizational networks "are about to become the new dominant form in the future replacing the formal hierarchical organization that has dominated the twentieth century."[3]

The remainder of this chapter is organized in eight sections: 1) Terminology; 2) Network Leadership and the H1N1 Influenza Epidemic; 3) Where Does Network Leadership Make a Difference?; 4) How Do Effective

Network Leaders Lead?; 5) Tips for Developing and Managing Trust and Connections; 6) How Is Network Leadership Learned?; 7) Emerging Opportunities for Network Leaders; 8) Challenges and Implications.

Terminology

In this chapter, we use the term *collaborative networks* to refer to two or more entities collaborating to achieve a shared goal, in which an entity can be an individual, an organization, or another collaborative network. There are, however, a number of other terms used in the field that also refer to these phenomena. Some synonyms that we have encountered are shown below.

Synonyms for *Collaborative Network*

Alliance: an association or union for mutual benefit, especially between organizations or countries.

Coalition: a set of individuals or groups in a community cooperating in joint action for a common cause.

Inter-organizational network: three or more organizations working together toward a common purpose; a set of three or more organizations linked to one another.

Organizational network: a set of people and organizations connected to an organization.

Social network: a set of people connected to one another.

Value alliance: a group of participants with aligned interests pursuing an outcome with value for each of them.

It is likely that in the next 10–20 years, more standardized terminology will develop to describe collaborative networks of different types. In the meantime, we recommend that network leaders use the terms that are the most comfortable for the people and organizations that they are supporting in their local context.

➢ *Network Leadership and the H1N1 Influenza Pandemic*

Why is leadership of collaborative networks of people and organizations—rather than of a single organization—important to think about? Is network leadership different from traditional organizational leadership? If so, then how? Our experiences during the H1N1 flu pandemic in 2009 provide a way to start answering these questions.

> *A Time-Sensitive Challenge*

Starting in 2008, with funding support from the United States (U.S.) Department of Homeland Security and the National Institute for Hometown Security, we were part of a multidisciplinary research effort to better understand how infectious diseases like influenza spread; how their diffusion can be tracked; and what interventions are most helpful in reducing the spread of the illness. The team we led was specifically focused on understanding and tracking the spread of infectious disease in schools at the primary and secondary levels.

As the H1N1 flu pandemic began to move across the world in 2009, scientists noticed that it spread quickly among school-age children. In addition, unlike most influenza strains that affect the elderly, H1N1 was causing higher than expected mortality in young people. For example, when the disease hit our area, big headlines appeared in newspapers when two formerly healthy middle school students tragically died as a result of H1N1. For these reasons, our research at the school level suddenly became highly relevant. Almost overnight, it became important to accelerate the tracking of the flu in the local schools, and to act quickly if needed to shut down schools, protect healthy children and their families, and take care of the sick.

The Importance of Collaboration

To bring about these results, many different organizations in both public and private sectors had to get involved and collaborate at local, state, national, and international levels.

Local organizations included several hundred public schools, which had some power over decisions as to when to send kids home or close the schools; public school district offices for each of several counties in our area; and many more private schools. They also included the mayor's office; the local public health department, which had the power to order quarantines; and the local police to maintain public order.

But as discussions continued, it turned out there were many other stakeholders to take into account as well. These included local physicians, hospitals, and pharmacies involved in vaccinating the public and treating patients; area employers who might need to act to stop the spread of disease in workplaces; area television, radio, and newspaper organizations who needed guidance regarding the dissemination of information in order to reduce public panic and potential for misinformation; and even shopping malls! It turned out that when sick kids were released from school or schools were closed, a surprising number of youngsters ended up at the malls, causing the disease to spread in yet another way—sometimes even more quickly.

Similar patterns of collaboration also emerged at the state level, as regulators, the governor, health, public health, law and order, and many other groups had to come together quickly to make decisions and take state-level actions to address this issue. This process included extensive coordination among state- and local-level actors.

In addition, on the national and international levels, major organizations, including the U.S. Centers for Disease Control and Prevention (CDC), the World Health Organization (WHO), national governments, vaccine manufacturers, airlines, and technology firms also had to collaborate to address this fast-moving challenge.

Not surprisingly, it turned out that the capacity of people and organizations to collaborate to address this shared challenge made a significant difference in how well communities, states, and nations fared during this crisis. For example, in some U.S. communities, there was a lack of coordination of activities between local schools and their districts and states. People didn't know whom to talk to or mistrusted one another, and were unable to agree quickly on a shared strategy. In other communities, the situation was exacerbated by media outlets that spread misleading or inaccurate misinformation, or by lack of coordination among public health officials, police, hospitals, physicians, and other entities. Fortunately, in many other communities, especially those with a track record of collaborating on other health-related issues, things went better.

➤ *Our Community's Experience*

In our community, a series of meetings were held among and between leaders of many different groups, with leadership provided by a few key people—including the well-liked and well-connected leader of our local public health department. A similar situation happened at the state level, with leadership provided by two groups: education leaders and health leaders, who came together (for the first time in many years!) to seek ways to pool resources to address the situation. The result: a generally effective response was launched.

But even in a community like ours, with a reasonably good track record in multisector collaboration and good state support, some barriers emerged that were difficult to overcome. For example, it turned out that sharing information about illnesses within a given school was very difficult. Each school tended to track health issues a bit differently, and the computer systems provided by the state were difficult to work with and even more difficult to change. Thus it was difficult to know exactly how quickly flu was spreading, and thereby to know when to close a school.

Fortunately, H1N1 proved to be far less virulent than initially expected, while vaccines proved to be reasonably effective, making this pandemic a kind of "warning shot across the bow." In a future situation, however, if diseases spread quickly through schools, the ability of multiple organizations from different sectors to collaborate could be a matter of life or death for many people.

➤ *Three Key Ideas*

This brief story points to three key ideas to keep in mind while reading the rest of this chapter.

1. Network leadership matters. The leadership of collaborative networks can make a difference—especially in situations in which many people and organizations need to collaborate to solve a complex problem.

2. Network leadership is different. Network leadership is different from organizational leadership. In organizations, a leader can require everyone to work together. In networks, however, there is usually no way to require that people and organizations come together. If people don't "feel like it," they simply just choose not to show up.

Thus to be successful, network leaders must bring different people and organizations together by using trust and persuasion. A major success factor is developing trusted relationships with key people and organizations over time, so that they can be called upon when a need arises.

3. Network leadership can be learned. Like most skills, network leadership is learned through a combination of study and experience. In our community, for example, our local director of public health effectively facilitated cooperation among many different people and organizations during the H1N1 crisis. His success was based on years of experience in collaborating in many different settings, combined with study and reflection about what works.

Where Does Network Leadership Make a Difference?

In the last section, we discussed how in the case of the 2009 influenza pandemic, collaboration among many organizations facilitated by network leaders mattered. But is this leadership the rule or an exception? A brief review of major types of disease that population health management addresses and the strategies that are used to address them—including the growing use of information technology to connect people and organizations in new ways—suggests that network leadership can make a difference in many places.

➢ *Infectious Disease Networks*

As the saying goes, infectious diseases know no boundaries. Whether it is malaria, smallpox, cholera, HIV/AIDS, mumps, measles, rubella, SARS, or hantavirus—in modern times, with every country on earth a plane-ride away and boats, trains, and cars crisscrossing the earth, infectious diseases can spread quickly. The potential for infectious diseases to spread quickly through neighborhoods, across communities, states, and nations, and around the world, points to a growing need for collaboration among many parties involved in protecting population health.

Some examples of organizations that may need to collaborate to address infectious disease health concerns include:

• Local, state, national, and international public health agencies;

• Transportation providers (e.g., planes, trains, buses, ships, taxis);

• Transportation hubs (e.g., airports, train stations, ports, bus terminals);

• Businesses that can facilitate the spread of disease (e.g., hotels, bars, theaters, nightclubs, sports arenas and stadiums, restaurants, shops, food suppliers);

• Hospitals, physicians, pharmacies, and other providers where patients go when they get sick; and

• Businesses that can provide immunization and/or protective gear.

In addition, as information technology systems improve, each of these organizations will have increasing opportunities to connect to local, regional, national, and international databases and information services to access more timely and complete information about the spread of disease and appropriate actions to take to address it. Thus another important area of collaboration is in the development of shared information systems that can support information exchange among different organizational-level systems.

➢ *Chronic Disease Networks*

Chronic diseases are so named because they are often slow to develop, and require treatment and care over a long duration. Chronic diseases include arthritis, hypertension, congestive heart failure, obesity, stroke, cancers, asthma, diabetes, chronic kidney disease, osteoporosis, and Alzheimer's disease, to name just a few.

To be effective, chronic disease care generally requires a whole-system implementation supported by networks of caregivers. These caregivers may include physicians, hospitals, community social support networks, home health care providers, and clinical professionals willing to act as partners or coaches. In addition, caregivers need access to health information and health information technology resources that are verified and relevant to the community context and patient situation. Knowledge-sharing, knowledge-building, and a learning community are integral to the management of chronic diseases.

Chronic disease management requires not only a focus on individual health care, but also on population health. Systematic approaches to managing chronic diseases across multiple settings of care for populations can reduce health care costs and improve quality of life by preventing or minimizing the effects of the chronic disease.

Chronic disease networks (CDNs) can be defined as networks of coordinated healthcare interventions and communications for populations with these types of diagnoses and conditions in which patient self-care efforts are significant. Many CDNs increasingly rely on such new technologies as health information exchanges, Web portals, apps, or social networking services to support their activities. Development of these CDN technologies is another important area in which inter-organizational collaboration is needed.

➤ *Social Disease Networks*

Social diseases are often referred to as lifestyle diseases. They are also called diseases of longevity or diseases of civilization because they appear with increased frequency as people live longer and as countries become more industrialized. Examples include atherosclerosis, asthma, some cancers, chronic liver disease, chronic obstructive pulmonary disease (COPD), type 2 diabetes, heart disease, metabolic syndrome, chronic renal failure, osteoporosis, stroke, depression, and obesity. Many of these diseases are also in the chronic disease category, but the difference is that they are all partially caused or can be exacerbated by social conditions. In addition, social diseases may include injuries caused by factors like firearms violence, domestic violence, rape, or exposures to environmental hazards.

Like people suffering from chronic diseases, sufferers of socially derived diseases may require care from caregivers of various kinds, including doctors, physicians, testing centers, and specialty service providers. Those providers also need access to sources of accurate, timely, verified information about the specific illness or condition—plus if possible, information about the social context influencing the illness. In addition, patients may need nonmedical care services and support from groups like homeless shelters, food banks, job training services, childcare services, social services, or law enforcement. Collaboration among healthcare, public health, and social support groups is an enormous challenge but also a great opportunity.

In addition, collaboration is required to address social disease determinants through the development and passage of new policies and regulations at local, state, national, and international levels. Passage, enforcement, and compliance with such regulation typically require collaboration among many different parties involved in patient care.

As an example, research in the area of social health disparities shows that income disparities (i.e., the difference in incomes between the wealthiest and poorest members of a social group) directly affect health and longevity.[4] Specifically, the lower the income status of a given population segment, the higher the illness and mortality rates will be for that population. In short: poverty kills. Furthermore, the greater the disparity between the poorest and richest segments of society, the greater the effect on illness and mortality for those at the bottom of the hierarchy. In short: high wealth disparities kill. A possible solution to this problem could be legislation to redistribute wealth in order to reduce the income gaps. To pass such legislation, however, support from many different individuals, business leaders, financial leaders, and politicians is usually required. One can anticipate wealthier individuals and organizations being asked to pay higher tax rates steadfastly resisting such a policy.

Another strategy to address social disease factors is the development of new information technologies. Such technologies can be used to measure the incidence and prevalence of different diseases; track their causes; and deliver personalized recommendations to help individuals protect and improve their health. For example, there are now several apps being tested that track the risk of an asthma attack for a given person based on local air pollution counts. If a risk is detected, a message is sent to the person alerting them to be aware, stay indoors, and make sure they have an inhaler available in case of an attack. These strategies too require collaboration across multiple contexts.

➢ *Population Health Research Networks*

We've now discussed diseases in three broad categories. So, on what diseases and in which categories should population health leaders focus? What can be done to address different diseases? What are the cures? Which illnesses are cheapest and easiest to treat? Population health research by researchers from all over the world is conducted to answer questions like these.

Several types of population health research exist, ranging from bench to bedside to the community. Bench research includes studies of genomes, biochemical factors, viruses, bacteria, and cells in the body, and the effects of different drugs and treatments. Bedside research involves the study of best practices of patient care "at the bedside." Community research involves the study of populations of patients across a community, and looks at effects of community-based interventions like cleaning up air and water pollution or reducing lead exposure for children. In each case, the job of population health research is to measure the incidence and prevalence of disease in given populations; identify the causes of those diseases; and develop treatments and interventions to reduce the impact of the given disease on a population.

Most of these kinds of research also require collaboration between multiple parties. Researchers must obtain funding from research funders—government, nonprofit, or private sector agencies. Researchers must then collaborate with multiple care providers, community organizations, and patients / consumers to gather information, run tests, and measure results. In many cases, such research may also require approval from government agencies or university oversight boards in order to run clinical trials. Thus here too, collaboration is an essential requirement for success.

The use of interconnected information technology networks to support collaborative health research is an increasingly important aspect of health research. Under the Patient Protection and Affordable Care Act of 2010 (ACA), for example, significant new funding is allocated to develop a nationwide network of interconnected "Big data" research repositories and analytic engines for health research. These include clinical data research networks (CDRNs) linked to large clinical healthcare providers with electronic health record systems, and patient-powered research networks (PPRNs) that are often founded by individuals or patient advocates to support research on a specific health condition such as different types of cancer, childhood asthma, or type 2 diabetes. Hundreds of millions of dollars are being provided to support development of these networks through the Patient-Centered Outcomes Research Institute (PCORI). *Population Health Policy Networks* Population health is typically governed by complex sets of laws and regulations passed by government agencies at local, state, national, and international levels. These laws are usually supported or modified through the workings of policy networks. Policy networks exist, or may develop, for policies related to virtually every major population health disease category out there. They typically succeed by bringing together a majority of stakeholders who collaborate to develop a specific policy that can pass. Collaboration based on relationships of trust is an essential aspect of success in this area as well. A number of new policy networks are emerging in relation to the Health in All Policies (HiAP) concept. Chapter 1 identified Health in All Policies (HiAP) as one of the themes of this book and discussed the importance of multisectoral partnerships in driving HiAP in policy making and applications. The 2012 *Health Affairs* article titled "Health in All Policies: The Role of the US Department of Housing and Urban Development and Present and Future Challenges" addresses this very point. It institutionalizes a cross-sectoral approach that encourages policy makers to weigh the health implications of policies that are not normally considered health-related.[5] Improving population health in the twenty-first century will require a HiAP focus on policy development. As organizational and network leaders in the public and private sector alike continue to grow and build collaborative efforts, technologies and processes will converge to produce new insights needed for this higher-level integrated approach to policy making and implementation. Policy networks of many types will need to be formed to develop effective policies that address the spectrum of challenges affecting the health and well-being of populations at community, state, and national levels.

How Do Effective Network Leaders Lead?

In the last section, we discussed many different types of collaborative networks that may be involved in addressing complex population health challenges. How do successful leaders of these kinds of networks lead? What is required for success? To fully answer these questions would require several books. Some of the basic ideas, however, are fairly straightforward. We offer the following as an orienting framework to get the reader started.

➢ *Leading through Power, Money, and Trust*

According to experts who study leadership, leaders at any level use three mechanisms, sometimes called *steering mechanisms*,[6] to achieve goals requiring coordination among multiple people and/or organizations. The first two are money and power (the carrot and the stick).[7] The third, which scientists are still learning about, is trust.[8] These three mechanisms can be thought of as a three-legged stool, as illustrated in Figure 2-1.

Figure 2-1. Three Mechanisms of Network Leadership

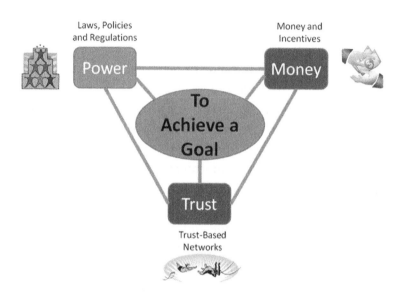

By intelligently leveraging all three mechanisms, network leaders can increase the likelihood of achieving the goals of improving population health for a given community.

➤ *Leading through Power (The "Stick")*

An initial instinct of many population health leaders facing the complexities of addressing a population health challenge requiring collaboration is to try to use the "stick"—the power of government to promote and ensure compliance with smart policies.

Typhoid Mary is a famous example of the use of state power to protect the health of the public.[9,10] Mary Mallon (1869–1938) was a cook infected with typhoid fever who had no symptoms. Over several years, outbreaks of typhoid were observed among customers in New York City who visited various restaurants where she worked. Based on then-current laws in New York State designed to protect the public from infectious diseases, the state intervened several times in efforts to stop Mary from infecting others. Mary changed her name, however; kept working as a cook; and continued to spread typhoid. Eventually, Mary was forcibly quarantined by the state and kept in isolation for the rest of her life. The story was widely reported by journalists. To this day it raises trenchant questions about individual rights versus state power: when and how should the state exercise power (e.g., imprison or restrain individuals) in order to protect the health of a broader population?

More recently, in the United States, a debate has emerged around questions of whether such religious organizations as Roman Catholic hospitals and universities whose leaders claim religious beliefs that do not support the use of artificial contraceptives for women should be required by the state to provide free access to such contraceptives as part of their employees' health benefits package. The ACA[11] says yes: compulsion is justified because access to free contraceptives has been shown to improve maternal and child health outcomes; reduce complications related to untimely or unwanted pregnancies; increase access to education and gainful employment for women; and reduce costs of maternal and child health for society. On the other hand, the idea of curtailing the religious freedom of a subset of the population to advance the interests of the overall population has engendered ongoing and contentious debate in the United States.

Both of these examples show how leaders in government and organizations can use power to change the behaviors of individuals in a population in order to improve public health for the good of the community. Government can require individuals and organizations to comply with certain regulations as a condition of living in the society; employers can require employees to comply with certain rules as a condition of their employment. These examples, however, also show how difficult it can be to attempt to use power to force people to do things they don't want to do. The examples point to an underlying tension between individual rights and freedom on the one hand, and societal laws and regulations that apply to everyone on the other. This tension exists because in the end, once laws are passed, government has the power to enforce those laws through lawful measures, including levying fines, shutting down businesses, or in extreme cases, putting people in quarantine or prison, as occurred with Typhoid Mary.

Because of this tension between individual rights and social obligations, getting new laws and regulations passed and/or enforced is often extremely challenging, at least in democratic societies. This difficulty is present because leaders in opposing political parties will typically take positions for or against such legislation in efforts to secure votes from portions of the population that are positively or negatively affected by the limitations of freedom being proposed.

Perhaps, after considering the use of power as a lever for change, a network leader may elect to tackle a few new regulatory issues or focus on enforcement of a select number of existing laws or policies. However, population health leaders will find many limitations to what can be achieved using power alone.

> *Leading through Incentives (the "Carrot")*

A second way to lead change is through money and incentives—the carrot. For a number of population health challenges, evidence supports the idea that when people and organizations are given the right information paired with the right incentives, they will do the right thing for themselves, their families, their neighbors, their employees, their communities, and even society as a whole. A good example is health insurance wellness discounts.

It is well known that such behaviors as annual wellness checkups, regular exercise, and not smoking are associated with better health *and* lower costs of health care. In recent years, various experiments by employers have shown that health-improving behaviors increase when employees are offered a discount on the monthly premiums they pay for insurance.[12] For example, a typical program might provide a $40-per-month discount for employees who don't smoke and do participate in a wellness program. The program also benefits the employer. The insurer provides the employer with a discount on annual insurance costs based on the number of employees participating in the wellness program. The discount is justified by an estimated reduction in health benefit claims calculated by the insurance underwriters.

Another example is the use of exercise apps like step-counters, which reward people who increase their walking and running activities. These apps automatically count the number of steps a person takes each day and feed them into an online database. People can then go online to see how many steps they take; compare themselves with others; look at trends over time; and receive special offers to join walking groups or special events like Saturday-morning hikes. These apps work in part by providing social recognition of healthy behaviors. They can also be linked to city-wide programs to improve health. For example, in at least one U.S. city, the mayor leads regular "walks for health" in which thousands participate. At the end of each walk, everyone can "plug in" their app to an online event dashboard.

Incentive-based approaches have also been used successfully to encourage hospitals, physicians, and other health care providers to take steps to improve the quality of care they provide to populations. For example, the ACA and the

2009 Health Information Technology for Economic and Clinical Health (HITECH) Act that preceded the ACA contained a number of incentive-based programs for eligible providers and hospitals that are making a difference. These programs include incentives of up to $40,000 per year per eligible provider for adoption of electronic health records (EHRs) in the Meaningful Use of EHRs program, and additional payments to physicians and hospitals that demonstrate the implementation of a successful patient health information exchange (HIE). Over time, the use of EHRs and HIEs is expected to increase the availability of accurate, complete, and timely health information at the point of care, thereby reducing medical errors caused by such occurrences as lack of information, duplicate tests, administrative errors, overdoses, and clinical workflow problems.

A fourth example is the new Medicare accountable care organizations (ACOs) authorized under the ACA.[13-15] In these programs government healthcare funding (e.g., Medicare) is tied to the overall improvement of the health of a designated group of 5,000 or more beneficiaries. A Medicare ACO must have a clinical integration program established as one of its foundational elements (e.g., the organizational integration of physician practices and provider organizations), and enroll a cohort of patients for whom it is responsible for everything from wellness visits to medication compliance to emergency department care to inpatient care. The Medicare ACO has opportunities to earn incentive revenue by working with patients to improve their wellness. For example, key factors for effective care of diabetic patients include regular physician visits, regular measurement of hemoglobin A1C levels, and effective management of insulin and diet. Failure to maintain this treatment protocol increases the risk of expensive emergency room visits and other serious health issues—including blindness, loss of limbs, and heart disease. Under Medicare ACO programs, a network of hospitals and physicians can work together to help patients manage their diabetes more effectively. Money is saved by reducing emergency room visits and expensive hospital-based procedures.

A portion of the financial savings is then paid to the Medicare ACO. This incentive allows the participating hospitals and physicians to earn additional revenue by sharing in both clinical and financial risk associated with working to improve the health of a population of patients.

➤ *Tragedy of the Commons*

Unfortunately, while there a number of areas in population health in which incentive-based approaches can be successful, there are also many areas in which money and incentives are not sufficient to achieve desired changes. One reason for this situation is sometimes referred to as the tragedy of the commons. This phrase comes from a study of a group of farmers who agree to share grazing land to save money.[16,17]

While each farmer intends to be a 'good neighbor,' each in practice puts more than his fair share of livestock in the common pasture, leading to systematic overgrazing. As a result, the pasture becomes progressively less fertile, leading over time to collapse of the shared resource and a loss of grazing land for everyone. Unsurprisingly, each farmer tends to blame the others for the problem, a phenomenon linked to what psychologists now call cognitive biases.[18]

Examples of Cognitive Biases
• *Anchoring bias*: the tendency to rely too heavily, or "anchor," on one trait or piece of information when making decisions.
• *Attentional bias*: the tendency to pay attention to emotionally dominant stimuli in one's environment and to neglect relevant data when making judgments about a correlation or association.
• *Availability heuristic*: the tendency to overestimate the likelihood of events with greater availability in memory.
• *Endowment effect*: the fact that people often demand much more to give up an object than they would be willing to pay to acquire it.

Cognitive biases mean that in many situations people do not perceive situations objectively and do not behave in ways that benefit the group over the individual. Short-term self-oriented thinking and behavior appears to be hard-wired into us.[19] For this reason, the mechanism of money and incentives by itself is often not robust enough to address population health challenges requiring cooperation among many different people and organizations.

Leading through Trust (The Network)

So far, in our discussion of mechanisms of leadership, we have considered the use of power (the stick) to require compliance with population health initiatives and of money (the carrot) to encourage voluntary support. Let us now turn to an emerging third way to achieve population health goals—leading by developing and leveraging trust (the network). Let us begin with some terminology.

➤ *What Is a Network and What Is Trust?*

In formal terms, a network is a set of nodes and links represented in a network graph (Figure 2-2).[20] Nodes can represent individuals, organizations, computers, or any other kind of object. The links represent connections between nodes.

Figure 2-2. Network Graph

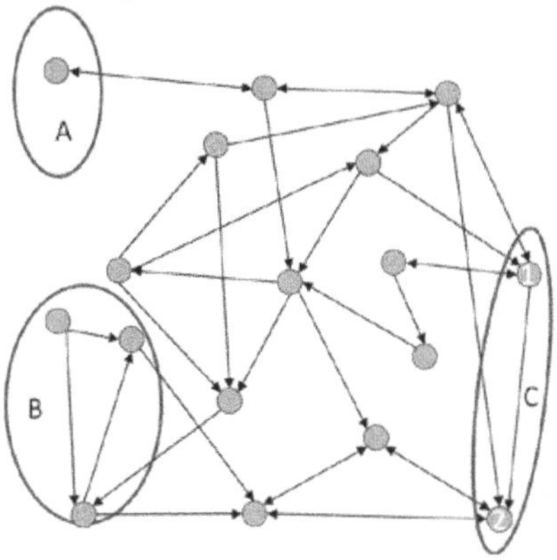

In human contexts, when individuals or organizations have stronger links or connections, scientists say they have more "trust."[21,22] Think about an individual you trust deeply. What makes them trustworthy? Perhaps you have known them for a long time. You probably know their first name and they know yours. You may have a sense they would be loyal to you in a pinch. You probably have a good idea of how they would behave in a challenging situation. You may know their friends and they may know yours. Your friends may confirm that this person is someone you can trust. Similarly, for an organization you trust, you might say with some confidence that its members would do the right thing for you in a pinch. They are reliable and have a good product or service. In a network graph, this kind of trust can be shown by two-way arrows. In Figure 2-2, which ellipse has nodes with the most trust connections? If you answered "C," you are correct.

➤ *What Is a Collaborative Network?*

A second important term is *collaborative network*. As mentioned earlier, a collaborative network involves two or more individuals, organizations, or other networks collaborating in order to achieve a goal none could achieve alone.[3]

Collaborative Network Examples
• Wikipedia
• A group of government agencies and private sector organizations collaborating to reduce air pollution in a community with high asthma rates.
• A group of consumer advocacy organizations and networks collaborating to lobby government to pass a new law to fund healthcare clinics for low-income families.
• A group of corporations collaborating to fund a community-wide wellness program for their employees.

A defining characteristic of a collaborative network is that no one individual or organization is in charge. By definition, these networks involve people and organizations working together collaboratively, based on connections of trust, in order to achieve a shared goal.[23]

➤ *A Collaborative Network as the Roots of a Tree*

Now that you have the definitions of networks, trust, and collaborative networks in mind, please take a look at Figure 2-3.[24] The image shows a collaborative network as a tree with three parts. The leaves represent money/resources. The trunk and branches represent such power as enabling laws/regulations and a governance structure. The roots represent the underground connections of trust among all the people and organizations involved in the collaborative.

Figure 2-3. Trust: the Roots of a Successful Collaborative Network

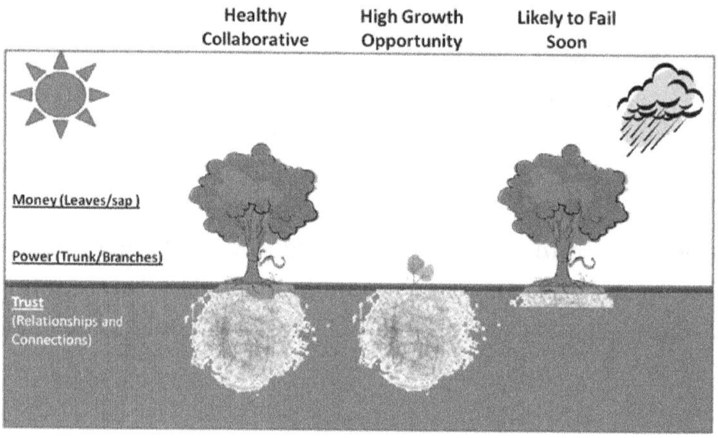

Just as a tree needs sunlight to grow, collaborative networks need money and resources to grow. Just as a tree needs a trunk in order to stand up and be stable, these networks need an empowering structure (laws and rules) to support them. And finally, just as a tree needs a root system to reach out and absorb such essential nutrients as water and minerals, collaborative networks need a 'root system' of people and organizations to reach out and gather up various elements needed to help the network succeed. In effect, people need to weave a network of trust—a root system to hold up the network tree.

As the image shows, a healthy tree will have a healthy root system (left side). A small tree with a strong root system is likely to grow very quickly (middle). And a big tree whose roots are not strong may easily topple.

Consider each of these trees as if it were a population health network. The first has high levels of money, power, and trust. It could be a childhood immunization program for a city that is amply funded by government and private health plans; authorized by an existing body of laws and regulations to make decisions through an effective governance structure in which area schools, pediatricians, hospitals, and others have a voice; and has earned *high trust* among many thousands of individuals and organizations who are used to working together collaboratively to achieve the shared goal of protecting children from infectious disease.

The second tree has very little money and power but a strong root network. Perhaps this one involves people in the same immunization network working to create a network for managing childhood obesity. They are seeking to leverage their strong root system to address a new and important health issue affecting many of the children involved in the vaccination program.

The third tree has large amounts of money and power but a weak root network. Perhaps the government in this case is trying to force participation in a vaccination program that includes gathering of private health information about which most people are uncomfortable. Perhaps there is an underground effort to sabotage the program or pass new laws to make it impossible to operate.

Take a moment and think about collaborations or networks in which you participate. What are the root systems like? Do these three kinds of trees exist in networks in which you participate?

Tips for Developing and Managing Trust and Connections

With the concept of a root system of trust in mind, let us now turn to some practical tips for developing and leading a collaborative network with a strong root system. Note: these are some of the more popular ideas covered in our Network Leadership course taken by graduate students at the University of Louisville.

➢ *Manage Social Capital*

Social capital is a general measure of the trust a person feels with reference to a population of others.[25] It is measured with a question like "How much do you think people can be trusted to do the right thing?"[26] It can also be measured for a particular population by asking a question like "How much do you think people in [company X, neighborhood Y, or government agency Z] can be trusted to do the right thing?" The lower social capital is among a group of people whose support is needed for a given population health initiative, the more time and effort it may take to build the trust needed for that group to succeed.

Leadership investments of time and effort to meet people face to face (digitally or in person) are ways to build social capital. Also, social capital spreads from person to person. Thus a shortcut to building social capital is to build trust with influential people trusted by the people with whom one wants to connect. On the other hand, it is important to be cautious: this process can cut both ways. Influential people who choose not to support you can make it more difficult for you to build the social capital you are seeking to develop with others.

➢ *Trust Takes Years to Build but Moments to Destroy*

A crucial point about trust is that it can take years to build but only moments to destroy. Can you think of anyone you trust implicitly whom you have not known for years? Conversely, has your trust in someone ever been irreparably broken in a moment? Have you ever found out that a person you trusted lied to you? Is there a chance that you would ever fully trust a person who lied to you twice? If you are interested in building population health collaboratives that require trust among many people, you should plan for it to take years to build. Also be aware that trust can be lost in a moment. You should manage your time, priorities, and communications accordingly.

➢ *Manage Bonding, Bridging, and Linking Capacity*

Leadership of collaboratives involving more than a few people involves management of three special types of trust sometimes called bonding, bridging, and linking capacity.[26]

Bonding Capacity

Bonding capacity is a measure of trust among such network leaders as directors and managers. Low bonding capacity is associated with ineffective decision making, technical errors, and communication breakdowns in a collaborative network. It can be measured by having each leader answer a question like "How much do you feel you can trust other members of this network's leadership group to do the right thing for the network?" Figure 2-4 illustrates three levels of trust that can exist between operational management and board level officers.

Figure 2-4. Bonding Capacity

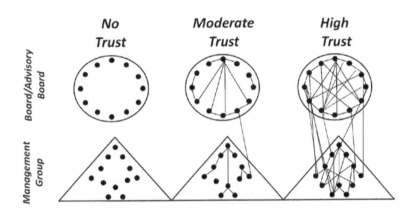

Bonds take time and effort to build and maintain. The more people who are involved in a leadership group, the more time and effort it will take to maintain high bonding capacity. This is why it often makes sense to start small with a few tightly bonded people and grow carefully.

Bridging Capacity

Bridging capacity is a measure of connections between network leaders and network participants (those served by the network). For example, in a community-wide child immunization network, bridges to such key stakeholders as pediatricians, hospitals, schools, and government agencies will be important to develop and maintain. Low bridging capacity is associated with low participation in the network. For example, if the local pediatricians felt no connection to the immunization network, they would be less likely to collaborate with others in the network to get more children immunized.

A good way to build bridging capacity is to include stakeholder leaders on an advisory board or council. In addition, media, press, and social networks can be used to build bridges between a network and potential members.

Linking Capacity

Linking capacity is a measure of connections between network leaders and such influential individuals or groups in the external environment as key legislators, political leaders, and major donors.

Low linking capacity can lead to failure to anticipate changes in the environment that can put a network at risk. Links can be built and maintained through the use of lobbyists, politically connected board members, or support of legislators. Links can also be developed by subscribing to newsletters or digital media reports that describe what is going on in the sectors of interest. Many new types of informational e-news services are coming into the market, offering free or low-cost information through the cloud about important people and groups in industries and sectors, government, and society at large.

➢ *Avoid Groupthink*

Groupthink is a pattern of high bonding with low bridging and linking.[27] Groupthink is associated with low innovation rates and sudden collapse. Cults and radical movements led by a single charismatic leader exhibit groupthink patterns. When almost everyone in a network looks to just one or two people for the truth and stifles dissenting viewpoints, groupthink is typically present in the network (see Figure 2-5).

Figure 2-5. Groupthink

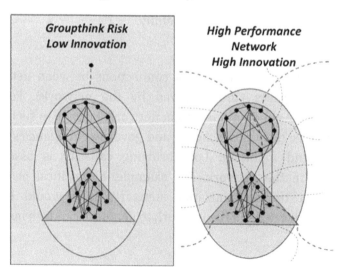

In general, a healthy network will minimize groupthink. It will encourage diverse bridges and links outside the network, and allow for respectful consideration of multiple viewpoints on important issues. Interestingly, stronger bonding capacity often reduces the degree to which team members feel threatened by diverse viewpoints, engendering increased idea sharing and innovation.

➤ *Use Information Technology to Lower Interaction Costs*

In today's increasingly interconnected digital environment, it is feasible to develop and maintain root systems without meeting face to face. Free global teleconferencing, videoconferencing, cloud-based information sharing, and the growth of social networking sites now support the ability to create and maintain trust connections between people and organizations located almost anywhere in the world.[28] Consider using IT to lower interaction costs needed to build and maintain social capital, bonds, bridges, and links.

However, as new IT tools and applications are adopted, users should be aware that in a new world of free, globally accessible technology, a second layer of digital trust has to be considered to protect the privacy and security of information and interactions. Make it a priority to engage experts in this field to assist your organization in the appropriate use of IT for your network.[29]

➤ *Minimize Complexity*

Another important tip is to minimize the complexity of your network. The more different types of entities (e.g., individuals, organizations, and other collaborative networks) with which you and your leadership team need to interact, the more time and effort it will take to establish minimal levels of trust and consensus needed to move forward. On the other hand, it is important to make sure there are ways to connect with representatives of all the key stakeholders involved in your network. It is important to consider ways to balance the tension between simplicity (and nonrepresentation) and complexity (requiring more time and resources to manage). One useful method is to create advisory boards that meet periodically. As mentioned earlier, advisory boards typically do not have formal input into decision making, but they do create opportunities to interact with and gather input from key stakeholders, resulting in higher levels of bonding, bridging, and linking capacity.

➤ *Consider Transformational and Transactional Leadership Styles*

The academic literature identifies two distinct styles of leadership that make a difference: transformational leadership and transactional leadership.[30]

Transformational leaders, as the term suggests, are successful in inspiring others to work together to achieve a radically new and different vision—to change the status quo. They tend to succeed by building passionate commitment to a new idea or direction, and encourage risk-taking, innovation, exploration, and collaboration to move people forward.

Transactional leaders, in contrast, keep the trains running on time, as the saying goes. A transactional leader sees to it that participants in an enterprise are doing their work on time, in tandem, efficiently, effectively, and appropriately. Reliability, stability, predictability, and operational excellence are adjectives that describe this type of leadership.

These two styles of leadership are not opposites. Transactional leaders with no vision of the future often lead people to nowhere, while people following transformational leaders with no capacity to manage day-to-day requirements often find they never get where they are trying to go. Rather, it is important for leaders to consider both types of leadership and select a leadership style appropriate to the situation at hand.

How Is Network Leadership Learned?

The last section discussed a number of skills, abilities, and bodies of knowledge needed by network leaders. Can these competencies be learned? And if so, how?

Network leadership, the ability to lead collaborations involving multiple individuals, organizations, and other networks, is like many complex skills, a learned skill. People are not born to lead networks. Network leadership skills are usually learned through a combination of education (formal and informal) and practice in actual leadership situations. There are many opportunities and pathways for leaders to refine their skills and for potential and aspiring leaders to develop their skills. Table 2-1 identifies a few educational pathways for strengthening essential leadership skills.

Table 2-1. Educational Pathways for Building Leadership Skills

University-based Education	Business (Continuing) Education	Other
MHA, MPH, MBA, PhD programs	Schools	Massive open online courses (MOOCs)
Certificate programs	Professional networks and associations	Peer-based learning programs
Online courses	Online learning	

In addition to formal and informal courses and classes, network leadership is learned through practice. At every stage in a professional's career, one should seek out opportunities to engage in leadership-level activities. One may start by serving as a team leader for a collaborative project in a community. At senior levels, one could end up in leadership roles for high-profile state or national collaboratives. Regardless of the level, the important thing is practice. Finding an opportunity to move from the classroom to the playing field is essential to putting the knowledge gained to use.

Emerging Opportunities for Network Leaders

Let us now turn toward the future. What opportunities for network leadership are emerging in population health? The following are a few of many areas of opportunity we see emerging for network leaders in the coming years.

Opportunity Area 1: Population Health Services

A growing number of network leadership opportunities can be identified by looking at the objectives of *Healthy People 2020*. The CDC tracks over 1,200 objectives in 42 topic areas.[31,32]

Goals of *Healthy People 2020*

1. Attain high-quality, longer lives free of preventable disease, disability, injury, and premature death;

2. Achieve health equity, eliminate disparities, and improve the health of all groups;

3. Create social and physical environments that promote good health for all' and

4. Promote quality of life, healthy development, and healthy behaviors across life stages.

These goals are being pursued by communities and states across the nation in efforts to create healthier communities. In virtually every case, success requires collaboration between for-profit, nonprofit, and government organizations. The final chapter of this book provides two case studies related to *Healthy People 2020* goals and objectives. One is related to addressing the challenges of childhood asthma and the second is focused on the high utilization of hospital emergency departments (ED) by the uninsured or underinsured. While the ACA will potentially divert some of the high utilization of ED services, the problem is likely to persist due to cultural and accessibility factors for certain segments of the population.[33]

Opportunity Area 2: Health in All Policies

A second area of opportunity is the HiAP approach discussed earlier in this chapter, focused on improving various social policies (e.g., housing and urban development, labor and employment, environmental concerns) in order to achieve direct and indirect positive effects on the health and quality of life of the citizens of each community. Success in this area requires leadership from network leaders who can weave together the interests and perspectives of many different population groups and organizations, including consumer advocacy groups; healthcare organizations; employers; politicians and government agencies at local, state and national levels; and those who can also understand the interconnectivity of policies at different levels. Success in this area will often involve the implementation of policies that make incremental improvements rather than radically changing how things are done.

Opportunity Area 3: Population Health Research Networks

Population health research networks are a third area of opportunity for network leaders. As discussed earlier, hundreds of millions of dollars of new investment in population health research and the information technology to support it are being made available as part of U.S. healthcare reform. Success in this area involves the development of collaborative relationships among multiple parties involved in research, including again, consumer advocates, health care providers, researchers, government agencies, and health research regulators at local, state, national, and international levels. In addition, success will be driven by collaborations between hundreds of different population health research data systems.

Opportunity Area 4: Clinically Integrated Networks (CINs)

Many new network leadership opportunities are also emerging as a result of new provisions in health care reform incentivizing the development of clinically integrated networks (CINs).[11] As noted by Flareau, Yale, and colleagues in their 2011 work titled *Clinical Integration: A Roadmap to Accountable Care,* second edition, CINs are

> Legitimate collaborations of otherwise competing providers (hospitals and/or physicians) organized in a way that improves efficiencies in care

delivery (including quality improvement and cost reduction) in a way that outweighs any potential anticompetitive effects.[34]

CINs are closely connected with accountable care organizations (ACOs) discussed above,[18] and patient-centered medical homes (PCMHs), defined as networks of physicians collaborating to improve patient care. In each case, they involve networks of providers collaborating in efforts to improve healthcare outcomes for the overall populations they serve. Successful CINs, ACOs, and PCMHs earn additional reimbursements from CMS and other payers.

Clinical integration among physicians and provider organizations is governed strictly by the Federal Trade Commission (FTC) and the Department of Justice (DOJ),[35] based on legislation designed to limit monopolistic trade behavior by local networks of hospitals and providers. Therefore, network leaders need to consider regulatory boundaries carefully when they design and build new CINs.

A case example of a successful new CIN comes from BayCare Physician Partners in Florida:

Case Study: BayCare Physician Partners

The Tampa Bay region of Florida (Tampa, Clearwater, and St. Petersburg) has a population of over 4.2 million people. Meeting the healthcare needs of this population is of the utmost importance to physicians and care provider teams in the region. BayCare Physician Partners, LLC, is a clinically integrated network (CIN) and wholly owned subsidiary of BayCare Health System, an integrated delivery network of 11 acute care hospitals, outpatient centers, and ancillary services headquartered in Clearwater, Florida. The foundation of this physician-led organization, one of the first CINs organized in the state of Florida, is grounded in the technological and managerial infrastructure developed over a number of years to support launching the CIN. In 2010 assessments and planning were initiated for the multiyear clinical and cultural transformation necessary to form the CIN under collaborative physician leadership, with the goals of improving population health services, care coordination, communication between and among physicians, and ultimately health outcomes for the citizens of the Tampa Bay region.

To create the new CIN, a Physician Steering Committee of 21 physician leaders, two-thirds of whom were independent, was formed. Together they worked collaboratively to develop and present a strategic and tactical plan to the BayCare Health System Board of Directors. The CIN is led by Bruce Flareau, MD, who serves as executive vice president of BayCare Health System and president of BayCare Physician Partners, LLC.[36] The network development strategy is centered on delivering high-quality care to the population served while lowering the total cost of care. With the strategic plan approved and later with the leadership team

Case Study: BayCare Physician Partners

assembled, the next critical task was to recruit affiliated and nonaffiliated physicians into the new network. Within a single year's time over 1,140 physicians were recruited to support the launch of the new CIN.

BayCare Physician Partners officially commenced operation in January 2013. The organization is in its infancy but has already made achievements in the local market, having established a new payment model under a collaborative care agreement with Aetna, Blue Cross Blue Shield, and Cigna that supports physicians in assuming accountability for the quality and cost of covered members' overall health care experience.[37] The structuring of agreements such as this requires meeting the clinical integration objective of the 1996 Statements of Antitrust Enforcement Policy in Health Care by the Federal Trade Commission and the U.S. Department of Justice, which is a guiding regulatory requirement for CINs and ACO programs.[38] Key to meeting this requirement is the need to establish an active and ongoing program to evaluate and modify practice patterns by the network's physician participants; establish mechanisms to monitor and control utilization of health care services to control costs and ensure quality of care; and adoption of technologies and data to assist in realizing such efficiencies.

Through its alignment with BayCare Health System's vision of advancing superior health care by providing an exceptional patient-centered experience, BayCare Physician Partners focuses on three strategic imperatives of the health system (i.e., patient-centered experience; one standard of care; and top decile performance and financial stability) to improve care coordination and delivery of services for the patients of BayCare. The vision of BayCare Physician Partners focuses on:

➢ An integrated, employed, and independent physician-hospital enterprise with shared governance;

➢ Support of a pluralistic model in a variety of physician practice models;

➢ Meeting federal guidelines for joint contracting, and

➢ Acknowledging the importance of measuring and reporting clinical and operational quality measures.

As BayCare Physician Partners moves forward, it will have a strategic focus on improving the use of data analytics and care coordination to help manage risks and establish best practices for other provider organizations. Strengthening connectivity among physician practices and across the spectrum of care settings is important to help close the gap experienced in care coordination, not only in the Tampa Bay region but throughout the nation. BayCare Physician Partners is structured around a physician-led business model with a balance of employed and

Case Study: BayCare Physician Partners

independent physicians from across the geographic area. It focuses on continuous improvement of services to meet the needs of the communities they serve at the population health level.

CINs, ACOs, and PCMHs are part of the evolution of the U.S. healthcare system's care delivery model toward a more network-centric national architecture. The BayCare Physician Partners case exemplifies the type of initiatives implemented across the country in the early twenty-first century to advance the quality of care delivered in communities to improve health at the population level.

Opportunity Area 5: Community Health Management Systems

Last, the concept of community health management systems (CHMS) is an exciting field of opportunity. As described by Steven Shortell, the CHMS could be a network comprising the local health department, community organizations, ACOs, CINs, local hospitals, physician practices, and other provider entities.[39] The CHMS would be organized as a local, publicly accountable, quasi-administrative entity similar to public accountability boards for electric power utilities.

A CHMS would have three functions: 1) to assess and prioritize the health needs of the population from a multisectoral approach; 2) to organize the community's assets, resources, and competencies to deliver the needed services; and 3) to be held clinically and fiscally accountable for the resulting health outcomes. It would deliver an annual report to relevant political bodies in the community. The success of CHMSs depends on the availability of relevant population-based metrics for health outcomes and on payment incentives that encourage integration of the multiple sectors involved in population health.

Challenges and Implications

The topics discussed in this chapter have raised and addressed many questions about the challenges network leaders may face as they participate in population health networks.

Most population health initiatives will have varying community contexts—geographic, political, economic, organizational, social, and technological. Networks can be formed and led in each of these contexts; and the skills, experiences, and abilities of those who lead the networks can all be traced back to several factors noted throughout this chapter.

Because of these varying contexts, there will be a number of challenges for network leaders to address in any network. These challenges include:

- *Alignment*: Network collaboration must be aligned both internally and externally.

- *Legitimation*: The collaboration must gain legitimacy and credibility within the community. Legitimation is all about building social capital in order to be successful.

- *Centralization*: The collaboration can gain legitimacy by understanding its centrality in the political environment of the community.

- *Comparative advantage*: Every collaborator has a core competency and comparative advantage. Collaborations fail because individual collaborators either overestimate or underestimate their comparative advantages and fail to recognize their core competency.

- *Education*: The concept of network leadership is evolving and is different from individual or organizational leadership. The kind of leadership that is needed, the kind of collaboration that can succeed, and the stage of development of the collaboration—all three must be considered in each network situation.

- *Transaction cost measurement and management*: Forming a collaborative network has transaction costs associated not only with its formation, but also with its operation. What are they? How are they measured? When all costs are considered, are the potential results worth the investment required?

- *Selection of collaborators*: The process of selecting collaborators, including tradeoffs and timing, needs to be explored more fully. As Collins noted in his 2001 classic *Good to Great*, it is critically important for leaders to apply a high degree of rigor in the selection of team members to enable an organization to achieve its goals.[40]

- *Use of information and communication technology (ICT)*: Many new types of ICT are coming into the marketplace each year, including cloud-based globally accessible information storage, processing, and retrieval tools; big-data tools; and free communications tools including audio, video, videoconferencing, webinars, private virtual networks, and social media.

Staying abreast of new ICTs will be a critical factor in the success of many network leaders and the networks they serve.

These challenges and implications serve as reminders for people interested in leading networks of all sizes, shapes, and configurations. Each leader has a multitude of issues to grasp and address to be successful in leading the way to improved quality of life for the population in their community.

CHAPTER 2 DISCUSSION QUESTIONS

Discussion questions are provided for team building or class exercises. Answers for all questions are provided in Appendix C.

Question Number	Question
1	What is a collaborative network? Give an example.
2	Why is collaboration increasing in population health? Give an example.
3	How is network leadership different from traditional organizational leadership?
4	Why is network leadership important? What difference can it make?
5	What are the three steering mechanisms (i.e., the three-legged stool) that leaders can use to effect change? Give an example of how and where each is used in population health.
6	How can social capital be measured? Give an example.
7	What is groupthink? Give an example.
8	What is an example of an emerging area of opportunity for network leadership in population health?

CHAPTER 2 SUMMARY

- In today's increasingly interconnected world, collaboration among and between many different people and organizations is becoming increasingly important.
  - Example: collaborating to protect the public in the 2009 H1N1 influenza pandemic.
- Collaboration is required to address most population health challenges in infectious, chronic, and social disease categories.
- Network leaders lead through three mechanisms: the three-legged stool of power (the stick), incentives (the carrot), and trust (the network). A growing body of science shows the importance of trust (the network) to achieve goals.
- A collaborative network is defined as two or more individuals, organizations, or other networks collaborating to achieve a goal they can't achieve alone.
- Collaborative networks have root systems. Healthy root systems have high levels of social capital, high bonding, bridging and linking capacity, and low levels of groupthink. When root systems break down, trees topple.
- Network leadership is a learned skill: formal education and "learning by doing" are pathways to success.
- There are many opportunities for network leadership in population health. Opportunities include *Healthy People 2020* service areas, health in all policies initiatives, population health research networks, clinically integrated networks (CINs), and community health management systems (CHMSs).

CHAPTER 2 REFERENCES

1.   Leavitt M, McKeown R. Introduction. *Finding allies, building alliances: 8 elements that bring—and keep—people together.* San Francisco, Calif.: Jossey-Bass; 2013:3.

2.   Benkler Y. *The wealth of networks: how social production transforms markets and freedom.* New Haven, Conn.: Yale University Press; 2006.

3.   Raab J, Kenis P. Heading toward a society of networks: empirical developments and theoretical challenges. *J Manage Inquiry.* 2009;18(3):198-210.

4.   World Health Organization. Social determinants of health. 2012; http://www.who.int/social_determinants/en/. Accessed December 25, 2013.

5.   Bostic RW, Thornton RLj, Rudd EC, Sternthal MJ. Health in all policies: the role of the US Department of Housing and Urban Development and present and future challenges. *Health Aff (Millwood).* 2012;31(9):2130-2137.

6.   Habermas J. *The theory of communicative action.* Boston, Mass.: Beacon Press; 1984.

7.   Williamson OE, Masten SE, eds. *The economics of transaction costs.* Cheltenham, UK: E. Elgar Pub; 1999.

8.   Powell WW. Neither market nor hierarchy—network forms of organization. *Res Org Behav.* 1990;12:295-336.

9.   Chan KY, Reidpath DD. "Typhoid Mary" and "HIV Jane": responsibility, agency and disease prevention. *Reprod Health Matters.* 2003;11(22):40-50.

10.   Brooks J. The sad and tragic life of typhoid Mary. *Can Med Assoc J.* 1996;154(6):915-916.

11.   Doherty RB. The certitudes and uncertainties of health care reform. *Ann Intern Med.* 2010;152(10):679-682.

12.   Naydeck BL, Pearson JA, Ozminkowski RJ, Day BT, Goetzel RZ. The impact of the Highmark employee wellness programs on 4-year healthcare costs. *J Occup Environ Med.* 2008;50(2):146-156.

13.   Centers for Medicare and Medicaid Services. Accountable care organizations. 2013.

14.   Peterson M, Muhlestein D, Gardner P. *Growth and dispersion of accountable care organizations: July 2013 update.* Leavitt Partners; 2013. http://leavittpartners.com/wp-content/uploads/2013/08/Growth-and-Disperson-of-ACOs-August-20131.pdf Accessed June 10, 2014.

15.   Helfgott AW. The patient-centered medical home and accountable care organizations: an overview. *Curr Opin Obstet Gynecol.* 2012;24(6):458-464.

16. Hardin G. The tragedy of the commons. The population problem has no technical solution; it requires a fundamental extension in morality. *Science (New York)*. 1968;162(3859):1243-1248.

17. Ostrom E, Burger J, Field CB, Norgaard RB, Policansky D. Sustainability: revisiting the commons: local lessons, global challenges. *Science*. 1999;284(5412):278-282.

18. Kahneman D. *Thinking, fast and slow*. New York, N.Y.: Farrar, Straus, & Giroux; 2011.

19. Simon HA. Models of bounded rationality. Boston, Mass.: MIT Press;1997.

20. Scott J. *Social network analysis: a handbook*. London, England: SAGE Publications; 2000.

21. Borgatti SP, Foster PC. The network paradigm in organizational research: a review and typology. *J Manage*. 2003;29(6):991-1013.

22. McEvily B, Perrone V, Zaheer A. Trust as an organizing principle. *Organization Science*. 2003;14(1):91-103.

23. Provan KG, Fish A, Sydow J. Interorganizational networks at the network level: a review of the empirical literature on whole networks. *J Manage*. 2007;33(3):479-516.

24. Thornewill J. *Arizona Health Information Exchange Governance and Collaborative Capacity Assessment*. St. Luke's Health Initiatives and GroupPlus, LLC, http://azhie.groupplusllc.com/; May 28, 2010.

25. Putnam RD. Bowling alone: America's declining social capital. *J Democr*. 1995;6:65-78.

26. Halpern D. *Social capital*. Cambridge, England; Malden, Mass.: Polity;2005.

27. Burt RS. *Brokerage and closure: an introduction to social capital*. New York, N.Y.: Oxford University Press;2005.

28. Google. Google Apps for Business. Everything Your Business Needs. https://www.google.com/enterprise/apps/business/benefits.html?section=together. Accessed December 25, 2013.

29. Tang ZL, Hu Y, Smith MD. Gaining trust through online privacy protection: self-regulation, mandatory standards, or caveat emptor. *J Manage Inform Syst*. 2008;24(4):153-173.

30. Sturm M, Reiher S, Heinitz K, Soellner R. Transformational and transactional leadership - A meta-analytical examination of their relationship with leadership effectiveness. *Zeitschrift für Arbeits- und Organisationspsychologie*. 2011;55(2):88-104.

31. Koh HK. A 2020 vision for healthy people. *N Engl J Med*. 2010;362(18):1653-1656.

32. US Centers for Disease Control and Prevention. *Healthy People 2020* overview. http://www.cdc.gov/nchs/healthy_people/hp2020.htm. Accessed August 20, 2013.

33.   Kangovi S, Barg FK, Carter T, Long JA, Shannon R, Grande D. Understanding why patients of low socioeconomic status prefer hospitals over ambulatory care. *Health Aff (Millwood)*. 2013;32(7):1196-1203.

34.   Flareau B, Yale K, Bohn JM, Konschak C. Clinically integrated networks. In: *Clinical Integration: A Roadmap to Accountable Care*. Virginia Beach, Va: Convurgent Publishing;2011:18-21.

35.   US Department of Justice and the Federal Trade Commission. *Statements of Antitrust Enforcement Policy in Health Care*. Washington, D.C.: US Department of Justice and the Federal Trade Commission; 1996.

36.   President of BayCare Physician Partners recognized nationally [press release]. *Reuters*. December 19, 2012.
http://www.reuters.com/article/2012/12/19/baycare-president-idUSnPnDC29357+160+PRN20121219. Accessed April 14, 2013.

37.   Aetna and BayCare to introduce collaborative care in Tampa [press release]. *BusinessWire*. December 17, 2012.
http://www.businesswire.com/news/home/20121217006345/en/Aetna-BayCare-Introduce-Collaborative-Care-Tampa#.U4Pd4fldW_c. Accessed April 14, 2013.

38.   Flareau B, Yale K, Bohn JM, Konschak C. The joint statements. *Clinical Integration: A Roadmap to Accountable Care*. 2nd ed. Virginia Beach, Va: Convurgent Publishing; 2011:125.

39.   Shortell SM. Challenges and opportunities for population health partnerships. *Prev Chronic Dis*. 2010;7(6):A114.

40.   Collins J. First who then what. In: *Good to Great*. New York, N.Y.: HarperCollins; 2001:42-64.

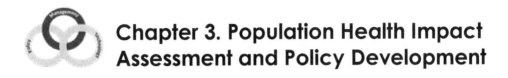

Chapter 3. Population Health Impact Assessment and Policy Development

Susan Olson Allen, PhD

Raymond Austin, MD

"The intellectual equipment needed for the job of the future is an ability to define problems, quickly assimilate relevant data, conceptualize and reorganize the information, make deductive and inductive leaps with it, ask hard questions about it, discuss findings with colleagues, work collaboratively to find solutions and then convince others."

Robert B. Reich
(1946 –)
Professor of public policy and political economist

Chapter 3 Learning Objectives

- Understand what a health impact assessment is and its methodology.

- Know where health impact assessements were first adopted internationally.

- Give two examples of past health impact assessements done in the United States.

- Identify the main barriers to wider adoption of health impact assessments in the United States.

- Be able to articulate the policy implications of the use and application of health impact assessements.

Introduction

This book discusses the needs and problems that face population health management in modern society from a systems perspective. There are several factors that can contribute to poor health across multiple dimensions—social, economic, political, physical, and environmental.Each of these can affect the health of individuals and the community as a whole.[1,2] Throughout society, government agencies, healthcare and public health organizations, and community stakeholder groups identify problems that affect the physical health and well-being of various population segments of their cities and regions. Over periods of time that range from days to years, solutions can be envisioned and implemented to try to make improvements. But how do we know whether the proposed solutions are effective in improving the population's health? How do we evaluate how well our solutions are working, or whether there might be a better way to manage those issues?

One approach to this challenge is the adoption of health impact assessments (HIAs) as a methodology to evaluate new programs, policies, and projects that can affect the health and well-being of the residents and stakeholders in a community. Originally based on the methods and techniques of environmental impact assessments (EIAs), HIAs have evolved into a valuable evaluation method of their own. Their wide-ranging uses include assessing policies, programs, and projects. They have been instituted in Europe and Australia since the late 1990s, and to a lesser extent in North America over the past decade. In United States (U.S.) cities in which HIAs have been implemented, such as San Francisco, Los Angeles, Trenton, and Atlanta, they have proved to be a valuable evaluation method for strengthening awareness of the effects or consequences that may result from various initiatives.[3-5] Within the course of evaluating any program, project, or policy with an HIA, it is important to recognize that

> . . . the HIA process should employ both qualitative and quantitative methods of research, and that the assessment itself should accordingly be based on both qualitative and quantitative data.[6]

Quantitative evaluation (i.e., statistical comparison of changes in health status, economic impacts, changes in the rates of crime in a community, etc.) provides insights that can be used in comparison with existing standards, statistics, and quantitative goals. Qualitative evaluations can include extraction of narrative feedback from interviews and surveys of stakeholders that yield descriptive insights; and most importantly from rigorous reviews of literature identifying pertinent evidence that can contribute to the theoretical justification for or potential negative impact of the program, project, or policy under study in the HIA.[6,7]

As one of the central themes of this book is technological innovation, there is a continued need for new analytic tools to use in HIAs to help forecast the positive or negative effects on population health from new social, environmental, or economic interventions.[8] The insights gained from analytic tools (e.g., such policy surveillance systems as the National Cancer Institute's State Cancer Legislative Database or SCLD) can aid policy and decision makers in managing expansive literature reviews, and evaluating potential effects of policy and built-environment changes in their effects on the social determinants of health for a community.[9] As the United States continues to move forward with HIAs, the use of advanced analytics tools and Big Data resources will only strengthen the quantitative and qualitative evaluations that support these emerging efforts to support community-level decisions.

The first two chapters of this book introduced a number of critical issues for understanding total population health as it exists and evolves in any community or nation's ecosystem. Health determinants, definitions of population health, network leadership, technological innovation, and the importance of Health in All Policies (HiAP) are some of the underpinning factors reviewed. Just as the authors of the first chapter noted that researchers and practitioners in accountable care organizations use data mining to identify care practices that result in better outcomes, HIAs can serve as tools to assist community decision makers in developing informed choices to improve the health and wellness of their community's population.

HIAs can be used to identify or define community-level problems in the Population Health Ecosystem model, as illustrated in Chapter 1 (Figure 1-2).

Figure 3-1. Population Health Ecosystem from Chapter 1

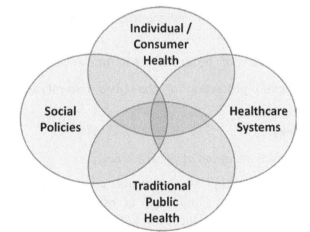

Health care systems might use HIAs to assess a policy decision (e.g., short-term benefits of covering wellness programs versus long-term costs of foregoing the coverage). Traditional public health government agencies or organizations have found HIAs to be a valuable methodology to evaluate a program, project. or policy changes that can impact a community.[10] They may be used to assess a policy (e.g., whether a local health department should provide immunization services); a program (e.g., whether a smoking cessation program is cost-effective to conduct relative to its success rate); or a project (e.g., the health effects of placing an apartment building near an expressway).

An example of a project HIA is the following case study of the Louisville Loop initiative. The initiative is one of the strategic efforts of the City of Louisville to improve the interconnectedness of parklands across the Louisville, Kentucky, area.[11]

The Louisville Loop Health Impact Assessment (2012)

The Louisville Loop is part of a comprehensive land-use plan for the City of Louisville. It is the centerpiece of a long-term plan to expand and improve parkland and environmental education. The Louisville Loop will eventually become a paved trail of more than 100 miles around the community. In 2011, Louisville Mayor Greg Fischer committed to complete the Loop and focus on connecting people by foot, bike, and public transit to community gathering places, schools, workplaces, natural areas and commercial centers. Expected benefits of the Loop include:

- Strengthened opportunities for economic development;

- Increased mixed use of the parklands;

- Improved connectivity of neighborhoods, schools, and retail businesses throughout the parks system;

- Improved quality of the air and the natural environment; and

- Strengthened protection of the city's natural assets, culture, and history.

Summary Findings:

a) Primary benefit is increased physical activity.

b) Other benefits include: More natural green space and its positive environmental impacts; improved access to parks; improved social interaction; and possible reduction in automobile use.

Barriers to Greater Benefits:

The Louisville Loop Health Impact Assessment (2012)

The primary barriers are safety and accessibility. In some cases, safety concerns, whether real or perceived, will prevent the Loop from being used. Second, lack of maintenance and lack of awareness that the Loop exists on the part of the public that the Loop exists may discourage use of the Loop and thereby limit its accessibility.

Key Recommendations:

a) *Improve interconnectivity*.

   i.   The Olmsted Parkway routing should be developed, as it has the highest concentration of vulnerable populations and provides a nexus of connections to all parts of the city and the Loop.

   ii. Avoid passing the Loop through areas prone to high levels of particulate matter, such as industrial plants and heavily travelled roads; or otherwise provide air monitoring with possible warning systems when the air is unhealthy, and provide control measures to mitigate the pollutants.

b) *Improve maintenance*. The Metro Council, working in conjunction with neighborhood leaders, community groups, and Friends of the Loop, could assist Metro Parks in overseeing and implementing maintenance.

c) *Green space buffer zones*. Landfills, brownfields, and Superfund sites could be reused for the Loop and its connectors, but safeguards and monitoring must be in place to ensure safety.

The Louisville Loop HIA provided insights about ways to improve connectivity in a metro area and maximize such opportunities to improve the health of the community as increasing physical activity and improving air quality. This project serves as an example of several HIAs that have been conducted across the country. One of the key challenges is evaluation of follow-up actions taken in regard to recommendations made. Many HIAs are conducted on programs, projects, or policies (e.g., interventions) that can take many years to realize the post-implementation effects. Resolving this challenge can in many cases require adoption of HIAs as part of local or county government activities; an example may be found in California with the extensive use of HIAs by the San Francisco Department of Public Health.[10] The time gap between the implementation of any intervention and the point at which its impact can be evaluated often creates a significant barrier to acquiring the resources and funding needed to fully evaluate post-implementation effects.

Historical Background

While HIAs have been recognized for quite some time as a valuable methodology in many countries, especially in Europe, they started being implemented in the United States only as a tool to identify the spectrum of issues for consideration in proposed health or social policy issues and related projects. In 1999 the European Centre for Health Policy produced the Gothenburg Consensus Paper.[12] The paper was widely considered to be one of the first major works to define and give structure to HIAs. The international group of partners defined an HIA as

> . . . a combination of procedures, methods and tools by which a policy, program or project may be judged as to its potential effects on the health of a population, and the distribution of those effects within the population.[12]

This definition is still the standard used today to shape and develop many HIAs. Another notion of the Gothenburg Consensus Paper still used as a basis for the development of HIAs is the values set put forth in the paper. They are

> . . . *democracy*, emphasizing the right of people to participate in a transparent process for the formulation, implementation and evaluation of policies that affect their life, both directly and through the elected political decision makers;
>
> *equity*, emphasizing that HIA is not only interested in the aggregate impact of the assessed policy on the health of a population but also on the distribution of the impact within the population, in terms of gender, age, ethnic background and socio-economic status;
>
> *sustainable development*, emphasizing that both short term and long term as well as more and less direct impacts are taken into consideration; and
>
> *ethical use of evidence*, emphasizing that the use of quantitative and qualitative evidence has to be rigorous, and based on different scientific disciplines and methodologies to get as comprehensive assessment as possible of the expected impacts.[12]

The Gothenburg Consensus Paper thus provided both the foundation and the structure on which many HIAs are based today. The methodology has been expanded and refined, but the initial tenets of HIAs as conceived by the contributors to the paper have remained consistent.

Conducting an HIA

As HIAs continue to become a more widely accepted practice in the United States, tools used to conduct HIAs continue to be developed and honed. One excellent source of best-practices examples is the San Francisco Department of Public Health, which has conducted more comprehensive HIAs than any other public health department in the nation and is generally considered a leader in the field in the United States. In a 2011 *Health Affairs* article, Bhatia noted the challenges experienced by the department with predictive factors for HIAs and how department policy analysts developed multivariate models to help estimate future changes in determinants of health.[13]

A number of formats and level of detail can be embodied within an HIA, but three types to understand include:[14,15]

- *Rapid-cycle Assessment:* quick-turnaround HIAs (perhaps a 1–2-day workshop);

- *Intermediate Assessment:* analysis that engages more in-depth assessment work; and

- *Comprehensive Assessment:* the most extensive and rigorous degree of analytical work.

The type of HIA to be conducted depends on several factors. First is the scope and depth of the HIA necessary to assess the issues the HIA is to address. Second is the amount of time between when the HIA is to be conducted and when the decisions about the policy, program, or project must be made. Third is the amount of resources available in terms of both people and money.

Rapid-cycle HIAs typically take only a few days to conduct, and usually examine existing knowledge, both in terms of expertise from the various fields involved with the issues and information gleaned from previous HIAs. Intermediate HIAs are more in-depth investigations than rapid-cycle HIAs, and generally take a few weeks to perform. They involve reviewing existing knowledge as do rapid-cycle HIAs, but also involve experts from the various fields in terms of their opinions and expectations as well as researching and analyzing new information. Comprehensive HIAs normally take several months to complete, and involve the same elements as intermediate HIAs, but also incorporate a review of the available evidence base as well as gathering and analyzing new information.[15]

There are five essential steps to conducting the HIA in using this approach. During the course of every HIA, factors can be evaluated that cover economic issues, social and community effects, and political implications. The steps are: 1) *screening*, which determines whether an HIA would be useful in the assessment of a policy, program, or project; 2) *scoping,* which determines which health impacts of the policy, program, or project should be assessed and which populations are potentially affected by those health impacts; 3) *assessment* of the health impacts in terms of magnitude, direction, and certainty; 4) *reporting* of the findings to decision makers; and 5) *evaluation* of the impact the HIA has had on the decision making process.[16] Figure 3-2 illustrates the process.[12]

Figure 3-2. Approach to Health Impact Assessments

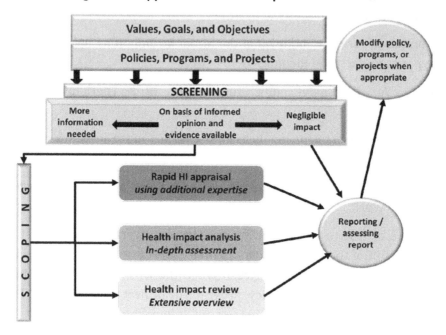

The Healthy Development Measurement Tool (HDMT) is perhaps one of the best-known and most widely used instruments for use in HIAs in the United States. Developed by the San Francisco Department of Public Health in 2007, it is revised and expanded on a regular basis.[17] The HDMT has been made available online and contains both community health indicators and a checklist pertaining to a wide range of issues affecting a population's health. Its scope is broad but systematic, with measures covering areas that include but are not limited to transportation, education, housing, community, and health systems; and the methodology is systematic in its approach.[18,19] Because of its ability to standardize its indicators, the HDMT is used in many HIAs for definitions of the variables being employed in HIA studies.

In the 2003–2009 timeframe, the European Commission's Directorate-General for Health and Consumer Affairs funded the development of a new tool for evaluating the impact on health determinants from changes to various policies instituted by different European countries. The new tool was called DYNAMO-HIA.[20] This new Web-based application brought additional quantitative evaluation capability to the HIA process for evaluating population-level health impacts. The developers of DYNAMO-HIA aimed at making the tool technically accurate for modeling the health effects on a community's population from policy interventions using epidemiological evidence at the European-country level. Acknowledging that predictive validity for such a tool as DYNAMO-HIA is difficult to achieve when it often takes several years for the effects of policy change to be realized, the developers stated that the results from modeled scenarios were intended to serve as a "decision-support tool" for future policy and community decision makers.[21,22] They operationalized the technical accuracy and the effectiveness for HIA into six criteria: real-life population, dynamic projection, explicit risk-factor states, modest data requirements, rich model output, and general accessibility. To date, DYNAMO-HIA has been used primarily at the national level in Europe, although its developers maintain that it could be used at the regional and local levels and in other countries. Examples of HIAs that have employed DYNAMO-HIA include assessing the effects of increased obesity among the Dutch population, and European Union-wide improvements in population health following a price increase on alcoholic products.[21]

Revisiting the Louisville Loop HIA

The Louisville Loop HIA was conducted by employees of the Louisville Metro Department of Public Health and Wellness (LMPHW) as well as an LMPHW consultant as part of a certification program offered in an HIA class. The project team conducted the HIA over a four-month period and included the HIA steps of screening, scoping, assessment, and reporting. Time limitations of the classes in the HIA certificate program did not allow for evaluation of the effects of the HIA on the decision making process. The primary data used in the assessment on health determinants and disparities were derived from the Centers for Disease Control and Prevention's (CDC) Selected Metropolitan/Micropolitan Area Risk Trends (SMART) Behavioral Risk Factor Surveillance Study (BRFSS) 2010 data set.[23]

The project team effectively demonstrated application of the HIA methodology. In this case, the HIA project team screened the project by determining that the Louisville Loop had the potential to have a positive impact on the health of the residents of the Metro Louisville area. The team then scoped the project by looking within the community and establishing that there were 15 determinants of health to be addressed; and then developed scoping worksheets for each determinant to evaluate the positive or negative effects on health for those determinants. Four major areas of potential health impacts for the community included: access, physical activity, safety, and environmental impacts. Identification of the determinants led to the team's creation of the pathway diagram in Figure 3-3.

Figure 3-3. Health Determinants Pathway Diagram for the Louisville Loop Project

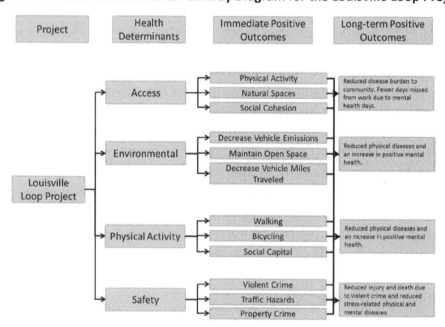

In the course of the HIA, the major impacts of the Louisville Loop were identified as (a) opportunities to increase social interaction and reduce social isolation of the residents; (b) improve access to parks and places for physical activity; and (c) highlight the importance of safety throughout the parks with shared roads and trails that have high traffic volume (i.e., more than 21 percent of nonfatal injuries occurring at intersections).

Improving Community Awareness of Population Health Challenges with HIAs

HIAs can serve as useful tools to aid community and policy decision makers in identifying challenges related to health determinant issues faced by members of their community, state, or country. They can elevate a community's understanding of health risks or impacts that may arise from implementation of new policies, programs, or projects; and provide new insights into health behavior-related issues, socioeconomic factors, crime and safety issues, and environmental/infrastructural elements that will be positively or negatively affected. One example cited in the literature is the HIA conducted on the city of Baltimore's TransForm Baltimore zoning code rewrite initiative released in April 2010.[24,25] In summary, a multidisciplinary team conducted the HIA between 2009 and 2010; it produced several findings. The primary methodologies used were interviews with participants in the zoning code rewrite process (and residents); literature reviews; and detailed analysis of the original and revised zoning codes. One noteworthy outcome of the interviews conducted as part of the HIA was that while the initial motives for the TransForm Baltimore initiative were "economic and non-health goal"-oriented, the HIA helped raise the awareness of the health and social determinant implications with the zoning code rewrite process.[24] Along with many projects conducted by the San Francisco Department of Public Health throughout the past decade, this HIA offers another strong example of the positive benefits that can be achieved to support efforts to improve population health in both urban and rural communities moving into the twenty-first century.

Policy Implications

The HIA approach provides a potentially very useful means of developing and evaluating policies related to promoting and managing population health. At a very basic level, policy development is the process of developing plans for actions aimed at carrying out some type of intervention intended to achieve identified desired objectives and goals. The policy analysis process is described as developing and understanding the policy making process and the development of knowledge necessary for making, implementing, and evaluating interventions.[26]

As a tool to support policy making and policy evaluation, HIAs can be incorporated into the evaluation processes in the early stages of the policy development prior to regulatory approval. The HIA can be applied to 'trial runs' or the review of existing similar or related policies. HIAs can be used to produce evidence-based policy recommendations for changing or refining policy objectives, as well as the procedures for measuring and evaluating outcomes of policy interventions.

The 'when and how' (i.e., the timing and use) of HIAs as a tool of policy development and evaluation is largely determined by the context, nature, and time frame of the policy matter under consideration. In this manner the HIA can be used to help guide decision making related to policy development and implementation as well as the evaluation of policy results. The context and nature of a policy intervention are significant in terms of the intended target that is most relevant to the identified problem addressed by the policy action. The policy focus of an intervention could be individuals, groups or segments, a community, or a society as a whole. The behaviors and actions of each of these could have significant implications regarding the application and details of the HIA.

Additionally, the HIA effort would need to carefully consider the choice of means and criteria for determining how the impact of a policy would be carried out. The means for determining the impact assessment of a policy may involve the assessment and measurement of a combination of such factors as the economic costs, the productivity gains and losses, and the distribution of costs and benefits, as well as the politics and values of key stakeholders involved in a policy intervention. The HIA can be further affected by more complex assessment measures like quality of life and longevity, both of which are commonly used measures related to matters of population health. Policy intervention efforts may be guided by such overarching value approaches as market justice and social justice, which may also need to be considered in the HIA policy process.

Although HIAs are often thought of largely in terms of their use in evaluating the results of policies after they have been implemented, they are also useful as a decision-support tool to policy makers. The results of quantitative and qualitative assessments of social and health determinant factors can bring added value and visibility of important issues that need to be considered in the early stages of any local, state, or federal policy making process.

Policy implications are important to consider in almost every HIA, no matter whether the purpose of the HIA is to assess new zoning codes for land use, new housing projects, park development, or policies that influence certain types of commerce. A final policy consideration is whether the HIA should be incorporated into an EIA or whether it should be a stand-alone document. This consideration is particularly significant in the United States, where EIAs are conducted only for large projects at the federal level. Engaging appropriate stakeholders at each level of policy making (e.g., local, state, and federal) to determine whether to make this integration of HIAs and EIAs a regulatory requirement could lead to more meaningful consideration of the merging of these methodologies as the need and benefits have been demonstrated previously.[5]

Conclusion

In closing, two final factors concerning HIAs are leadership and technology. New Web-based and automated tools continue to be needed for the advancement of HIAs in the United States. In the coming years, as HIAs become more widely accepted in the United States, new predictive analytics tools will aid researchers and policy makers in refining these evaluations of the potential health impacts of new policies, programs, and projects. Last is the issue of leadership. The nature of HIAs often requires multisectoral engagement of partners and collaborators. Solving community challenges related to social determinants of health can involve multiple variables that include economic, environmental, zoning and planning, public health, medical care, and legal issues. Getting the right leaders involved at the right time can make a tremendous difference in maximizing the value of insights to be derived from any health impact assessment.

For the next decade and beyond, as society continues to recognize the interconnectedness of health and wellness for the population of each community, such innovative tools as HIAs can enhance decisions made about new policies, programs, and projects. Ultimately, engaging competent leaders and new technologies will help advance and strengthen HIA initiatives and lead to healthier communities for the next generation in the twenty-first century.

CHAPTER 3 DISCUSSION QUESTIONS

Discussion questions are provided for team building or class exercises. Answers for all questions are provided in Appendix C.

Question Number	Question
1	Which city public health department in the United States is providing best practices in HIAs for the United States?
2	What is DYNAMO-HIA and how can it be used in the United States?
3	From the Louisville Loop HIA example, what health determinants were identified as being the most important or impacted in the community?
4	What are the two key components to the San Francisco Public Health Department's Healthy Development Measurement Tool (HDMT)?
5	What is an HIA and what are its five components?

CHAPTER 3 SUMMARY

- A health impact assessment (HIA) is a methodology that employs both qualitative and quantitative methods of research, and specifies that the assessment itself should accordingly be based on both qualitative and quantitative data. Its five steps are: screening, scoping, assessment, evaluation, and reporting.

- The Healthy Development Measurement Tool (HDMT) is perhaps one of the best-known and most widely used instruments for use in HIAs in the United States as developed by the San Francisco Department of Public Health in 2007. The HDMT is available online; it contains both community health indicators and a checklist pertaining to a wide range of issues affecting a population's health.

- The HIA approach provides a potentially very useful means of developing and evaluating policies related to promoting and managing population health.

- HIAs can serve as useful tools to aid community and policy decision makers with identifying challenges related to health determinant issues. They also can elevate a community's understanding of health risks or impacts that may arise from the implementation of new policies, programs, or projects.

- Leadership and technology are two important factors that will contribute to the advancement of HIAs moving into the twenty-first century.

- There are three types of HIAs: rapid-cycle assessments (perhaps a one- or two-day workshop); intermediate assessments; and comprehensive assessments.

- HIAs originated in Europe after the 1999 publication of the European Centre for Health Policy's release of *Health Impact Assessment: Main Concepts and Suggested Approach – Gothenburg Consensus Paper*.

CHAPTER 3 REFERENCES

1. Kent J, Thompson S. Health and the built environment: exploring foundations for a new interdisciplinary profession. *J Environ Public Health.* 2012;2012:958175.

2. Schulz A, Mentz G, Johnson-Lawrence V, et al. Independent and joint associations between multiple measures of the built and social environment and physical activity in a multi-ethnic urban community. *J Urban Health.* 2013;90(5):872-87.

3. UCLA Health Impact Assessment Group. Health impact assessment of modifications to the Trenton Farmer's Market (Trenton, New Jersey). Los Angeles, Calif.: UCLA Fielding School of Public Health;2007.

4. Georgia Institute of Technology. *Atlanta BeltLine Health Impact Assessment.* Atlanta, Ga.: Georgia Institute of Technology;2007.

5. Bhatia R, Wernham A. Integrating human health into environmental impact assessment: an unrealized opportunity for environmental health and justice. *Environ Health Perspect.* 2008;116(8):991-1000.

6. Love K, Pritchard C, Maguire K, McCarthy A, Paddock P. Qualitative and quantitative approaches to health impact assessment: an analysis of the political and philosophical milieu of the multi-method approach. *Crit Public Health.* 2005;15(3):275-289.

7. Mindell J, Biddulph J, Taylor L, et al. Improving the use of evidence in health impact assessment. *Bull World Health Organ.* 2010;88(7):543-550.

8. Cole BL, Shimkhada R, Fielding JE, Kominski G, Morgenstern H. Methodologies for realizing the potential of health impact assessment. *Am J of Prev Med.* 2005;28(4):382-389.

9. Brownson RC, Royer C, Ewing R, McBride TD. Researchers and policymakers: travelers in parallel universes. *Am J Prev Med.* 2006;30(2):164-172.

10. Dannenberg AL, Bhatia R, Cole BL, Heaton SK, Feldman JD, Rutt CD. Use of health impact assessment in the U.S: 27 case studies, 1999-2007. *Am J Prev Med.* 2008;34(3):241-256.

11. Ballard M, Hannon L, Rhodes M, Walfourt N. Executive summary. *The Louisville Loop Health Impact Assessment.* Louisville, Ky.: University of Louisville, School of Public Health and Information Sciences Health Impact Assessment course;2012.

12. European Centre for Health Policy. *Health impact assessment: main concepts and suggested approach—Gothenburg consensus paper.* United Kingdom: HIA Gateway, West Midlands Public Health Observatory;1999.

13. Bhatia R, Corburn J. Lessons from San Francisco: health impact assessments have advanced political conditions for improving population health. *Health Aff (Millwood).* 2011;30(12):2410-2418.

14. Forsyth A, Slotterback CS, Krizek K. Health impact assessment (HIA) for planners: what tools are useful? *Journal of Planning Literature.* 2010;24(3):231-245.

15. Blau J, Ernst K, Wismar M, Baro F, Blenkus GM. The use of health impact assessment across Europe. In: Stahl T, Wismar M, Olila E, Lahtinen E, Leppo K, eds. *Health in all policies: prospects and potentials.* Helsinki, Finland: Finnish Ministry of Social Affairs and Health;2006. 209-230.

16. Dannenberg Al, Bhatia R, Cole BL, et al. Growing the field of health impact assessment in the United States: an agenda for research and practice. *Am J Public Health.* 2006;96(2):262-270.

17. Farhang L. *Making the case for health in urban development: using the healthy development measurement tool.* San Francisco, Calif.: San Francisco Department of Public Health;2009.

18. Forsyth A, Slotterback CS, Krizek KJ. Health impact assessment in planning: development of the design for health HIA tools. *Environ Impact Assess Rev.* 2010;30(1):42-51.

19. San Francisco Department of Public Health. Sustainable communities index: measures. 2013; http://www.sustainablecommunitiesindex.org/webpages/view/39. Accessed February 10, 2014.

20. European Commission's Directorate-General for Health and Consumer Affairs. *Annual newsletter Dynamo-HIA 2009.* Rotterdam, The Netherlands: European Commission's Directorate-General for Health and Consumer Affairs;2009.

21. Lhachimi SK, Nusselder WJ, Smit HA, et al. DYNAMO-HIA—a dynamic modeling tool for generic health impact assessments. *PLoS One.* 2012;7(5):e33317.

22. Veerman JL, Mackenbach JP, Barendregt JJ. Validity of predictions in health impact assessment. *J Epidemiol Community Health.* 2007;61(4).

23. Centers for Disease Control and Prevention. SMART: BRFSS city and county data and documentation. 2010; http://www.cdc.gov/brfss/smart/smart_2010.htm. Accessed December 9, 2013.

24. Johnson Thornton RL, Greiner A, Fichtenberg CM, Feingold BJ, Ellen JM, Jennings JM. Achieving a healthy zoning policy in Baltimore: results of a health impact assessment of the TransForm Baltimore zoning code rewrite. *Public Health Rep.* 2013;128(Suppl 3):87-103.

25. Baltimore City Department of Planning. Planning / Transform Baltimore. Zoning Code Rewrite Documents. 2010; http://www.baltimorecity.gov/Government/AgenciesDepartments/Planning/TransformBaltimore.aspx. Accessed December 8, 2013.

26. McLaughlin CP, McLaughlin CD. *Health policy analysis—an interdisciplinary approach.* Burlington, Mass.: Jones and Bartlett Publishers, LLC; 2008.

Chapter 4. Understanding the Numbers: The New Demographic Realities and the Future of Population Health

Ronald T. Crouch, MA, MSSW, MBA

"We're all better off, when we are all better off."[1]

Eric Liu and Nick Hanauer

*The Gardens of Democracy:
A New American Story
of Citizenship, the Economy and
the Role of Government*

Chapter 4 Learning Objectives

- Understanding the demographic trends taking place around the world.

- Gain insights on the demographic trends taking place globally, in the United States, and in regions and states.

- Understanding the role of racial and ethnic diversity in demographic trends.

- Comprehend the role of longevity in demographic trends.

- Application of demographic trends to the implications for population health.

Introduction

The United States of America (U.S.), as well as the world at large, is undergoing major demographic shifts that will affect our healthcare delivery system and how we think about population health. The world, as well as the United States, is experiencing two simultaneous demographic revolutions as populations become more diverse and experience the major demographic force of an aging population.

The child, adolescent, and younger adult populations in the United States are becoming more diverse as the non-Hispanic white population declines in real numbers while the minority population experiences population growth in real numbers. Our overall child, adolescent, and younger adult populations, however, are growing very slowly. Immigration is the only factor causing some growth in these populations, as fertility rates among all major race and Hispanic-origin native-born populations are at or below the replacement fertility rate of 2.1 children per family.[2]

At the other end of the age spectrum, we are experiencing a longevity revolution in our mature adult population. In 2013, our mature adult population, the Baby Boomers, has grown dramatically. The population of Baby Boomers, born between 1946 and 1964, is our largest age cohort. A statistic incorrectly reported is that our younger population is our largest population cohort in raw numbers. Yes, it is larger than the Baby Boomer population in the late 1940s to the mid-1960s; however, the population in the Baby Boomer cohort is also now larger as immigration has increased the size of that age cohort as well. The young-old population, now between the ages of 68 and 82, is a smaller population cohort; they were born in the baby bust of the 1930s and early 1940s when the United States had to cope with the Great Depression and World War II. The old-old population, born before 1930 and now aged 80 and over, is growing significantly as well; it is a larger population cohort than the young-old, and the old-old's life span is increasing. We have not yet really experienced the aging revolution, but as the Baby Boomers age into the young-old age cohort, that population cohort will explode.

These new demographic realities are starting to and will have an increasing impact on health care and public health policy as well as the delivery of health care and traditional public health services. The United States must develop the leadership in both the public and private sectors that will be needed to allocate the resources necessary to move from a *sick care model* of health care delivery to a *health and wellness care model* of delivery. It will require stressing an investment in wellness for keeping people healthy; ensuring that the physical environment people live in promotes health through clean air and water; providing safe and secure surroundings that promote the well-being of all; addressing policies that communicate and manage both individual and societal responsibilities; and utilizing advances in technology to enhance delivery of quality health care as a first priority and sick care when needed.

We need to understand the economics of our current and future healthcare systems. If you do what you have always done, you'll be where you've always been. Unfortunately, the current healthcare delivery system cannot survive economically over the long term on the basis of where it has been. We also need to understand the differences in healthcare issues related to income, race or Hispanic origin, and longevity. We need to address these differences to better serve the health needs of our population.

World Demographic Trends

In 1800 the world population reached one billion persons. It took another 130 years, to 1930, to reach a second billion; and just 30 years to reach three billion persons in 1960. Since 1960 the world has added another one billion persons every 12 to 14 years, reaching 7 billion in 2011. The United Nations population projections have been revised downward over the years as fertility has declined in both developed and developing countries; however, declining fertility rates have slowed in recent years in some countries.[3]

The recent United Nations report, *World Population Prospects: The 2012 Revision*, projects the world's population to reach 8.1 billion by 2025, 9.6 billion by 2050, and 10.9 billion by 2100 under the medium-variant projection. Population growth in the past has been driven by fertility, however, and the increasing growth of the young cohort; but future population projections indicate that most growth will be due to the worldwide longevity revolution. The high-variant projection predicts that fertility will remain mostly a half-child higher than in the medium-variant; while the low-variant projection predicts that fertility will be a half-child lower than in the medium-variant. Global fertility rates are projected to drop from 2.53 children per woman in 2005–2010 to 2.24 children per woman in 2045–2050, and below the replacement level of 2.1 children per woman to 1.99 children per woman in 2095–2100 in the medium-variant. The 2095–2100 projected replacement level of 1.99 children per family would result in the world's population starting to decline over time, with only the older population growing if longevity continues to increase.

If, however, the world's population changes according to the low-variant United Nations model, the world population would reach only 8.3 billion in 2050 and start falling to 6.8 billion by 2100. In reality, changes in fertility, longevity, the global economy, economic development in developing countries, urbanization, global warming, natural and manmade disasters, and epidemics are all factors that affect the future world population and certainly involve many unknowns. The health of the population that is affected by policy, management, and technology is also influenced by these factors.

Under the medium-variant projections, most of the 3.7 billion growth that is projected to occur between 2013 and 2100 will be in the 15 to 59 age cohort, with a growth of 1.6 billion; and the 60 and over age cohort, with a growth of 1.99 billion. These two age cohorts will account for 97 percent of global growth, with only 3 percent of the population increase being people under age 15. The developing countries will experience the vast majority of global growth and be shaped more and more by increased longevity. Global life expectancy is projected to increase from 69 years in 2005–2010 to 76 in 2045–2050, and to 82 years in 2095–2100. The global population aged 60 and over is expected to more than triple by 2100, and the global population aged 80 and over is expected to increase by almost sevenfold. These trends will vary by developed and developing countries, as will the effect on the health of the consumer population in each of these nations. The United Nations also states that 66 percent of the world's older population, age 60 and over, now live in developing countries. This percentage is projected to increase to 79 percent by 2050 and 85 percent by 2100.

The urbanization of the world population is also increasing dramatically, having reached a crossover point in 2005, when more people lived in urban areas than rural areas. Projections are that by 2050 the urban/rural ratio will be two people in urban areas for every one person in a rural area; and by 2100 the urban/rural ratio will be six people in urban areas for every one person in a rural area. The United Nations attributes increased urbanization to agricultural modernization and the demand for paid labor in urban areas, with women benefiting the most from paid labor opportunities. Urban areas offer better educational opportunities, greater access to health care, and freedom from traditional norms, according to the United Nations. From the perspective of population health, urbanization will lead to significant environmental impacts through efforts focused on the spectrum of social determinants of health growing in importance. If the process of urbanization is handled well, the outcomes could be very positive but if not, the health of the population could be at risk.

United States Demographic Trends

Only three developed countries are experiencing most of the developed world's population growth: the United States, Canada, and Australia, according to the United Nations population projections. According to Ben Wattenberg, an American demographer and political commentator, this growth results from their being "Settler Nations" that allow immigration from other countries. Wattenberg states

> America is becoming a universal nation, with significant representation of all human hues, creeds, ethnicities and national ancestries. Continued moderate immigration will make us an even more universal nation as time goes on.[4]

All three countries have projected that fertility rates will fall below the replacement level of 2.1 children per woman between 2010 and 2015, to 1.97, 1.66, and 1.88 respectively. The United Nations and U.S. Census Bureau numbers for 2011 report a fertility rate of just 1.89 for the United States, down dramatically from the high fertility rate of 3.8 in the 1950s, when the postwar Baby Boom (1946–1964) took place.[3,5] From a population health perspective the good news is that the teen birth rate is at a record low, as is the birth rate for women in their early twenties. The United States is also seeing a falling preterm birth rate and a falling rate of low-birth-weight births.

For most of its history, the United States was a country in which each younger generation was larger than its predecessor, and the country's population pyramids really were pyramid-shaped. The shape of the population structure started to change, however, after the Baby Boom that followed World War II. In the 1950s and 1960s many schools had to schedule double sessions, and portable classrooms were needed to accommodate the larger Baby Boomer generation. The question in 1952 was where did all these new first-graders come from? Of course they were born in 1946, six years earlier, at the start of the Baby Boom, but educational officials did not see the wave coming and it lasted for 18 years. In 2012, 60 years later, for some reason those first-graders entered their sixties and were now moving into their Medicare and Social Security eligibility years. It appears to be a biological rule that the Baby Boomers get 10 years older every decade. A later section will discuss the longevity revolution in greater detail.

We are now seeing the squaring and inverting of the United States' population pyramids for its overall population, as the Baby Boomers continue to age and the younger population has limited growth due to lower fertility rates. When the population pyramids are broken down by race and ethnicity, we see wide differences. The Baby Boomers have had a significant impact on how we approach strategies and policies to improve the health of the population. Everything from health information technologies to public and private health insurance to the balance of inpatient to outpatient services offered throughout the country has been influenced and will continue to be shaped by the progression of the Baby Boomer population segment. The resulting changes will also be discussed in greater detail in a later section.

Demographic Trends by Region and State

Like the rest of the world, the United States is experiencing the urbanization of its population. Census Bureau maps show most rural counties in the Midwest losing population between 2000 and 2010, especially in Illinois, Iowa, Kansas, Nebraska, North Dakota, and South Dakota.[6] The Southern states of Alabama, Arkansas, Mississippi, and West Virginia are showing similar urbanization trends. In addition, some states in the Northeast, including Maine, New York, and Pennsylvania, show population loss in their rural areas. In many of their rural counties, the death rate now exceeds the birth rate. The Census Bureau recently released data reporting that the death rate for non-Hispanic whites in the United States exceeds the birth rate for non-Hispanic whites; and a number of these states with declining rural populations have high percentages of non-Hispanic whites.[7]

The United States population, according to the 2010 Census, totaled 308,745,538 persons, with the Northeast's population being 55,317,240 and 17.9 percent of the total population. The Midwest's population of 66,927,001 is 21.7 percent of the total population, while the South's is 114,555,744 and 37.1 percent of the total and the West's is 71,945,553 and 23.3 percent of the total population.

Population growth varied significantly by region and state between the 2000 Census and the 2010 Census.[6] The overall national population growth was 27,323,632 or 9.7 percent. Population growth was higher than the national average in the South, 14,318,924 or 14.3 percent, and in the West, 8,747,621 or 13.8 percent, while it was significantly lower in the Northeast, 1,722,862 or 3.2 percent, and in the Midwest, 2,534,225 or 3.9 percent. Within the states, growth rates went from a high of 35.1 percent in Nevada to -0.6 percent in Michigan— the only state that lost population between 2000 and 2010. California, the state with the largest population, 37,253,956, grew near the national average at 10.0 percent. Our second largest state, Texas, 25,145,561, grew at double the national average, at 20.6 percent; and our third largest state, New York, 19,378,102, grew at one-tenth the national rate, at just 2.1 percent.

Tables 4-1 and 4-2, Sample Population Change by Age, 2000–2010, show an example of population change by region coupled with a change between the states with the largest (Texas) and smallest amount of change (Michigan) and the state of Kentucky's change from the 2000 Census to the 2010 Census by age cohorts. Within population age cohorts, the United States experienced very different growth trends across regions and states.

Table 4-1. Sample Population Change by Age, 2000–2010 (numbers)

Area	< 18	18–24	25–44	45–64	65+
United States	1,887,655	3,528,634	-2,905,697	19,536,809	5,276,231
Northeast	-714,591	682,793	-1,792,933	3,115,042	432,551
Midwest	-519,558	310,4310	-1,852,414	3,832,628	763,259
South	2,221,854	1,520,693	388,715	7,731,944	2,455,718
West	899,950	1,014,838	350,935	4,857,195	1,624,703
Greatest Change (Texas)	979,065	374,088	587,534	1,823,700	529,354
Least Change (Michigan)	-251,699	41,752	-518,421	531,052	142,512
Kentucky	28,553	10,943	-67,895	252,563	73,434

Table 4-2. Sample Population Change by Age, 2000–2010 (percentages)

Area	< 18	18–24	25–44	45–64	65+
United States	2.6%	13.0%	-3.4%	31.5%	15.1%
Northeast	-5.5%	14.4%	-11.0%	25.6%	5.9%
Midwest	-3.1%	5.0%	-9.7%	26.9%	9.2%
South	8.7%	15.5%	1.3%	34.9%	19.7%
West	5.3%	16.1%	1.8%	36.2%	23.5%
Greatest Change (Nevada)	29.9%	38.5%	22.6%	50.7%	48.2%
Least Change (Michigan)	-9.7%	4.5%	-17.5%	23.8%	11.7%
Kentucky	2.9%	2.7%	-5.6%	27.2%	14.5%

Source: U.S. Census Bureau, Population Division, Decennial Census 2000 and Decennial Census 2010. Table data prepared by Research and Statistics Branch, Office of Employment and Training, Kentucky Education and Workforce Development Cabinet.

All four regions had their largest population growth in the Baby Boom age cohort, ages 45 to 64, which grew nationally at 31.5 percent. Within regions, growth rates varied slightly, from 25.6 percent in the Northeast and 26.9 percent in the Midwest to 34.9 percent in the South and 36.2 percent in the West. There was also significant growth in the 65+ population, which grew nationally at 15.1 percent but varied significantly within regions, from 5.9 percent in the Northeast and 9.2 percent in the Midwest to 19.7 percent in the South and 23.5 percent in the West. What are the implications for the South and West, which have the fastest-growing older populations that also have the highest health care expenditures? These implications will be discussed in detail in a later section.

As the United States' mature adult workforce ages, the population between the ages 45 and 64, and the population of older adults 65+ grew significantly.

This increase was not the case for the young adult workforce population between the ages of 25 and 44, which declined by -3.4 percent as the youngest Baby Boomers joined the older Baby Boomers in the mature adult workforce age population. There were significant declines in the 25 to 44 age cohort in the Northeast, -11.0 percent, and the Midwest, -9.7 percent, while there was limited growth in the South of 1.3 percent, and in the West of 1.8 percent. The population of children grew only slowly, at 2.6 percent across the United States, with significant declines in the Northeast of -5.5 percent and the Midwest of -3.1 percent, compared to growth of 8.7 percent in the South and 5.3 percent in the West.

There were major differences by state, with the child population declining in several large states: by -9.7 percent in Michigan, -7.8 percent in New York, and -5.5 percent in Ohio. California, where the population of childbearing age is two-thirds minority, grew only by 0.5 percent or one-fifth of the national average. Some larger states in the South had significant growth rates in their child populations: 16.6 percent in Texas, 16.2 percent in North Carolina, and 14.9 percent in Georgia.

The native-born fertility rate, 1.84, is below replacement level; only immigration kept the U.S. child population growing, with a foreign-born fertility rate of 2.19.[8] In addition, as educational levels increase, fertility rates decline. Only women with less than a high school diploma are at or above replacement level with a fertility rate of 2.56, while high school graduates are only at 1.89, college graduates at 1.76, and those with graduate or professional degrees at 1.67.[8]

These regional and state trends have significant implications for public health when population diversity is considered. Much of the healthcare literature indicates that minority status, low educational levels, and poverty negatively affect access to health care, illness, and life expectancy. These intertwined variables are discussed in detail in the next section on diversity in demographic trends.

Demographic Trends by Race and Ethnicity

The report compiled by the National Center for Health Statistics and titled *Health, United States, 2011: With Special Feature on Socioeconomic Status and Health* looks at a wide variety of healthcare data, including births, health status, and access to health care based on the racial or Hispanic origin of the population.[9] The minority population in the United States is growing significantly while the non-Hispanic white population is experiencing little growth and is significantly smaller in the younger age cohorts.[10] The population in the United States grew by 27 million persons or 9.7 percent between the 2000 and 2010 census.

When this growth is broken down according to age, race, or Hispanic origin, the Census data reveal that all growth under the age of 45 occurred in the minority population in the United States. Overall, the African American population grew by 4,271,129 persons or 12.3 percent and the Asian population by 4,431,254 persons or 43.3 percent. The Hispanic population, which may belong to any racial group, grew by 15,171,776 persons or 43.0 percent, and the mixed-race population grew by 2,182,845 or 32.0 percent. These figures compare to a non-Hispanic white growth of only 2,264,778 persons or 1.2 percent; thus the United States is becoming a country in which the non-Hispanic white population will no longer be the majority population. The reader should notice that the Hispanic population accounted for the majority of population growth in the United States between 2000 and 2010. By themselves, these demographic trends should not be of importance to population health unless there are health care disparities based on minority status.

Both fertility rates and immigration are factors in the changing diversity in the United States with the overall fertility rate of 1.89 for the U.S. population. The fertility rate varies from 2.23 for Hispanic women and 1.97 for African American women to 1.78 for non-Hispanic white women and down to 1.71 for Asian women.[11]

Population Pyramid 4-1, based on the 2010 Census, shows the squaring of the total population in the United States, with the Baby Boomer generation being slightly larger than the younger adult population in their teens and twenties.

Figure 4-1. 2010 Population Pyramid: Total

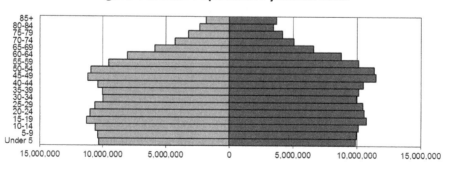

Moreover, the age cohort now in their late sixties and seventies was born during the baby bust of the 1930s and early 1940s, the period of the Great Depression and World War II, and is much smaller than the Baby Boomer age cohort. The left side of the pyramid shows the male population and the right side the female; from age 45 and above the female population of the United States increases its share of the age cohort as women live longer. This difference will be discussed in more detail in the next section.

The population pyramid for "Black Alone, Not Hispanic" shows a slightly larger population of younger African Americans, both male and female, in their teens and early twenties; however, when the male population ages 25 and above on the left side of the pyramid is compared to the female population on the right, the number of males starts declining as a ratio much sooner than it does for the total population pyramid.

Figure 4-2. 2010 Population Pyramid: Black Alone, Not Hispanic or Latino

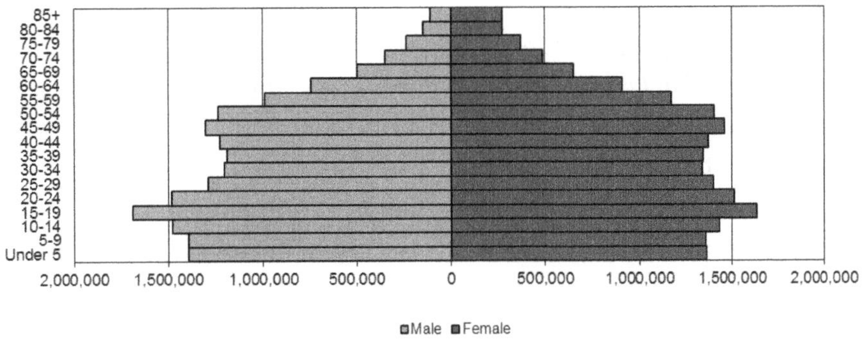

The death rates for homicides shown on Table 38 in the National Center for Health Statistics' 2011 report, *Health, United States, 2011, With Special Feature on Socioeconomic Status and Health*, indicate a much higher homicide rate for African American males than for any other racial or ethnic group. The overall age-adjusted homicide rate for males is 9.3 per 100,000; for the age cohort 24 to 45, it is 14.6 percent for 2008. Those rates are really half the rates of 1980, indicating improvement over time in the population health problem of homicide. The homicide rates are 3.9 and 5.8 respectively for the non-Hispanic white male population, and 10.5 and 15.2 respectively for the Hispanic male population, while they are dramatically higher for the African American male population, at 34.4 and 59.2 per 100.000. What is the public health cost of violence, particularly in the minority communities, combined with the lack of jobs, public transportation needs, high poverty rates, drug enforcement policies, and the fraying of the social safety net to serve at-risk populations? Today the cost is certainly higher than we want it, as it has a negative impact on population health across the United States. This high cost is yet another sign of the need for social policy (e.g., workforce, education, law enforcement, and housing) reform to respond to the challenges that confront the U.S. poor and minority populations.

The U.S. Census Bureau's 2011 population survey titled *Income, Poverty, and Health Insurance Coverage in the United States: 2011* shows a poverty rate for African Americans of 27.6 percent compared to an overall poverty rate of 15.0 percent. It also shows a median household income of $32,229 for African Americans compared to an overall median household income of $50,054. The survey further shows a 2011 uninsured rate of 19.5 percent for African Americans compared to an overall uninsured rate of 15.7 percent.[12]

The wealth gap grew during the recent great recession that began in 2008 as the wealth of African Americans and Hispanics declined with the fall in home prices. In 2010 white households, with an average wealth of $632,000, averaged six times the wealth of African American ($98,000) and Hispanic ($110,000) households.[13]

A July 2013 report by the Center on Budget and Policy Priorities titled *Various Supports for Low-Income Families Reduce Poverty and Have Long-Term Positive Effects On Families and Children* documents the importance of federal assistance in lifting people, including children, out of poverty and providing access to health care along with food stamps, childhood education, Temporary Assistance to Needy Families (TANF), tax credits for low-income workers, and child care assistance.[14] A popular phrase to describe the wisdom of relieving poverty in the near rather than the distant future is "pay me now, or pay him later." We cannot afford as a nation to be penny-wise and pound-foolish by not investing in long-term population health efforts across the board. The health of the population is directly affected by health and social policy decisions that create these types of federal assistance programs. Differing opinions of the effectiveness of the programs emerges and is often influenced by political positions. As a result, getting to the core effects of federal subsidy programs is sometimes difficult but essential to understand both the health and macro-economic impact on the U.S. and regional populations.

The population pyramid for Asians shows a dramatically inverted pyramid, with the young workforce adult Asians being the largest age cohort. The Asian child population is much smaller, and the fertility rates for Asian women are well below the replacement level at 1.71.[11] On the other hand, the Asian population has the fastest growth rate as mentioned earlier, but it is entirely due to immigration.[6]

Figure 4-3. 2010 Population Pyramid: Asian Alone, Not Hispanic or Latino

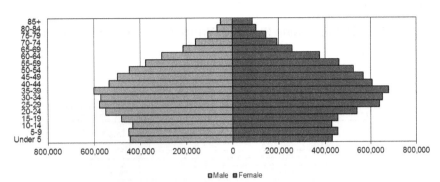

The median household income for Asians is the highest at $65,129; but the fact that larger Asian families share housing and have small numbers of children somewhat overstates their income.[12]

The population pyramid for Hispanics or Latinos shows the dramatic increase in the Hispanic population in the United States with each younger age cohort being larger than the preceding age cohort.

Figure 4-4. 2010 Population Pyramid: Hispanic or Latino

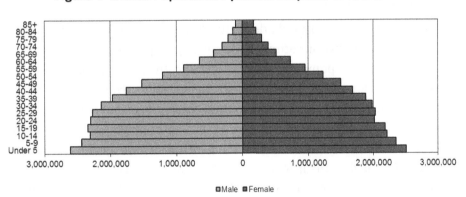

Only the Hispanic fertility rate is above replacement level at 2.23, but as the growing share of native-born Hispanic women account for a larger share of Hispanic births, the Hispanic fertility rate will decline. Just as was the case for the African American population, Hispanics have a higher poverty rate of 25.3 percent and a median household income of only $38,624. The survey also showed that Hispanics have an uninsured rate of 30.1 percent, the highest uninsured rate by far among the various racial and ethnic groups in the United States.

The population of non-Hispanic whites shows a significantly inverted pyramid, with 30 percent fewer young non-Hispanic whites as the non-Hispanic white Baby Boomers age and the fertility rate of non-Hispanic whites is below replacement level at 1.78.

Figure 4-5. 2010 Population Pyramid: White Alone, Not Hispanic or Latino

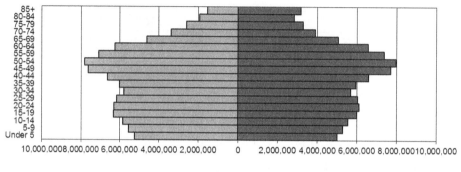

The poverty rate for non-Hispanic whites, 9.8 percent, is only about a third of the poverty rate for African Americans and Hispanics. The median household income of $55,412 is above the national household median income. In addition, the uninsured rate of 11.1 percent is significantly below those of African Americans and Hispanics.

These population pyramids do show that the United States is transforming into a country in which no ethnicity or racial group makes up a majority of the population. From a population health perspective, the higher poverty rates, lower median household incomes, and higher uninsured rates of the African American and Hispanic populations that currently exist in the United States mean that the challenges to population health management will continue to increase unless the economic well-being of these two groups improves. The controversial health insurance mandate that is part of the 2010 Patient Protection and Affordable Care Act (ACA) is a potential solution to the lack of health insurance coverage in these relatively poor minority groups; but as of this writing in 2013, the long-range impact and effectiveness of the landmark reform remains to be determined post-implementation. The educational, income, and wealth gaps will slow economic recovery until these gaps are addressed through social, educational, and workforce policies that will then take years to implement, operate, and evaluate. The racial divides within the United States and the resultant disparities do not serve the United States well. The consequences of not addressing these divides and disparities are affecting our country, as exemplified by racial profiling by law enforcement in some city and state jurisdictions and recent voter ID laws in some counties and states. Public education that addresses facts and not emotions, continued growth and maturation as a society, and grassroots work by community leaders and role models for youth in America is of critical importance.

From the recent U.S. Census Bureau report, *Overview of Race and Hispanic Origin: 2010,* Figure 4-6 shows the minority population as a percentage of the U.S. population. The figure indicates that the minority population is not evenly distributed across the United States; the Western coastal states, the states along the southern border north of Mexico, the Gulf Coast states, and the Southeastern coastal states have numerous counties whose population is 50.0 percent or more minority.

Figure 4-6. 2010 Minority Population as a Percentage of County Population[10]

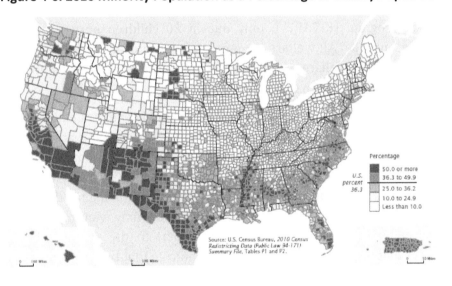

With limited exceptions, the Midwestern and the Northeastern states are much less diverse except in a few large cities. The reader should notice the large-population states of Illinois, Michigan, and New York, which the general public would believe have large minority populations; in fact they have limited minority populations outside their large urban areas.

As we look at our children's population, a growing concern at the population health level is the increasing numbers of children born to unmarried mothers. The July 2013 Child Trends Data Bank report titled *Births to Unmarried Women: Indicators on Children and Youth* states that children born to unmarried mothers are more likely to experience unstable living arrangements; live in poverty, and have socio-emotional problems.[15] In 1960 only 5.0 percent of children were born to unmarried mothers, but this percentage has increased several percentage points every five years, reaching 32.2 percent in 1995 when the Aid to Families with Dependent Children (AFDC) program developed as part of the New Deal legislation of the 1930s was dismantled and replaced with the TANF.

The common wisdom was that AFDC assistance was responsible for the increasing numbers of children born to unmarried mothers. Many so-called experts predicted that if the social safety net were reduced, more women would marry and the number of illegitimate births would decline. Between 1995 and 2000, however, the percentage of children born to unmarried mothers increased to 33.2 percent during a period of economic growth; and since the economic downturn of the 2000s, it increased again, to 40.8 percent in 2011. Data from the TANF program for the state of Kentucky, as an example, indicate that only 5.0 percent, or one in 20, children born to unmarried mothers in Kentucky receives welfare support through a program called Kentucky-Temporary Assistance Program (K-TAP). If only one in 20 children born to unmarried mothers receives K-TAP welfare support, this figure challenges the belief that the availability of welfare support is the primary cause of the increasing percentage of children born to unmarried mothers.

The U.S. Census Bureau's report titled *Social and Economic Characteristics of Currently Unmarried Women With a Recent Birth: 2011* stated that 57.0 percent of women with less than a high school education have nonmarital births compared to 49.0 who are high school graduates and 39.8 percent who have some college.[16] Only among women with a bachelor's or higher degree is the rate significantly lower, at 8.8 percent. While society may want to attribute the increase in births to unmarried mothers in part to the women's liberation movement that began in the 1970s, the data indicate that the problem is directly related to lack of education and low household income. Young adult women in their twenties account for 60.3 percent of unmarried births, not teenagers, who account for only 14.7 percent. These numbers are even more of a concern when the birth data show that births to teens and young women in their early twenties are at record lows.[5] Birth rates among unmarried women varied by state in the latest 2010 data, from a low in Utah of 19.3 percent to a high in Mississippi of 54.8 percent.[17] They also varied by racial and ethnic origin, with a rate of 29.0 percent among non-Hispanic whites; a rate of 53.4 percent among Hispanics; and a rate of 72.5 percent among African Americans.

One of the public health questions presented by the data is this: are the racial disparities caused by the declining middle-class economy, poverty, and lower educational levels rather than race and Hispanic origin one of the reasons for higher birth rates among unmarried mothers in the minority populations in the United States? Also, what is really driving the significant increase in unmarried births across population groups? The U.S. Department of Labor's Bureau of Labor Statistics July 2013 report indicated that U.S. job growth has been slow to recover from the recession of 2007–2009 and the majority of newly created jobs are part-time low-paying positions in the food and retail trade industries.

The report found that between March 2013 and July 2013, part-time jobs grew by 791,000 compared to 187,000 for full-time jobs.[18] The national minimum wage of $7.25 per hour would need to increase by $3.45, or nearly 50 percent to $10.70, to be at its 1968 level when corrected for annual inflation and cost-of-living increases over the past four decades. In addition, there are increasing numbers of major employers with new two- and three-tier wage systems in which new employees receive wages 50 percent lower, more limited benefits, and the evaporation of pension benefit plans, making the American Dream disappear. These trends are resulting in more full-time workers qualifying for food stamps, factory workers at or near the poverty level, and growing inability to afford health care.[19,20] All these macroeconomic trends are affecting the health of a nation and the social policies instituted over the past four decades. Along with societal changes, they have had a continued detrimental impact on population health in the United States. These factors and others cited throughout this book contribute to the need for a more comprehensive examination of social and health policies through a Health in All Policies (HiAP) approach to break down the complexities of our macroeconomic ecosystem and work toward more sustainable community change and improvement in many of these demographic realities in the next generation.

Are growing economic disparities and the resultant social inequalities leading to negative health outcomes, as seen in many of the population health measures noted throughout this chapter?

From the mid-1940s following World War II to the mid 1970s, we saw broad economic gains for most people in the United States as increases in wages followed increases in productivity. This period was called the Great Compression in a paper published in 1992. Have we lost the understanding that programs developed in the New Deal paved the way for a large and growing middle class and that "we're all better off, when we're all better off"?[21] Starting in the late 1970s the economic gains in the United States have gone to the wealthiest share of the population through the failure of trickle-down economics. In the book *What Went Wrong* George Tyler states,

> To be precise, economists Emmanuel Saez and Thomas Piketty have concluded that only five percent of earners enjoyed income gains exceeding inflation during the era since the 1980s, and most of that was concentrated in the earnings of the top 1 percent. That is why income disparity widened noticeably.[22]

Demographic Trends in Longevity

The good news is that we are living longer. The bad news is that we are living longer. The United States is in the midst of a longevity revolution in that its population growth is occurring primarily among people in the 45 to 64 age group, per the 2010 census data referenced earlier in this chapter, with a growth rate of 31.5 percent since 2000; and in the population of those who were 65 and older in 2010, with a growth rate of 15.1 percent since 2000.[2] Between 2010 and 2030 the 65+ population in the United States is projected to grow from 40.2 million persons to 72.1 million persons—an increase of 31.9 million persons or 79 percent.[23] The young-old population, ages 65 to 84, will grow by 28.9 million or 83.7 percent, as all the Baby Boomers move into this age cohort. The old-old population, age 85+, will grow by 3.0 million or 52.1percent. The major growth in the aging population will be in the young-old group during the period between 2010 and 2030.

Life expectancy varies by race and ethnicity, with the overall 2010 life expectancy for non-Hispanic whites of 78.8 years; for males, 76.4 years and females, 81.1 years; for African Americans, an overall life expectancy of 74.7 years; for males, 71.4 years and females, 77.7years; and for Hispanics, an overall life expectancy of 81.2 years; for males, 78.5 years and females, 83.8 years.[24] The long life span of Hispanics has been a point of discussion and debate over the years. It is referred to as the Hispanic Paradox due to the Hispanic population data indicating lower socioeconomic status and therefore shorter life expectancy. Explanations have ranged from Hispanic immigrants being healthier in general; the supportive nature of the Hispanic culture; lower rates of tobacco use; the so-called "salmon bias," in which immigrant Hispanics who become ill return to their home countries and are not counted in U.S. death statistics; or just incomplete data related to Hispanic mortality.

In addition, as we age, the ratio of women to men increases in the population. In 2010, there were 75.4 men for every 100 women aged 65 and over, while in the 85–89 age group there were only 55.1 men for every 100 women.[23] Census data record the number of persons 65+ living alone, and those numbers are primarily female. A related issue is that in earlier generations there were more multigenerational households as well as single-worker households in which caregivers were available to care for sick and aging family members. The number of multigenerational households has declined, and more families require two incomes to make ends meet. Given the disappearance of these transitional household factors, how will we meet the caregiving needs of an aging population?

Disabilities increase with age, with 24.7 percent of persons 65 to 69 having a severe disability, compared to a much larger 55.8 percent of persons aged 80 and over.[25] Overall disabilities also vary by racial or ethnic origin, with age-adjusted disability rates of 14.4 percent for Asians, 22.3 percent for African Americans, 17.8 percent for Hispanics, and 17.6 percent for non-Hispanic whites.

Interestingly, the major growth in the aging population between 2030 and 2050 will shift to the old-old, as the Baby Boomers move past age 85 and much slower growth occurs among the young-old.[23] The numbers show that after 2030 to 2050, the cohort in the 65 to 84 age group will grow very slowly, by only 6.2 million or 9.7 percent as the baby bust of the late 1960s and 1970s moves into that cohort. On the other hand, the population over age 85 will grow dramatically, by 10.3 million or 117.7 percent as the Baby Boomers all move into the old-old population.

The aging of the U.S. population—both the young-old and the old-old—will have major cost consequences as the Baby Boomers start receiving Social Security and Medicare, and the numbers in both programs increase dramatically. In 2009, the average Medicare-only expenditure for a person with medical expenditures was $9,540; for a person with Medicare and other public coverage it was $13,046.[24] These figures compare with health care expenditures of $3,285 for a person aged 18 to 44, and $6,266 for a person aged 45 to 64. As the United States population ages dramatically over the next 20 years, health care costs will go up dramatically as well unless we are able to provide more preventive care, including preventive services to reduce levels of disability and illness in later life. Preventive care can include:

- Addressing issues of economic well-being throughout a person's life;

- Public safety;

- A safe and clean environment;

- A strong social safety net; and

- Preventive health care services over a person's life span.

Our goal should be to have a country in which people live as "young" as possible as long as possible and die as "old" as possible as soon as possible. We need to continue to maximize health and minimize the prevalence of diseases and disorders to improve overall population health throughout the United States.

Demographic Policy Implications and Conclusions

The United States, like the rest of the world, is experiencing a major demographic revolution, as our country becomes more diverse and at the same time experiences a longevity explosion. This revolution will require that we understand both the health care challenges and opportunities. There is no one silver bullet or one single answer. It requires an open mind and a willingness to experiment and use multiple approaches to achieve the end result of ensuring the best healthcare and public health system for our population. Some important societal questions must be answered:[2]

- Is health care a public or private good/service?[3]

- Is access to health care a right or a privilege?[4]

- What are the personal and the societal responsibilities for ensuring the good health of the population?

We need to better understand the realities related to health care in the future, whether it is affected by race or ethnicity; the aging of the population; socioeconomic trends; the role of government in providing a social safety net and access to health care; cost factors; or innovations in science, technology, organizational structures, or policy.

Our current healthcare system relies too much on taking care of people after they get sick; there appears to be more profit in treating people when they get sick rather than making investments in keeping people well. The Urban Institute's Health Policy Center's 2011 article *The Role of Prevention in Bending the Cost Curve* mentions multifactoral community interventions including schools, the built environment, lifestyle choices, disease prevention, and others.[26] A July 2013 article in the *New York Times*, "Status and Stress," discusses the role of "status syndrome," in which the stress that kills is "characterized by a lack of a sense of control over one's fate" and a "learned helplessness." It raises the concern that inequality and poverty are disruptive and "get under the skin."[27] We live in a country in which many believe in survival of the fittest and that people are on their own, while others believe we are our brothers' and sisters' keepers. The answers to questions about health care are different at different points along the political spectrum.

The battle around the ACA is a battle between those who think high-quality health care is a right and those who think that individuals deserve only the health care they can afford. The ongoing debate over and implementation of the individual health insurance mandate holds many unknowns even at the time of this writing. Those who believe in the provision of health care as a right see a government ensuring everyone's access to high-quality health care as the fulfillment of delivering a general public good to an entire nation. A number of public health quality measures have been presented in this chapter. Issues of birth rates, regional population changes over years, aging of the population, prevalence of disabilities, and death rates are all examples of such measures. Recognizing the transgenerational effect of health and social policies implemented at the federal and state levels is critical to understanding the underlying forces that produced the trends and rates of occurrence in the measures presented in this chapter. As a nation moves forward in the twenty-first century, people should pay attention to where we stand today on the basis of these measures of health and social disparities and inequalities with a focus on making policy changes that result in needed improvements in population health.

CHAPTER 4 DISCUSSION QUESTIONS

Discussion questions are provided for team building or class exercises. Answers for all questions are provided in Appendix C.

Question Number	Question
1	What are the demographic trends taking place around the world?
2	What are the demographic trends taking place in the United States?
3	How do these demographic trends vary by region and state?
4	What are the consequences of racial and ethnic diversity and longevity in relation to public health?
5	Is health care a right or a privilege?

CHAPTER 4 SUMMARY

- The United States, as well as the rest of the world, is experiencing a demographic revolution as we become more diverse and our people live longer.

- There are major demographic differences between regions and states that will affect their futures.

- We are becoming a more diverse nation and we need to understand these realities.

- The longevity revolution changes all the rules as we face the future, and will require us to rethink issues like education, work, retirement, and others.

- People disagree about the roles of individuals and government, and the future we want.

- We cannot continue the current system of healthcare, which focuses on providing care after people fall ill rather than preventive care.

- We need a healthy debate about the future in which we can disagree with others and be respectful of different viewpoints.

CHAPTER 4 REFERENCES

1. Liu E, Hanauer, N. True capitalism. In: *The gardens of democracy: a new American story of citizenship, the economy, and the role of government*. Seattle, Wash.: Sasquatch Books;2011:117.

2. Crouch R. The changing face of America: diversity and longevity. *Views & Visions;*Fall 2011.

3. Wattenberg B. *Immigration is good*. Washington, D.C.: American Enterprise Institute;2002.

4. Population Division of the United Nations Department of Economic and Social Affairs. *World population prospects: the 2012 revisions*. New York, N.Y.: United Nations;2012.

5. Jarosz B. *Birth rate at record low for young women in the U.S.* Washington, D.C.: Population Reference Bureau;2013.

6. US Census Bureau. *Population distribution and change: 2000 to 2010. 2010 census briefs*. Washington, D.C.: US Census Bureau;2010.

7. Cohn D. *Why there are more deaths than births among whites*. Washington, D.C.: Pew Research Center;2013.

8. US Census Bureau. *Completed fertility for women 40 to 44 years old by single race in combination with other race and selected characteristics*. Washington, D.C.: US Census Bureau;2010.

9. US Department of Health and Human Services (DHHS), National Center for Health Statistics. *Health, United States, 2011: with special features on socioeconomic status and health*. Washington, D.C.: DHHS;2012.

10. US Census Bureau. *Overview of race and Hispanic origin, 2010*. Washington, D.C.: US Census Bureau;2011.

11. Hamilton B, Martin, J., Ventura, S. *Births: preliminary data for 2011*. Atlanta, Ga.: Centers for Disease Control and Prevention, Division of Vital Statistics;2011.

12. DeNavas-Walt C, Proctor, B., Smith, J. *Income, poverty, and health insurance coverage in the United States: 2011. Current Population Reports*. Washington, D.C.: US Census Bureau;2012.

13. Urban Institute. *Racial wealth gap divide is 3 times wider than income gap, threatening economic opportunity integrity*. Washington, D.C.: Urban Institute;2013.

14. Sherman A, Trisi, D., Parrott, S. *Various supports for low-income families reduce poverty and have long-term positive effects on families and children*. Washington, D.C.: Center on Budget and Policy Priorities;2013.

15. Child Trends Organization. *Births to unmarried women: indicators on children and youth*. Bethesda, Md.: Child Trends Data Bank;2013.

16. US Census Bureau. *Social and economic characteristics of currently unmarried women with a recent birth: 2011.* Washington, D.C.: US Census Bureau;2011.

17. Centers for Disease Control and Prevention. National Vital Statistics Reports, 61(1);August 28, 2012.

18. Davidson P. Many new jobs are part time and low-paying. *USA Today.* August 4, 2013. http://www.usatoday.com/story/money/business/2013/08/04/part-time-low-wage-jobs/2613483/. Accessed September 3, 2013.

19. Downs J. Rise in full-time workers receiving food stamps. *Courier Journal.* October 11, 2011. http://archive.courier-journal.com/article/20111012/BUSINESS/310120051/Rise-full-time-workers-receiving-food-stamps. Accessed June 13, 2014.

20. Uchitelle L. Factory jobs gain, but wages retreat. *New York Times.* December 29, 2011. http://www.nytimes.com/2011/12/30/business/us-manufacturing-gains-jobs-as-wages-retreat.html?pagewanted=all&_r=0. Accessed June 13, 2014.

21. Liu E, Hanauer, N. *The gardens of democracy: a new American story of citizenship, the economy, and the role of government.* Seattle, Wash.: Sasquatch Books; 2011.

22. Tyler G. Facing reality. In: *What went wrong: how the 1% hijacked the American middle class . . . and what other countries got right.* Dallas, Texas: Benbella Books;2013.

23. U.S. Census Bureau. *The next four decades: the older population in the United States: 2010 to 2050.* Washington, D.C.: US Census Bureau;2010.

24. U.S. Department of Health and Human Services (DHHS), National Center for Health Statistics. *Health, United States, 2012: with special feature on emergency care.* Washington, D.C.: DHHS;2013.

25. Brault M. *Americans with disabilities: 2010. Household economic studies.* Washington, D.C.: US Census Bureau;2012.

26. Waidmann TA, Ormond BA, Bovbjerg RR. *The role of prevention in bending the cost curve.* Washington, D.C.: Urban Institute Health Policy Center; 2011.

27. Velasques-Manoff M. Status and stress. *New York Times.* July 27, 2013. http://opinionator.blogs.nytimes.com/2013/07/27/status-and-stress/. Accessed June 13, 2014.

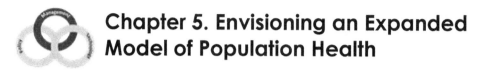

Chapter 5. Envisioning an Expanded Model of Population Health

Toward a Socio-Cultural-Ecologic Model Based on Resources and Relationships

Robert William Prasaad Steiner, MD, MPH, PhD

Barry Wainscott, MD, MPH, ABPM

"The purpose of Public Health is to maximize the health of a population, not to minimize disease."

Tom Wallace, MD, MPH
(1923–2004)
Former Director, Jefferson County Health Department
Louisville, KY

Chapter 5 Learning Objectives

- Comprehend the inherent differences between the traditional medical care model and the public or population health model.

- Realize the need for incorporating social determinants of health into how we assess, develop policies for, and assure the health of communities.

- Consider the interconnected policy implications of social policy change across health domains.

- Appreciate the global perspective of the social-cultural-ecological construct and the evolving need for adoption and incorporation of this model and vision.

- Recognize the potential benefits of adopting the conceptual notion of "positive health" as psychosocial relational and behavioral mechanisms to drive improvement in quality of life.

Introduction

Relationship-centered Population Health and Cultural Contexts

Population health is about how people in communities and other forms of social networks live their lives during normal social role activities, including work, school, and play, and at home with family, friends, and neighbors. It includes the relational qualities and functional capacities of individuals during the course of activities of daily living and the values that are present within those relationships. Qualities of relationships, values, and assumptions about the world in which we live all play a role in determining the cultural context of our lives.

We all make assumptions about the world in which we live. Being healthy in a community means that the social and environmental aspects of where we live, work, learn, and play, contribute to dynamic interactive relationships that promote health and well-being. Yet there are often unexamined, or implicit, cultural assumptions that are present which shape our relationships and the qualities of the world in which we live. We are often not even aware of these beliefs, attitudes, values, and sociocultural forces that interact and guide our lives within layers of social context—as individuals, within families, within communities, and as participants in larger societies.

We may make assumptions and judgments about the qualities of our relationships with friends and families, neighbors, and those we encounter in our daily activities. Such relationships have the potential to contribute to a subjective sense of health and well-being, and also to play a role in our decisions, motivations, and willingness to participate in community activities. Each of these factors can contribute to the social cohesion within a community. One premise of this chapter is that both our subjective senses of health and well-being, as well as our objective behaviors, are both directly and indirectly related to our health. Indeed, our notions of health are shaped by these ubiquitous cultural assumptions.

Yet these same cultural assumptions that bind people together within communities can also serve as barriers to common understandings among different people and groups, and as impediments to engendering friendly and productive relationships. Any lack of awareness of the cultural assumptions about our worldviews can become like a cocoon of invisible insulation that protects us from others, including those with different objective characteristics, like race, ethnicity, religion, wealth, education, social status, and even different worldviews.

Culture is like an invisible container, a cocoon in which we live in a comfort zone, based upon acceptance of what is familiar and aversion to what seems different or uncommon.[1,2] Social inclusions and exclusions and other forms of bias result from such processes. The tensions from such implicit and unexamined processes eventually contribute to health inequalities at the level of the community. Examining the cocoon of implicit assumptions and values may be one means to better address these kinds of population health concerns.

There is more to health than access to medical care. The qualities of the places where we live and the social environment in which we live are determinants of health. The emphasis in this chapter will be on the high-level conceptual perspectives of community health as a local variety of population health, more so than focusing on the detailed characteristics of the medical care system for individuals. Nonetheless, the authors intend to provide a complementary model for population health that embraces the systems of medical care.

We will first add a new dimension of positive health into the basic constructs for health promotion and population health, including applications for measuring and evaluating measures from generic health-related quality-of-life assessments in population health. The very nature of health promotion will be reexamined from the perspective of population health. This presence of positive health as a new dimension in population health will yield novel priorities that will need the development of new health policies to be sustained. We will then examine societal aspects of population health from the macro-perspective of the social collective, and how communities can be involved with transforming the cultural basis of health. Finally, we will link the approaches to the positive dimensions of health and quality-of-life assessments with health policy development and the social determinants of health at the macro-level, including a brief section on approaches to Health in All Policies (HiAP).

Evolving Paradigms of Science

The very nature of population health includes aspects of both the natural and the social sciences. A new paradigm of health is emerging to better describe the essential characteristics of population health and public health as a relationship-based science and art, one that is present as an ecology of sociocultural forces, environmental factors, and biologic phenomena. The new paradigm is not exclusive to one approach or another, but it does have a complementary nature that includes both natural and social sciences.[3]

Thomas Kuhn (1922–1996), a philosopher of science, spoke about paradigm change in the context of revolutions in scientific thinking.[4] For Kuhn, a paradigm is a framework for assessing causal relationships, a viewpoint through which the world is seen. He argued that all scientific works occur within a paradigm, and that revolutionary ideas will eventually force the collapse of any existing framework and so result in a new paradigm. The evolution of this new vantage point, or worldview, is what Kuhn called a "paradigm shift."

Social considerations can also be viewed as a component of the very nature of science. For example, one paradigm of current scientific practices is known as positivism. Positivism in science includes notions that the world of experience is governed by preexisting "truths" that can be discovered through investigative methods. Yet the Hungarian-born scientist, physician, and philosopher Michael Polyani (1891–1976) argued against positivism in science; he focused on the relations of scientists to their work as scientists and their role in society.

Polyani suggested that scientists are not driven by skepticism accompanied with skills in critical objective methods. Rather, he contended that scientists are socially oriented and steadfastly committed to established beliefs and dogmas within the scientific community. He argued that it is the social scientific community, not a rational scientific method, which is the determining condition for acquiring new scientific knowledge. Polyani contended that science is an inherently normative form of knowledge and that society gives meaning to science, rather than scientific investigations providing a newly uncovered "truth" to society. From this perspective, it seems that social considerations may influence the interpretation of scientific findings, perhaps even the acceptance of new approaches to the generation of knowledge, and even the means to address socially enmeshed health concerns.

Epidemiologic Transitions in Health and Health Care

Within this context, a brief review of the history of epidemiologic transitions may provide some insights into the nature of the ongoing scientific revolutions and paradigm shifts in population health. The nature and scope of causal relationships for health and disease changed in the United States during the past century. These major transitions also occur globally, in other nations as their economies and politics change and as cultures evolve.

Omran has described a series of epidemiologic transitions in health from a historic perspective.[5] The first epidemiological transition in the United States focused on infectious and communicable diseases at the turn of the twentieth century. At that time, most deaths and illnesses in the United States were attributed to tuberculosis, influenza, gastroenteritis, and diarrheal diseases. The growth and dispersion of public health sanitation measures, including clean water, sewage disposal, safe food, and better housing, all contributed to reducing the impact from these kinds of diseases. Although the relative magnitude of the impact from these categories of diseases in developed regions has diminished over the past decades, the burden of suffering associated with communicable diseases remains an important public health issue, especially at the global level.

A second epidemiologic transition in modern times includes increased attention to chronic diseases. During the 1970s, there was a heightened awareness of the increasing prevalence of cardiovascular diseases, cancers, arthritis, and others. These diseases not only affect mortality, they also have a high impact on morbidity, including limitations in functional status,[6] quality-of-life assessments,[7-9] and increasing costs for health care. The scope of concern for chronic diseases was not only for individuals as patients but also included families, employers, and other community aspects. The approaches to risk assessment and risk reduction in programs for chronic diseases occurred at the clinical level and also at the population level, including assessments of worksite health promotion programs. There is a rich literature and a complex array of implications and options for policy development for chronic diseases to promote healthier communities.[10,11]

A third epidemiologic transition exists, according to some experts.[23] Socially enmeshed health concerns are a more recent transition within the evolution of health issues within established societies. For example, as early as 1979, violence was first declared a public health issue in the United States, in the U.S. Surgeon General's report at that time. Emphasis on community engagement to address foundational issues that are present within socially enmeshed health concerns is the essence of community-based solutions for this current epidemiologic transition. The Healthy Communities approach to domestic violence in Romania, subsequently presented in this chapter, is one example of community-based policy solutions for a specific socially enmeshed health concern.

Each of the transitions represents a change in the focus on categories of societal ills, and each category of epidemiologic transition requires different methods to address the particular concern. From a medical care perspective for individuals with infectious and communicable diseases, antibiotics for treatment and vaccines for prevention make sense. Yet from a population perspective, sanitary measures directed toward water, food, and sewage offered a more efficient means of disease control to protect the health of the public.[12] Similarly, the biomedical model offers many medications, procedures, and interventions for treatment and prevention of select chronic diseases; yet additional social and economic benefits are afforded by the Americans with Disabilities Act, while some worksite wellness programs are associated with cost savings, decreased absenteeism, and increased job satisfaction.[13,14] Other effective means include mass media campaigns that address changing social norms toward healthier goals,[15] either directly or indirectly.[16]

Table 5-1. Summary Approaches to Epidemiologic Transitions

Epidemiologic Transition	Solutions for the Health Concerns	Methods of Management
Infectious and communicable diseases	Physical environment (sewers and water)	Sanitation and hygiene
Chronic degenerative diseases	Lifestyle modifications	Supportive physical and social environments
Socially enmeshed health concerns	Access to community resources	Community engagement linked with social health policy development

The next section will address select issues in the high-level conceptual perspectives on health and wellness, disease and illness, and individuals and populations within societies and cultures.

Field Models and Multidimensional Constructs of Health

One manifestation of the third epidemiologic transition for socially enmeshed health concerns includes an emphasis on field models of health.[17] In part, this approach serves as a means to portray multidimensional causality, the interactive nature of the social determinants of health, and upstream and downstream aspects of health policy development.

Marc Lalonde, the Minister of National Health and Welfare in Canada during the 1970s, spurred new ways of thinking about population health, as illustrated in Figure 5-1. He and his staff summarized the complicated nature of population health into four broad categories: human biology, environment, lifestyle, and the healthcare organization.[17] Accordingly, each and every category in this model is necessary for effective health promotion in Canada or anywhere on the globe.[18] This framework provided an opportunity for the realization that some of the determinants of health were outside the existing medical care systems.

Figure 5-1. Field Model of Health [19]

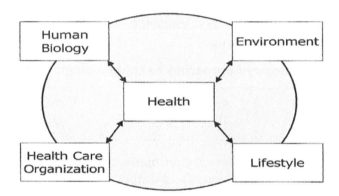

Lalonde recognized the need for target goals and measureable objectives, but this method was first accomplished at a national level in the United States with the publication of the first *Healthy People* report in 1979 from the Office of the U.S. Surgeon General.[20] By comparison, the World Health Organization (WHO) did not introduce measureable objectives until 1984. Finally, Lalonde acknowledged there was a possibility that misalignment of funds to favor medical care over the other social determinants of health may be detrimental to population health.

During the 1990s, Evans and Stoddart formally challenged many assumptions about the relationships between sickness and medical care.[21,22] They acknowledged that there is more to health than a collection of negative characteristics, and they introduced the notion of well-being into their model. Furthermore, they pointed to the obvious issues that had been long overlooked—that all human activity is associated with health consequences. They cited studies about stress and the new concepts of social gradients of health from studies of multiple national populations. Furthermore, they included positive health and well-being as components of their new model, as well as interacting and interdependent factors for health, disease, and health care. Interactions between components of the model, including both positive and negative feedback loops with direct and indirect effects, were a basic part of their model. The model extended the interactions to include reciprocal relationships for well-being with both the social and physical environment.

Positive health and health policy development and evaluation merged within the PRECEDE-PROCEED model.[23] Health-related quality-of-life (HRQL) assessments become the starting point for assessing the social diagnosis of any community of interest. Accordingly, measures of HRQL become the starting point for health policy development and the endpoint for assurance of the effectiveness of the new policy,—as illustrated in Figure 5-2, adapted from the classic text by Green and Kreuter.[23]

Comparing the results from disease-oriented research using national data with similar results that focus on the field models of the social determinants of health shows some interesting results. Historic landmark articles by McGinnis and Foege in 1993 showed the relationship between disease-specific mortality rates and select risk factors at a national population level.[24] Mokedad and associates replicated the pattern of findings about measures of impact for mortality with behavioral risk factors, using data from the year 2000.[25]

Patterns of behavioral and lifestyle risk factors for fatal diseases emerged from these two studies. Heart disease and cancers accounted for the majority of deaths. When the same data sources were examined for behavioral causes associated with the outcomes, tobacco smoking, poor diet, and lack of physical activity showed the largest impact. The translation from disease to underlying behaviors was associated with a change in priorities, and a shift in awareness and attention to address these health issues.

Figure 5-2. PRECEDE-PROCEED Model for Health Policy Development and Evaluation

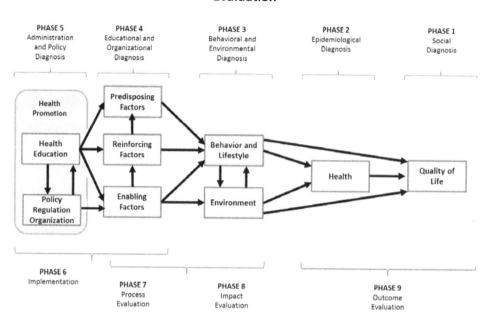

The relationships between prevalent causes of death and common behavioral risk factors became readily apparent from these reports. There were implications for health promotion and policy development at the local level.[10] From this perspective, lifestyle modification in the social and cultural context became the primary issues of concern for population health. Others contend that policies that support the production rather than consumption of unhealthy commodities are the major issue of concern.[26]

Galeo and associates provided a report of summary evidence about the impact of social factors on mortality.[27] They found that risk estimates for deaths associated with social factors were as potent as risk factors measured from the leading pathophysiologic, or disease-oriented models. Multilevel analyses of structural social risk factors were reported, showing high impact for low educational attainment, poverty, and reports of low social support. Higher levels of impact were present for each social risk factor among respondents older than age 65. Among reported community-based area-level measures, racial segregation and income inequalities impacted most heavily upon mortality. Again, the translation from disease to social health issues was associated with a different set of priority health concerns to address them.

The magnitudes of the social risk associations for mortality are nearly as potent as risk factors for the more traditional disease-oriented model. Other authors support the findings related to the potency of social factors with health. Woolf described "social policies as health policies" in a poignant editorial.[28] Satcher and associates estimated that more than 83,570 excess deaths each year could be prevented in the United States if the African American/white mortality inequity were to be eliminated.[29] Woolf estimated that correcting racial and ethnic disparities in education-associated mortality rates would save eight times as many lives as medical care during the same period.[30]

Social Gradient of Health

The social gradient of health is based upon the works of Sir Michael Marmot and the Whitehall studies of British civil servants, especially the Whitehall II studies.[31-35] Marmot and Wilkinson synthesized and integrated information from multiple sources into concepts known as the social gradient of health. These studies demonstrate that as the adequacy of the social resource base declines among civil servants, so too do measures of health status and well-being. The decrements in health are present not only among the poorest poor as compared to the richest rich. Rather, there is a gradient such that even vice presidents of a company will likely show decrements in health when compared to those who are positioned at categorically higher administrative levels, like CEOs and presidents. There is a gradient of health that includes all people living within a community, such that people with lower social standing, less wealth, or even lower class status are typically less healthy than those with more resources or higher social standing.

The social determinants of health have become more prominent in the medical literature, showing high relative impact upon measures of population health status. WHO defines the social determinants of health as:

> ... the circumstances in which people are born, grow up, live, work and age, and the systems put in place to deal with illness. These circumstances are in turn shaped by a wider set of forces: economics, social policies, and politics.[36]

More specifically, if a person's standing in socioeconomic status (SES) is pictured as a ladder, those lower on the ladder can be expected to have shorter life expectancies and the presence of more disease, more ill-health, and less subjective well-being compared to those who are higher on the SES ladder.

Marmot stated a profound approach toward improving population health: The aim is to improve health of individuals by creating healthier societies.[37]

Rather than focusing on the behavioral and attitudinal changes among individuals, he suggests that we should attend to changing a society as a whole, and so influence those that live within that social unit. Marmot, Wilkinson, and others have championed the view that geographic, demographic, and social indicators all influence our health.[38-42]

Marmot's approach to healthier communities begins with the collective aspects of society as a means to influence the behaviors, attitudes and motivations of individuals. This approach begins with the notion that the capacities of people to lead lives that they value are determined by social conditions. From this perspective, it is useful to see social disadvantage and manifestations of poverty as lack of empowerment. Health promotion efforts as generated through the Healthy Cities/Healthy Communities models[43,44] are guided by core values of equity, participation, social justice, interdependence, intersectoral action, community participation, and innovative public health policies.[45] As such, these activities are expected to be enabling and empowering. If these factors are not present, then the very spirit and definitions of health promotion have been violated.

Some models of socio-cultural-ecologic approaches to population health suggest that culture change may be an effective means to attend to the multiple determinants of developing health promotion programs.[46] Likewise, approaches based on complexity and network theory are more recently proposed as avenues for effective societal change toward healthier communities.[47-50] In other words, the health of a community depends upon the very presence of its residents and how they embody the values that they hold dear, not only for themselves, but on behalf of the entire community in which they live.[51] It is the interactions of individuals with their own internal values and how they embody that process, as well as the manifestations of their interactions with others within the community, that engender a cohesive emergent unit called "society."

Marmot cites the following statements as contributing factors to the social gradient of health[41]:

1. Health follows a social gradient;

2. Stress damages health;

3. The health impacts of early development and education last a lifetime;

4. Poverty and social exclusion cost lives;

5. Stress in the workplace increases risk of disease;

6. Job security improves health; unemployment causes illness and premature death;

7. Social supports and supportive networks improve health;

8. Alcohol, drug, and tobacco use are influenced by the social setting;

9. Healthy food is a political issue; and

10. Healthy transport means walking and cycling and good public transport.

Psychosocial mechanisms whereby people compare their status with that of others are active within the social gradient. The psychosocial comparison approach emphasizes hierarchy and social distance as determinants of health. Health inequalities, especially in developed nations, are strongly influenced by the citizens' interpretation of their status in society.[52,53] At an individual level, people tend to compare their status with others, and they may react with feelings of worthlessness, shame, and other negative reactions if they are lacking appropriate external or internal resources.[54]

These psychosocial comparisons of relative worth can then lead to a psychobiology of stress and compensatory behaviors that threaten health. At the community level, social comparisons of disparities can lead to mistrust and loss of social cohesion. Wilkinson in the United Kingdom and Kawachi [55-57] and Kennedy [58,59] are advocates of this ideological position in the United States. The psychosocial comparison model may be considered the subjective complement to the more objectively oriented approaches of the materialists and neomaterialists. Raphael provides a concise summary of these three approaches.[60]

This model for managing population health may include the medical care model, but the community (societal) health components are not causally driven by measures of disease or illness. Rather, measures for community health as the collective aspect of public health depend upon comparative measures of social standing, including status and material wealth. These include, for example, differences between measured social resources (e.g., education, employment status, income, and the like) for specified groups on a social gradient.

The patterns that emerge are that a lack of any given social resource, whether that resource is objective in nature (e.g., income, educational attainment, etc.) or subjective (e.g., sense of belonging, empowerment, confidence, self-efficacy, etc.), is each associated with decrements in health.

Social risk is then a measure of a lack of social resources—one that is often translated into lack of opportunity within the context of society.

Social resources can serve as both opportunities and as indicators of risk. Social resources and social risk are complementary to the disease-oriented definitions that have driven classical epidemiology and the causality of disease. Social risk in the context of resources can be used to extend the biomedical model to a bio-psycho-social-cultural model, in which comparative differences between people within the same or similar communities become the social risk factor of interest—one that is based upon available resources and opportunity.

Community-based Approaches to Socially Enmeshed Health Concerns

Effective solutions for socially enmeshed health concerns will likely encompass different strategies than interventions for medical care. From such a perspective, it appears that the personal medical care system is necessary—but insufficient—to assure a healthy community, especially when socially enmeshed health concerns are prominent.

The issue of domestic violence is a good example for consideration. Once a person is injured and seeks medical treatment of physical injuries from domestic violence, it is not ethical or reasonable to send the typically female victim back home to the same abusive environment. Nontraditional personnel and community resources are needed to provide optimal care for victims and families in such situations. Shelters, advocates, police protection, courts, lawyers, judges, and other community assets all play a role in the solutions to this form of a socially enmeshed health concern.

Addressing existing power structures within a given society were necessary approaches for success with the Healthy Community Partnership in Constanta, Romania, exemplified by the case report description below. Healthy Cities and Healthy Communities are formal approaches for initiating and sustaining improvements in community health, with an evidence base that successes are possible.[43,61] The Romanian project utilized a train-the-trainers model. This approach was one of the factors associated with success of this project, since the trainees continued to reside within Romania, and they were nearly always present to serve as advocates for the cause of the project.

Making a Healthier Community: The Constanta – Louisville Partnership, 1998–2002

Constanta, Romania is a port city on the Black Sea with a population of 350,000 residents; Constanta County has a population of 720,000. In 1998, the Constanta Department for Health Promotion and Health Education and similar departments from six counties in Romania submitted proposals to the American International Health Alliance (AIHA) to participate in a Healthy Communities Partnership with a selected city in the United States. AIHA first selected Constanta to participate in a partnership. The competitive grant proposal developed by the team from Louisville, Kentucky, was then selected to participate with the Constanta team. AIHA specified that a formal Healthy Communities approach would be used by the partners to develop methods for improving women's health.

Partners from Constanta included: the Constanta County Health Directorate, especially the Department for Health Promotion and Health Education, the Medical School at the Ovidius University, with the Mayor's Office and Constanta City Hall. The Louisville partners included: the University of Louisville, the Jefferson County Health Department, and the Humana Foundation. Numerous nongovernmental organizations (NGOs) for women's health issues in Romania also participated.

The Constanta and Louisville partners developed exchange programs and training-the-trainers models to demonstrate practical methods for engaging the community to empower Romanian citizens to improve women's health. During the course of the partnership, eleven exchanges took place, seven to Romania and four to Louisville.[62] These collaborative efforts demonstrated processes for developing local partnerships to represent the community-based commitments toward improving women's health in Constanta.

The Constanta team then engaged in community health improvement processes (CHIP). They began with an analysis of strengths, weaknesses, opportunities, and threats (S-W-O-T) of the community and the social context of Constanta. This analysis was followed by multiple focus groups in schools, worksites, nursing homes, and other community sites. Public service radio announcements, newspaper articles, and television shows highlighted the collaboration.

A scientific survey was designed, using Romanian translations of standardized questionnaires to assess health-related quality of life, depressive

Making a Healthier Community: The Constanta – Louisville Partnership, 1998–2002

symptoms, and behavioral health issues. The survey was completed by more than 1,300 female residents of Constanta between the ages of 16 and 90 years. The results from focus groups, surveys, and statistical data provided information for a representative group of women to use consensus development methods to determine the major public health priorities for the Constanta County community. They elected to focus on domestic violence (DV) as the priority health concern.

Programs for prevention, monitoring, and combating domestic violence in Constanta were developed jointly with the Louisville team. Each Louisville team member provided training to their professional peers from Romania, with a goal of establishing a network of community services for the victims of domestic violence in Constanta. The training and consultations were based on a model of networked community services for domestic violence projects that had been previously funded in the Greater Louisville metropolitan area by the U.S. Department of Justice. The premise for this approach was that if all organizations and providers who served victims of domestic violence could be linked in networks of coordinated and integrated services, then more complete medical, social, and legal support services could be provided to victims and their families. It was envisioned that an integrated approach to managing cases of DV might be associated with better outcomes.

The Office for Women was opened by the Constanta Community Foundation in 2000 with financial support from the Humana Foundation. Members of the Constanta team organized and initiated a community-wide public education campaign to increase awareness of the incidence, impact, and costs of domestic violence. Volunteers handed out brochures about DV and pins and pens with the motto "Live Safely." They established a hotline for victims of domestic violence in Constanta. The Office for Women now provides free legal advice and counseling to female victims of domestic violence, and provides some support services within the courts.

New laws and regulations about domestic violence were passed in legislative efforts in Bucharest, the capital of Romania. These programs became a model for a specific law to prevent and combat domestic violence that was adopted for the first time at the national level in Bucharest in 2003. A National Agency for Family Protection was developed with specific departments in each

Making a Healthier Community: The Constanta – Louisville Partnership, 1998–2002

county of Romania. This national legislative approach became a model for similar projects in other counties, with support from the United Nations Fund for Population Activities (UNFPA). The Romanian team leaders later served as consultants for addressing domestic violence issues in neighboring Eastern European nations. The results and details about the processes for CHIP were disseminated in Europe, the United States, and Africa.[62,63]

Declining trends in numbers of cases of domestic violence prosecuted each year serve as an indicator of the emergence of new cultural norms in women's health in Constanta and Romania. A decade of success was celebrated in Louisville in 2010, when members of the Board of Directors of the Constanta Community Foundation offered commemorative medals to all partners from the United States and Romania who were involved in the Constanta–Louisville Healthy Communities Partnership.

There are other formal approaches available for improving community health, with each model utilizing community engagement and participation and each with an overall goal of improving select indicators of community health. Exemplary models include Health Impact Assessment (HIA); Mobilizing for Action through Planning and Partnerships (MAPP), developed by the National Association of County and City Health Officials (NACCHO); and the CDC's Planned Approach to Community Health (PATCH). HIA is a multidisciplinary process that has roots in environmental assessment, but it can be used for population health assessments.[64-66] MAPP can help communities to prioritize public health issues and identify resources for addressing them.[67,68] Similarly, the PATCH model helps state and local health departments to partner with community groups.[69] There are other useful models (e.g., the CDC's Assessment Protocol for Excellence in Public Health; APEX-PH).[70]

The evidence base to support policy approaches to address health equities and the effectiveness of interventions toward social justice is in early phases of development. The CDC's Guide to Community Preventive Services[71,72] is intended to complement the clinically oriented U.S. Preventive Services Task Force (USPSTF) Guidelines. The Community Guide is designed to address public and organizational policies; health issues within the built environment, such as schools, housing, and worksites; and population health issues at macro-perspectives of communities, states, and nations. For example, the Community Guide topic for Health Equity includes evidence for the following topics:

education programs and policies; culturally competent health care; and housing programs and policies. More specifically, policy statements about children attending kindergarten and housing assistance for the poor have a sufficient evidence base to allow recommendations within these three broad areas. The Community Guide methods for evaluation include cost-effectiveness analyses, unlike their clinical counterpart from the USPSTF.

Health and Disease Examined as Multidimensional Constructs

One main premise of this chapter is that health and disease are multidimensional constructs that are both interdependent and interactive. We posit that health is a construct which is positively oriented and resource-based, while disease is a construct focused on a biomedical model of disease, which is consistent with problem-solving methods that are present within the development of most medical interventions. Traditional models of health represent disease and wellness as extremes on a linear continuum. Yet these traditional linear models lack construct validity; and at best, they are incomplete. It is important to include indicators of positive health as well as of disease and illness to assure the construct validity of the new models.

From the perspective of the biomedical model, successes of medical interventions are measured as relative reductions in the magnitude of both the clinical signs and patient-reported symptoms of disease—to a near zero-experience—such that neither signs nor symptoms are present; or they may be present at a minimal level that is tolerable to the patient as a result of a successful medical intervention.

A Patient Case Example

A patient with a minor acute illness, a presumed case of acute otitis media (AOM), sought medical care from her primary care physician. The patient based her provisional diagnosis on the presence of subjective symptoms, including the discomfort of an earache and the presence of dizziness, as well as the more objective signs of a low-grade fever, diminished hearing, and a discharge in her external canal.

The family physician confirmed the diagnosis of acute otitis media (AOM), and prescribed an oral antibiotic and a short course of a decongestant. A follow-up appointment was made.

The patient then completed the course of antibiotics and returned for a

A Patient Case Example

follow-up appointment. The physician asked how things were going, and the patient replied, "I feel great today! Thank you for helping me." The AOM had resolved and there were no complications or residual effects. No preventive exams were due.

After the medical encounter, the patient began a process of reflection about the medical encounter. She reviewed the events with her primary care physician and wondered whether the physician could validly be credited with the fact the patient had reported a statement of subjective well-being – "I feel great today!"

After considerable reflection upon the situation, the patient decided that the best answer to that question was *no*! The physician *cannot* be given credit for the patient's proclamation of well-being. The rationale for this conclusion is presented below in Figure 5-3.

Both positive and negative dimensions in health provide opportunities for examining means to enhance health for both individuals and communities. The negativities that are inherently present within signs and symptoms can be alleviated partially or totally through medical interventions. Success in medical care is assessed as reductions in the magnitude of signs and symptoms to a near-zero clinical experience. Yet the positive aspects of life experiences are not well considered in disease-oriented biomedical models. Positive aspects of health are more likely to be encountered in the bio-psycho-social approaches developed in family medicine.

Examining Positive Health, Including Fitness and Subjective Well-being

The familiar aspects of disease and illness remain within the model proposed in this chapter. These measures are complemented by additional dimensions, including the positive aspects of fitness and subjective well-being, also known collectively as wellness.

Tom Wallace, MD, MPH, the former director of the Jefferson County Health Department in Louisville, Kentucky, succinctly stated, "The purpose of Public Health is to maximize the health of the population, not to minimize disease."[*] This axiom of population health requires a construct that can differentiate true health status from disease prevalence. It also requires that explanatory models

---

[*] Personal communication between Tom Wallace and Robert Steiner in 1995.

of public health should have the capacity to differentiate the factors related to positive health status from those associated with risk factors for disease.

It is possible, and indeed likely, that the causal factors for dimensions of positive health are different from the factors associated with negatively oriented disease status. Likewise, interventions to remedy the impact of disease are likely to be different from tonics to improve wellness, and consequently to counter the detrimental effects of disease and illness, or at least to buffer them to make the existing situation more acceptable.

From the case example above, a statement of subjective well-being (SWB), such as "I feel great today," is an expression of the presence of internal resources that operate at an experiential level to produce a sense of positive health. These expressions of positive health were merely obscured or overwhelmed by interactions with the illness experience. The physician and treatment removed the metaphoric cloud of the illness experience, but the physician did not necessarily directly alter the positive resource base of the patient other than through the presence of a trusting professional relationship between physician and patient. Figure 5-3 below shows a model with interactive axes for positive fitness and wellness that is a complement to the negativelyoriented model of disease-illness.

Figure 5-3. Multidimensional Model of Health:

A Positive Axis for Wellness and Fitness Complements the Negative Aspects of Disease and Illness in the Traditional Biomedical Model

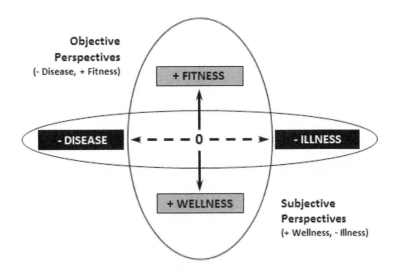

Quality of Life Assessments Include Positive Indicators of Well-being

We propose that health is a construct that is different from disease. Health is a construct that is positively oriented and resource-based (see Figure 5-4). We posit that the attributes of positive health, also known as wellness, include both subjective well-being and objective physical fitness. These indicators of positive health cannot be assigned within the format of the disease-oriented biomedical model.

Wellness is a positively oriented construct that is independent yet interactive with the negatively oriented components of the disease-illness model in medical care. Furthermore, the wellness model contains both subjective and objective aspects, and it is dimensionally congruent with its negatively oriented complement—objective disease status and the patients' illness experience.

One application of the positive dimensions of life, including both objective and subjective assessments, is found within the construct and measurements for quality-of-life assessments. Health-related quality of life (HRQL) assessments are a specific area of study within such disciplines as social epidemiology, sociology, psychology, and health policy. Guyatt and associates noted that the concepts for health status, functional status, and HRQL were often used interchangeably.[73] A variation of the HRQL construct, adapted from Haas[74] and illustrated in Figure 5-4, shows domains for objective and subjective dimensions that are all clearly related to an embedded concept of quality of life.

Figure 5-4. An Exemplary Construct for Health-Related Quality of Life to Examine the Domains

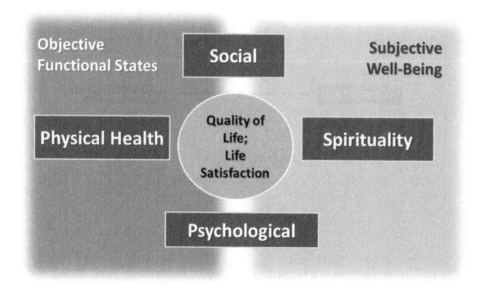

Patrick and associates defined HRQL as:

> Health-related quality of life is the value assigned to duration of life as modified by the impairments, functional states, perceptions, and social opportunities that are influenced by disease, injury, treatment or policy.[75]

Seligman provided a definition of well-being as "people's positive evaluations of their lives, including positive emotions, engagement, satisfaction and meaning."[76] This definition contains at least two independent components: positive emotions that are experienced and measured as utilities, while the measures for life satisfaction in multiple domains and scales for the meaning of life are evaluative in nature.[77] Other researchers include measures of happiness and negative emotions, and also provide examples of questions for use in surveys.[78]

There is no universal agreement about the domains for HRQL assessments. For example, spiritual domains are contained within this proposed construct. The domain of spirituality, however, is not present within the WHO definition of health. The WHO made a landmark definition of health in their constitution that was enacted in 1948, as below:[79]

> Health is a state of complete physical, mental and social well-being, and not merely the absence of disease or infirmity.

Amendments were offered to the WHO definition in 1998, such that "health" might be redefined to include an additional dimension and other new characteristics:[80]

> Health is a *dynamic* state of complete physical, mental, *spiritual* and social well-being, and not merely the absence of disease or infirmity. [*Emphasis added by authors.*]

This amended definition of health was not, however, formally adopted by the WHO. Apparently the medical doctors at the WHO regional meeting supported the idea that health should be kept within the natural sciences, and that health should not be part of disciplines in which culture, traditions, and beliefs play a role.[81] Obviously, this historic decision is not consistent with the position of the authors of this chapter.

The development of measurement questionnaires for assessing HRQL have spanned more than four decades.[82] Earlier questionnaires, like the Sickness Impact Profile[83] and Quality of Well-Being[84] scales are oriented toward eliciting objective, observable measures, like symptoms and functional limitations, with no inclusion of measures for the positive dimensions of well-being. The Dartmouth CO-OP Charts presented a series of pictograms to better serve people with lower levels of literacy and elicit their responses about functional status,[85] and the charts included a ladder for a single-item measure of overall quality of life assessments. During the 1990s, short questionnaires became more prominent, like the Short Forms (SF), including SF-12, SF-6 and others, each derived from the RAND Medical Outcome Study.[86,87] Additional questionnaires have emerged from longer questionnaires as well as shorter HRQL questionnaires to reduce response burden that have also been developed and utilized.[88,89] Many of these HRQL questionnaires are now proprietary, and so require legal permissions and fees to be paid prior to using the measures for research.

There are both generic and disease-specific varieties of validated and reliable HRQL questionnaires.[73] There are different methods of valuation, including preference-based and utility-based methods. Systematic variations are present between different approaches to utility-based methods for weighting responses.[90] Comparisons between national populations are available for many HRQL measures.[91]

The predictors of HRQL among those with morbid conditions will likely be different from the HRQL scores and predictors that are causally associated with mortality. In other words, the policies to reduce deaths from disease are likely to be different from the policies to improve quality-of-life assessments among the living. Likewise, the balance of numbers of positively and negatively oriented indicators in HRQL questionnaires is rarely considered in analyses of results about quality of life. Similarly, systematic differences may be present between questionnaires generated from HRQL measures that were derived from standard gamble methods, time tradeoff, or willingness-to-pay approaches. These differences may be one reason why comparisons of results from preference-based measures of HRQL can yield different results on the same research subjects.

There are multiple metrics for impaired quality of life, including HALYS (health-adjusted life years), QALYS (quality-adjusted life years), and DALYS (disability-adjusted life years).[92] When HRQL metrics are used to assess the impact of morbidity upon the living rather than as predictors of death, then different disease priorities of interest will likely be present. For example, Verbrugge and Patrick conducted such a study.[6] They reported that arthritis, visual impairments, and hearing impairments each had weights for limiting daily activities among the elderly that were comparable to the weight of indicators for such fatal diseases as ischemic heart diseases and lung diseases like COPD. The authors conclude that "nonfatal conditions do not receive health services care commensurate with their prevalence and impact," and that such findings reflect the longstanding, unbalanced attention given to fatal conditions in research and medical care. In short, the priorities for those who are living with chronic diseases seem to be different than the list of diseases associated with mortality.

The applications of these findings lie within the realm of socio-cultural-ecologic models of population health for health policy development. Multiple studies show that the highest negative correlations with measures of life satisfaction ratings are in people with mental health issues.[93-95] Diener suggested that including measures for subjective well-being in health policy discussions may favor the development of public policies that favor wellness and may also improve services for those with mental health needs.[96]

The Centers for Disease Control and Prevention is consistently using HRQL measures in the Behavioral Risk Factor Surveillance System (BRFSS) and the National Health and Nutrition Examination Survey (NHANES).[97] Other HRQL measures are available in national databases, and national norms for multiple HRQL questionnaires have been assembled as resources for comparison.[91] *Healthy People 2010* explicitly included HRQL within the first overarching goal: to increase quality and years of healthy life. Within the drafts for *Healthy People 2020*, quality of life is integral to each of four overarching goals:

- Attain high-quality, longer lives free of preventable disease, disability, injury, and premature death.

- Achieve health equity, eliminate disparities, and improve the health of all groups.

- Create social and physical environments that promote good health for all.

- Promote quality of life, healthy development, and healthy behaviors across all life stages.

It is apparent that measures of HRQL have a large and often unexamined potential as indicators of novel solutions in multiple arenas for health policy development. Yet despite the presence of encouraging social health goals from multiple national documents over past decades, formal assessments of HRQL with indicators for positive health are not yet commonly measured by most local providers and agencies of traditional public health in the United States.

Refining Definitions of Public Health and Population Health

Understanding patterns of health that extend beyond disease into the social determinants of health invokes newer models of public health that have been developing over several decades. Socio-ecologic models of public health have been presented before.[17,20,98,99] This part of the chapter will take a position that just as the biomedical model has been complemented by the introduction of the bio-psycho-social model into primary care arenas,[100] so now disease-oriented population health models may be complemented with socio-cultural-ecologic models. The socio-cultural-ecologic models of public health may include newer metrics, including indicators of positive physical fitness and subjective well-being (SWB), and other key concepts for assessing qualities of social relationships as primary determinants of health.[101]

Such an expansion of the model for population health may require a critical review of the definitions and applications of basic underlying concepts of health. For example, health promotion may be examined from the perspectives of either goals or methods. If health promotion in the medical model is examined from the perspectives of goals or purpose, most health education is a category of risk assessment and risk reduction, since the alleviation of signs, symptoms, and consequences of disease seems to be the main intention. When focusing on process and methods, however, health promotion efforts in population health seem to be different from the secondary levels of disease prevention or health promotion (DP/HP) in medical care. Whereas health promotion in the medical model focuses on educational and motivational interactions to assist patients in making behavioral changes, the proposed model for positive health in the context of population health is about promoting equality in access to such community resources as housing, food, safety, education, and the like. Social risk in this sense is the lack of socially normal community resources.

Thus the presence of the social determinants of health and socially enmeshed health concerns makes the interpretation of health promotion a bit different when considered from the perspective of population health. The goal of large community-oriented health campaigns for awareness of such cardiac risk factors as blood cholesterol levels seems to be geared toward increasing risk awareness as a means to reduce cardiac morbidity and mortality. As such, many community campaigns that appear to be health education may actually be part of the secondary level of DP/HP.

The presence of a positive axis for health and well-being, however, allows for different interpretations of the appropriate categorization of these kinds of efforts. By focusing on the appropriate use of available community resources to assist with educational attainment or improve access to housing, food, health care, or other basic needs, these factors may assist in upward social mobilization, or they may serve to make a difficult social situation more tolerable. As such, improving access to the use of available community resources is more in line with the first level of DP/HP at the population health level. The best measures for outcomes are formal quality-of-life assessments, especially those that include positive indicators of well-being. The focus for this categorization is on the accessible social resource base within the community and includes positive indicators of well-being.

Figure 5-5. Comparing and Contrasting Approaches: Individual Disease-Oriented Medical Care and Resource-Based Community Health

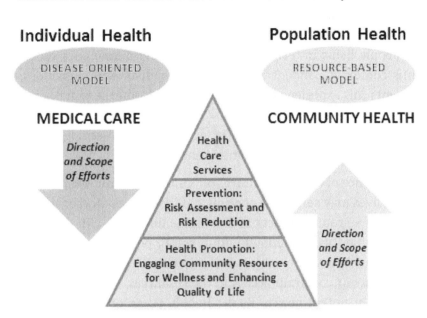

Population Health Management within the Context of Culture

Population health management is a set of strategies with a focus on the health resources, needs, and concerns of groups within designated communities, and how to enact those strategies to achieve the goals and objectives. Population health is in essence a relational issue between people and organizations within the context of their socio-cultural milieu.[102] It is not only an assessment of objective, material and structural indicators about social capital, social class, income, education, employment, wealth and the like, but it also includes the perceptions and comparative relationships that determine the influence of these factors on health.[103,104] These socio-cultural-ecologic influences that occur at the macro-level of society influence the qualities of our relationships and the qualities of life that we experience.

Both social and ecological perspectives have been central to public health concepts and methods from the earliest formulations and applications.[37,105] Kartman eloquently states,

> ... the ecology of human disease must start with the social fabric—and once that becomes clearly defined, the matters of public health can be delineated and analyzed in terms of their interrelationships in that social fabric. The

starting point is not a disease or the prevalence of infection, and it is not epidemiology—it is the social unit.[106]

Population health is a social good that may be viewed as a series of complex adaptive responses, engendered through interdependent network relationships, among people living in a shared culture and environment. As such, population health is context-dependent and culturally relative. And it includes subjective assessments of experiences of objective and interpersonal circumstances. Complexity and network sciences provide novel means for understanding and relating to the emerging aspects of a socio-cultural-ecologic construct that embodies the web of life as population health.[107]

The presence of implicit "culture" or "cultures" within which individuals live their daily lives may serve as a concept and label for the forces that link persons together into a group that acts as a cohesive unit.[108] Health of both individuals and communities are embedded within social, political and economic systems that shape our behaviors, values and attitudes. These systems and forces may either facilitate or constrain access to the resources, clinical and social, that are necessary to maintain health. Public Health, as an organization with political means for initiating legislative and regulatory initiatives, and Boards of Health with explicit missions to act as the voice of the community as advocates for population health, is one means to address the macro-perspectives of population health.

Culture is like an emergent property of the collection of agents in a society. An emerging model of population health may be envisioned that includes the interactive characteristics of organizations and groups of people within the context of networks of social and environmental forces. These social forces shape the human experience, including health and quality-of-life assessments.[105,109] An organizational network approach is posed in which stewardship of the qualities of network relationships and within aspects of community health depend upon intangible qualities that are present and generated during the course of these same interpersonal relationships.[110] The dynamics of the both the unexpected[111] and the novel nature of emergent phenomena[112] make possibilities for prediction less likely.

Clearly relationships, social networks, complexity and emergence are all factors within public health as it impacts society. The premise for total public health or population health is that how we live our lives within the context of communities does influence the qualities of life and health outcomes, and those social health policies can influence health status and qualities of life among individuals and groups.

From the perspectives of this chapter, health is a resource to maintain daily ongoing processes for active living. It is through the diversity of many collaborative relationships, each instilled with motivations to bring benefit to all encountered, that the health of the whole society will improve.

Examining the Collective Nature of Public Health

Traditional public health may be defined as the formal set of organizations with authority to exercise legislated and regulatory laws within a defined geopolitical area to manage the health and health-related conditions of the population of all resident citizens, including all visitors and transients who may be within that region at any time. As such, traditional public health is the formal, politically sanctioned, organizational approach for maintaining and improving community health. It includes one important approach to improving population health that is supported by government regulations, ordinances and the force of law. The Institute of Medicine (IOM) in the *Future of Public Health* defined Public Health as:

> What we, as a society, do *collectively* to assure the conditions in which people can be healthy.[113] *[Italic emphasis added by authors]*.

The word *collectively* is a key word in the definition. The collective aspect of people living within a society is greater than the sum of the aggregate of individuals. The implications of the word *collective* is that social relationships can bind disparate groups into cohesive unions as organizations, neighborhoods, communities, societies, and the like. One influence of such binding social network forces of a collective is to foster collaboration and cooperation.[114]

The collective aspects of public health are historically associated with the works of Emile Durkheim (1858–1917), one of the founding fathers of modern sociology.[115] He developed the perspective of "structural functionalism" with the notion that sociology should study phenomena attributed to society-at-large, rather than being limited to the combined actions of individuals.[116] His works are still applicable to current social health concerns, including divisions of labor and class conflict, race, education, law, deviance, religion, and other facets of modern life.

Others define population health from the perspective of the aggregate of individuals rather than the collective. For example, Kindig defined population health as "the aggregate health outcome of health-adjusted life expectancy of a group of individuals, in an economic framework that balances the relative marginal return from the multiple determinants of health."[117] He also defined population health as "the health outcomes of a group of individuals, including the distribution of such outcomes within the group".[118] Most epidemiologic studies use a methodological approach that implicitly addresses the characteristics of the aggregate of individuals rather than attending to the more pervasive aspects of the collective.

The collective nature of public health implies the presence of some unifying factors or forces that bind individuals together as a unit within the context of everyday living in a given society.[119] A unifying factor may be a type of social network force, such as social capital, that can form an invisible link between one person and another, and between groups.[120-126] Dynamic network models of health based in part on social capital and cybernetic systems with feedback loops fit with this approach.[109] The use of indicators of social capital demonstrate that relational and subjective indicators are necessary when considering research about population health, health promotion, social health policy development, and health service research.[104,127] Socio-cultural-ecologic approaches to population health are one means to better understand the emerging spectrum of global health.

Collective explanations emphasize the importance of shared norms, cultural traditions, social values, and interests; and so add an anthropological perspective to the social, economic, psychological, and epidemiologic perspectives for evaluating health.[128] These perspectives will necessarily open newer areas for study that have received less attention in previous transitions, including ethnicity, religion, politics, shared histories, domestic division of labor, appropriate social roles, and so on. The characteristics of the material infrastructure of a neighborhood and community are important, as are the perceived characteristics of the neighborhood and peer comparisons of self-rated and quality of life assessments.[103] In short, the relational aspects of people with and within the context of society must be considered for valid outcome measures in population health.[127]

Historic Evolution of Health Promotion

This section of the chapter provides an overview of the threads in the evolution of health promotion occurring in a long series of meetings spanning decades. There are both individualistic and social approaches to health and disease.

Public health strategies that emphasize the individual as the unit of focus may highlight utilization of the biomedical model and the disease-oriented approach. Structuralists' approaches to population health are more likely to emphasize the social determinants of health and disease. Merging approaches to population health that favor social justice with approaches that favor the more traditional market-driven forces is an ongoing tension in public funding for public health and for prioritizing categories of services for improving population health.

The series of WHO-sponsored health promotion conferences have served to redefine and alter the scope of practice for health promotion over a series of decades. The WHO and UNICEF jointly sponsored a conference in 1978 that described health as a human right, and further declared a goal of achieving "Health for All" people by the end of the century.[129,130] The conference affirmed access to basic health services as a fundamental human right. Concerns with social inequalities in health were emphasized in the WHO declaration of Alma-Ata in 1978.[130]

Health care was to be reoriented away from hospitals to be more intensely focused on the community, including new community health centers and more community health workers. Health services were to go beyond medical care to include agriculture, food, industry, education, and housing.[131] This reorientation brings to light an important concept from that conference: Health cannot be attained by the health sector alone. In developing countries in particular, economic development, antipoverty measures, food production, clean water, sanitation, housing, and environmental protection all contribute to health and have the same goal of human development.

Actions from several sectors in a given society would be required to achieve the goals, including health sectors, as well as social and economic sectors. The approach was intersectoral, involving agriculture extension officers, schoolteachers, women's groups, youth groups, ministers of religion, and the like.

The WHO's Ottawa Charter in 1986 has had a profound influence on health promotion. It championed the view that health promotion is a key concept to achieving health goals internationally. The WHO-sponsored Ottawa Charter for Health Promotion described health as:

> . . . the extent to which an individual or a group is able, on the one hand, to realize aspirations and satisfy needs; and on the other, to change or cope with the environment. It is a *positive concept emphasizing social and personal resources*, as well as physical capacities.[132]

[Italics emphasis added by authors]

and

Health is . . . seen as a resource for everyday life, not the objective of living.[133]

The Ottawa Charter steered health promotion toward social and ecologic approaches to health promotion that address the structural determinants of health within societies. Simply stated, the charter identifies prerequisites for health as peace, shelter, education, food, income, a stable ecosystem, sustainable resources, social justice, and equity.[134] Likewise, the Ottawa Charter took health promotion efforts away from the dominant health education models that mainly targeted changes in individual behavior.

The Ottawa Charter changed the context for health promotion, so that well-being, community participation, and empowerment are all included, as well as ecologic sustainability and interdependency among various community agencies. The charter defined community-oriented strategies for health promotion, including the creation of supportive environments for health; strengthening community advocacy and actions for health through healthy public policy development; development of personal lifestyle skills for better health; and reorientation of health services.

The Jakarta Conference on Health Promotion in 1997 urged international action on poverty.[135] Poverty was identified as the major threat to health. The Jakarta Conference reinforced the positive dimensions of health; the concept of health as a resource; and health as a means rather than an outcome. The notion of empowerment through community engagement and participation is present in this charter.[131] The WHO's global strategy Health for All by 2000[136] considered primary health care (PHC) as a means for universal coverage of such basic services as educational methods for preventing and controlling prevailing health problems. The methods extended to the community through community health workers, including attention to the promotion of food security and proper nutrition; adequate safe water supply and basic sanitation; maternal and child health, including family planning; vaccination; prevention and control of locally endemic diseases; appropriate treatment of common diseases and injuries; and provision of essential drugs.

Within the plans for Health for All by 2000, the qualities of delivered health services were to be improved by focusing on vulnerable populations, community engagement, and collaborative intersectoral activities that would promote comprehensive PHC. With the PHC model, the emphasis changed from the larger hospital to that of community-based delivery of services with a balance of cost-effective preventive and curative programs. The community, through its leaders, was to be involved in the planning and implementation of its own health care services through community-based Primary Health Committees. Where Western-trained doctors and nurses were not available, community representatives and village health workers were to be trained to serve within the healthcare system. Health and health care were to be part of community life rather th~ ~mmodity for those with more wealth and resources.[136]

Some exper~ ~id not achieve the intended goals for several reaso~ ~xperts and politicians in developed countries to ac~ ~nities should plan and implement their own health~ ~ economic philosophy led to the replacement of co~ ~y a more limited notion of selective primary health care (~ ~ealth Sector Reform" based on market forces and the economic bene~ ~etter health. Professional organizations became the antagonists of community participation in setting priorities for health decision making. Rather, the agendas were set and monies made available to attend to interventions for one or two specific diseases. These authors claimed that it was time to abandon economic ideologies about socially enmeshed health concerns and community engagement, and to focus on determining methods that will effectively provide access to basic (disease-oriented) health care services for all people.[138]

The focus on eradication of select specific diseases through strategies known as structural adjustment policies by the World Bank became the preferred method of intervention for this group.[138] Top-down leadership models prevailed over bottom-up strategies intended to engage and empower the communities in need. The limited or false premises proposed by the World Bank and the International Monetary Fund, which stated that the production of better population health is usually achieved through improvements in healthcare, were once again in place.[139] The Global Fund, a series of public-private partnerships, including funds from the Bill and Melinda Gates Foundation, served as a financial agency for treating diseases like malaria, tuberculosis, and HIV/AIDS in specific countries by using select technologic approaches while not attending to the broader socio-cultural-ecologic and more removed determinants of health, such as income, education, housing, and the like.[140] These perspectives were contrary to the positions of prior WHO Charters.

Several core messages remained the same in the Bangkok Charter of 2005 while others changed. The Bangkok Charter proposed to make the promotion of health central to the global development agenda. It reiterated the core responsibility for health for all of government; provided a key focus on communities and civil society; and added a requirement for good corporate practice.[141,142] Perhaps, however, reflecting the changes brought by Health for All by 2000, the language of the Bangkok Charter 2005 was distinctly different from the tone of the earlier WHO charters.[134] For example, there was a shift in emphasis from the humanitarian workings of democracy for social justice to favor the language of the more technocratic aspects of law and policy work designed to increase opportunities for disease treatment. The Bangkok Charter changed perspectives from representing people in communities to a focus on consumers in a healthcare system. Likewise, the document redirected the focus from workers to employers.

Recently, the WHO's Commission on Social Determinants of Health (CSDH), under the direction of Professor Sir Michael Marmot, provided reports in 2007 and 2012.[143,144] The final report from the CSDH suggested an ambitious series of actions to close the gap in health inequities between population sectors within a single generation. The actions include immediate investments to make changes in social policies, economic arrangements, and political actions. The CSDH suggests focusing on the very shape of societies[145] and encouraging active participation of all people as a means to empowerment and toward meaningful change within the fabric of society itself[146] as a means toward a healthier society that will engender healthier individuals.[37] The CSDH made three overarching strategic recommendations for policy development: to improve daily living conditions; to tackle the inequitable distribution of power, money, and resources; and to measure and understand the problems and assess the results of the proposed actions.[146]

Health Policy Development

Socioeconomic disparities are an aspect of population health that is consistent with the Institute of Medicine's (IOM's) definition of public health. In other words, income inequality is tied to the collective aspect of the public health society. Policies that affect redistribution of funds, from wages to taxation, access to health care and similar topics, will in turn affect the health of a society.

Evidence indicates that increases in life expectancy are more likely linked to improved living conditions than to improved health care services.[147,148] Clinical care delivery is responsible for only about 10 percent of premature mortality and health status, while the major causal factors include genetic predispositions (30 percent) and behavioral patterns (40 percent), with each influenced by social circumstances (15 percent) and environmental exposures (5 percent).[10,149] The capacity of the healthcare sector to improve population health and health equity is strongly influenced by other sectors within any society.[150,151] By this logic, investments in new medical interventions will likely increase health inequities, since the interventions are more likely to reach more advantaged groups before, if ever, trickling down to those with fewer opportunities and resources.[152,153]

Race and ethnicity receive attention as major factors for premature death and lack of health.[154] Others cite social class status, accompanied by the relative contributions to health status of education, income, and occupation as major factors that are often unmeasured and so ignored as contributing factors to premature death and lack of wellness within American societies.[155] Health policy development is a major means of influencing community health status,[113] and a major means of influencing population health outcomes and quality-of-life assessments.[23] Legislative approaches are one avenue for development of new social health policies, but organizational policies that influence the lives of people at worksites, schools, and other community sites can influence social norms and health behaviors. The basic premise is that the social determinants of health are the social characteristics in which living takes place, and they can be modified by health policies that can reshape social norms, values, and behaviors.[156,157]

Societies in which inequalities abound are also more likely to suffer from an increased prevalence of other social problems, including low educational performance, violence, higher rates of imprisonment, bullying, unwanted teen births, reduced social mobility, lower levels of social capital or trust, and longer working hours. Whereas these are behavioral outcomes, their presence provides evidence that these very psychosocial processes are indeed associated with inequality. The apparent connection between increasing economic inequality and the erosion of social capital hints at the possibility of revitalizing civil society through fixing the upstream problem of maldistribution in incomes, or the more upstream factors that cause this maldistribution.[125]

Marmot cites six generic categories of social health policies to address inequalities. Each is in accord with the principles of social justice. He presented them in *Fair Society, Healthy Lives*:[158]

1. Give every child the best start in life;

2. Enable all children, young people, and adults to maximize their capabilities and to have a sense of control within their lives;

3. Create fair employment and good work for all;

4. Ensure healthy standards of living for all;

5. Create and develop healthy and sustainable places and communities;

6. Strengthen the role and impact of preventing illness.

Most population health strategies still focus on downstream methods that focus on individual behavioral changes—for example, changing to healthier diets, increasing physical activity levels, and reducing the number of people who use tobacco. These kinds of efforts persist despite increasing evidence that these downstream approaches are generally ineffective.[159] Indeed, some authors claim that individualization of risk is likely to be dependent on prevailing political and economic ideologies rather than based on evidence.[160]

Upstream activities may be a more effective approach for policy development to address health concerns that are socially enmeshed. Upstream policies are macro-perspectives of the sociocultural context that provide a means to develop culturally appropriate approaches for processes that advance new social norms. Upstream strategies are summarized in the WHO documents titled "Levelling Up."[150,161]

Marmot notes that policy makers need to consider two strategies concurrently to enable meaningful progress.[158] One strategy is to use a targeted strategy to focus on people at the bottom of the gradient, using the humanitarian principle that the greatest efforts and resources of a society should be allocated to those people in greatest need. Marmot clearly states, however, that attention to people at the bottom of the social ladder will not sufficiently reduce inequalities. He suggests that this approach should be complemented with an approach involving policies with universal application across the entire social gradient. The concurrent approaches to policy development, with both applications targeted to specific groups in need and others applied to all of society, is known as "proportionate universalism."[158,162]

Whitehead clearly states that "population health policies should have the dual purpose of promoting health gains in the population as a whole and reducing health inequities,"[163] and that the "objective of reducing health inequities constitutes an integral part of a comprehensive strategy for heath development, not an alternative option."[158] Whitehead provides commentary about the challenges of implementing large-scale national strategies using upstream methods.[163] She cites the essence of common political arguments—that such broad policies are simply too expensive; and on the other hand, that inaction cannot be afforded. Navarro discusses a more political perspective on the social determinants of health—that the issues related to the resultant growing disparities in health and inequalities in social class status are mostly about the politics of people in power relationships rather than the health effects of social inequalities themselves.[164]

Wilkerson makes important observations about the nature and impact of poverty. He states that health remains closely associated with deprivation but that the relationship is based on relative changes rather than absolute values. Accordingly, health is influenced by differences in relative income differences between groups of people within the same society, not by the absolute level of the average incomes for each society as a whole.[165] Thus the healthiest countries are those with the least variability between the richest rich and the poorest poor.

The importance of this finding regarding relative income is that it is a social concept that cannot be applied at the individual level. Societies, not individuals, have income distributions. There is evidence that points to possibilities that there is a threshold magnitude of difference in categories of available resources (wealth, income, education, housing, food, and the like) between social gradient categories for the richest, when compared to the poorest groups in a community, may be associated with the very sustainability of that society as a whole. Large disparities between social classes may serve as an indicator of increasing social deviance and impending social unrest or increasing civil disobedience. Indicators of well-being within community groups may serve as buffers for the critical differences between these extreme groups and serve to soothe the impact of the loss of social capital and cohesiveness within larger societies. Further research is needed in this content area.

The CDC has updated a series of indicators tied to the socioeconomic environment and health status,[166] as in Table 5-2 below.

Table 5-2. CDC's population health status indicators: Socioeconomic environment

Number	Socioeconomic Indicators for Assessing Population Health Status
1	Poverty rate
2	Unemployment rate
3	Average household income
4	Affordability of single-family home
5	Bankruptcy and foreclosure rates
6	Percentage of households on public assistance
7	Percentage of single-parent households
8	Percentage of children receiving free or reduced-price lunches
9	Concentrated disadvantage and concentrated affluence scales
10	Percentage of adults older than 24 years with less than a high school education
11	Percentage of adults older than 18 years with less than an eighth-grade education
12	Public high school graduation and dropout rates
13	Percentage of third- and tenth-grade students at grade level in reading
14	Percentage of tenth-grade students at grade level in math
15	Racial segregation
16	Density of voluntary organizations
17	Voter registration and turnout

Varieties of Health Policy Development

Public policies can influence health in at least three different ways.[167] Laws and regulations that influence infrastructure directly affect the social determinants of health, while interventional policies provide direct effects on health. Incidental laws and policies can influence income, education, housing, and the like, and so have an indirect or buffering impact on health outcomes.

The presence of new dimensions within the construct of health and population health provides new opportunities for generating effective health policies. Two types of policies will make a difference in curtailing premature mortality and reducing health disparities: policies that affect the steepness of the socioeconomic ladder, its length, and the distance between its rungs; and policies that buffer the adverse consequences of living lower on the ladder.[168]

For example, Sheldon Cohen proposed a buffering hypothesis for social support as an inter- and intrapersonal resource that can aid in alleviating the harmful effects of stress.[169] Social support can buffer the effect of stress on a given outcome.[170] Cohen has teamed with other social scientists to extend the buffering hypothesis to domains involving health policies. There are policies that have a direct influence on outcomes, and those that influence change through indirect means or through buffering.[145]

Policies that influence the steepness of the steps on the socioeconomic ladder are polices with potential to affect health and well-being directly. Policies in this genre include educational, financial, and skills-training approaches for appropriate individuals or groups. All the direct approaches provide means to increase opportunities for residents in a given community. The redistribution of resources at the community level in accord with social justice models is a means to operationalize this approach. In other words, all policies with direct impact or influence provide means that increase opportunities for a target group to improve access to needed resources for a valued level of life in the community.

Health and disease are complementary constructs, one positively oriented and one negatively oriented, respectively. Each construct is interdependent with the other, and these two constructs interact with one another. The interaction of two independent measures means that buffering, also known as effect modification, is possible. One application of this model (Figure 5-5) is that the presence of interdependent and interacting natures of health and disease means that a person may be both sick and well at the same time.

The utility of this model (Figure 5-5) may be evident in an example. People with such chronic diseases as cancer may survive with the disease for a considerable time. During this time, the cancer may produce or be associated with some signs or symptoms that impair functional capacities or quality of life. On the other hand, the person may maintain skills, talents, and personal characteristics, for example, which bring delight to either self or others. Thus disease-illness and wellness-fitness models are not mutually exclusive constructs. They coexist and the measures interact statistically with one another.

This is the basis of the stress-buffering model for policy development, based in part upon the early works of Sheldon Cohen.[169-172] In this model, the presence of positive health resources can lessen the negatively oriented burden of suffering attributed to a stressor, for example, like the onset of disease-illness, or even the loss of a loved one.[13-15] Buffering, or effect modification, of deficiencies in social health resources can be used as a strategy in health policy development, especially when measures of positive health are present in evaluations, surveys, and scientific reports.

Policies that buffer the adverse conditions of living lower on the ladder (social gradient) without necessarily changing the location of a person or group on the social status ladder include at least three different kinds:

Policies Affecting the Physical and Social Environment

- Improve traffic safety

- Reduce crime

Policies Affecting the Workplace Environment

- Limit exposure to physical hazards and toxic chemicals

- Limit psychosocial strains in workplaces

- Increase opportunities for control over work demands

Policies for Healthier Environments and Opportunities That Enable Healthy Behaviors

- Ban smoking in public areas

- Improve nutrition in school lunch programs

- Ban sale of soft drinks and junk foods in schools

Public Policies Address Well-being to Improve Population Health

Subjective approaches to health policy and quality of life assessments began in the United States with landmark studies by Campbell[173] and Andrews and Withey;[174] others provide historic reviews of measures and applications of well-being.[175] Socioeconomic disparities are an aspect of population health that is consistent with the IOM's definition of public health. In other words, income inequality is tied to the collective aspect of the public health of a society. Policies that affect redistribution of funds, from wages to taxation, access to health care and adjustments to the cost of living and the like, will impact upon the health of a society. The influence and potential effects of greater equality within societies reach far beyond our typical notions of outcomes related to access to interventions for disease-oriented medical care. Market forces for a profit-driven form of capitalist economy seem to be at odds with changes that are needed to support a model of social justice. Pluralism in the democratic processes may be both a source and a source of possible solutions for the expression of these competing values.

Newer studies have provided a context for understanding the impact of poverty on the lives of people. "[I]n rich countries and poor, poverty means not participating fully in society, and having limits on leading the life one has reason to value."[38] Policies that buffer, as listed above, can help people to tolerate or accommodate their life situations better than if these policies were not present.

Health in All Policies to Improve Population Health

Health in All Policies (HiAP), a concept introduced in Chapter 1, is becoming an accepted approach for improving population health. HiAP is a collaborative approach to improving the health of all people by incorporating health considerations into decision making across sectors and policy areas.[188] Thismethod for addressing the social determinants of health can be easily adapted for the Healthy Communities and Healthy Cities approaches for improving population health.[43]

In the HiAP approach, the responsibility for addressing solutions to the social determinants of health falls to many nontraditional health partners, such as housing, transportation, education, air quality, parks, criminal justice, energy, and employment agencies. HiAP is not so much about content as it is about the values that underlie and motivate the processes for improving health. Marmot and associates clearly state that, "[a]ction on the social determinants of health must involve the whole of government, civil society, local communities, business and . . . agencies."[189] There are efforts in the policy arena for development for HiAP.[190]

HiAP is an approach to public policies across sectors that systematically takes into account the health implications of decisions; seeks synergies; and avoids harmful health impacts in order to improve population health and health equity. The Harvard sociologist David Williams states during the CDC-sponsored video, *Unnatural Causes...is inequality making us sick* (2008):

> Housing policy is health policy, educational policy is health policy, anti-violence policy is health policy, and neighborhood improvement policies are health policies. Everything that we can do to improve the quality of life of

individuals in our society has an impact on their health and is a health policy. In other words, there is no magic bullet in the policy arena that will take care of socially enmeshed health concerns. Rather, current evidence and recommendations suggest that cohesive, coordinated and persistent efforts over time and across traditional boundaries for social sectors should be attempted for optimal outcomes.

Methods for HiAP include intersectoral action in areas related to education, housing, transportation, environment, inequities, and other areas related to the material and structural aspects of life. Others suggest that governance is clearly a part of the solution, as per the Adelaide Statement on HiAP (2010), with its emphasis on "moving towards shared governance for health and well-being."[191] HiAP is likely to be a common theme in global health during the next years, and the content of this approach may likely influence local approaches to population health. Louisville, Kentucky, has made HiAP a major approach for improving population health, according to the *Healthy Louisville 2020* report released in February 2014.

Discussion

The introduction of new dimensions of positive health and well-being in a relationship-based construct for population health is akin to exploring a new world order. Many new possibilities for assessing health status and developing new health policies are present as a result of the new dimensions. Habitual tendencies, however, will likely lead community groups to revert to old ways of addressing negativity—focusing on problems and problem-solving orientations while attempting to attend to the needs of individuals within the medical model as patients, clients, and consumers. The medicalization of the public health approach has been construed as a socially normal process, made possible by the prominence of the disease-oriented biomedical model. The biomedical model is useful when appropriate, but it is not the only way to address socially enmeshed health concerns in population health.

The social determinants of health and the social gradient of health are ubiquitous and are causally related to health outcomes. Within this chapter, we have examined some basic assumptions about the nature of health and disease, not only for individuals but also for groups of people as communities and neighborhoods. In other words, the nature of population health and the solutions for socially enmeshed health concerns are complex. Attempts to find solutions to complex problems require appropriate methods. Using reductionistic methods and linear solutions for complex issues may not be valid or effective. It is likely that population health will remain a complex balance between resources and stressors, between the objective and subjective needs of people, each and all within the context of common social units—families and neighborhoods, states and nations.

Marmot states that fairness is at the heart of all social health policies. The patterns of inequity,

> . . . the unequal distribution of health-damaging experiences is not in any sense a 'natural' phenomenon but is the result of a toxic combination of poor social policies and programs, unfair economic arrangements, and bad politics.[146]

He continues that health inequalities result from social inequalities, and the concerns about health status require action on all the social determinants. Focusing solely on the most disadvantaged will not reduce inequalities sufficiently. Rather, action is needed across the whole of the social distribution. These are principles for social health policy development.

The view of public health from the perspective of the collective is simply different from the current perspectives of population health that promote the aggregate of the members of a defined community as the units of analyses. As such, the solutions for many socially enmeshed health concerns and global health issues extend beyond any one form of logic or method within any community.

Complexity is a paradigm that can contribute to health promotion and to public health paradigms for population health.[192] Complexity and nonlinear dynamics are means to expand awareness beyond the current culturally sanctioned limits—to include novel aspects of the same situation that were simply not considered in prior analyses or conversations when undertaken using conventional methods. Yet there are limits; the very nature of emergence makes it difficult if not impossible to predict the future of such efforts accurately.

Rather, the human agents representing communal interests must adapt to the continually changing social environment and competing priorities. Similarly, scientists within the field of epidemiology may need to work more closely with scientists from other traditions, including sociology, anthropology, political science, macroeconomics, ethics, and law. These collaborative approaches will likely better address research and measurement issues from the societal and cultural perspectives, and they may be more likely to overcome political barriers to progress.

A socio-cultural-ecologic model for population health, as developed in this chapter, provides a perspective from the collective aspects of society. The emphasis lies on giving more attention to the social good while respecting the rights of individuals. Communities can identify and better utilize existing resources as parts of their potential solutions for socially enmeshed health concerns.

Collaborative communities can foster new ideas, and proposals can be forged among local agents from multiple diverse organizations. From the perspectives of complexity, such interactions allow the foundations for new social health policy solutions to emerge, each with the potential to benefit many in the community. Potential solutions will likely require well-motivated people who are each interested in providing benefits to others, who will then engage with communities of interest to elicit potential solutions with them. An emphasis on uplifting the social good, as defined by participating members of local communities, must be given high priority.

Conclusion

All sciences are based on theories. Both science and theories are limited by the constraints imposed by their respective measures. Scientists make models to represent the situation they are investigating, each in accord with their often implicit assumptions, beliefs, and worldviews. The models are often presented mathematically, with an implicit and pervasive sense of order and logic. Yet the models that scientists create are always simplifications of real-world phenomena, perceptions, and experiences. In this sense, George Box has aptly stated (paraphrased), "Essentially, all models are wrong, (although) some are useful."[193]

Some observers suggest that a paradigm shift has already occurred within modern science. For example, the focus on the nature of reality as phenomena (ontology) is shifting toward a greater emphasis on the study of human interaction with the phenomenal world (epistemology). More simply, the content of scientific investigation (i.e., the "what") is yielding more to the process of knowing (i.e., the "how"). The results and implications are radical. Complexity suggests that we are living in a participatory universe of self-organizing hierarchies of networks rather than in a world of clockwork mechanisms in which we just happen to reside! Such a change is a paradigm change.

We close this chapter with a visual metaphor about changing paradigms in science, viewed as potentials and possibilities for improving population health; see Figure 5-6. The purpose of science for improving population health is to provide a means for understanding the world in which we all live. The purpose of science is not necessarily to grasp new self-existing truths about the phenomenal world, especially those ideas that seemingly exist as phenomena that are seemingly independent of human awareness. Rather, science can be a means, a tool, to a better understanding of the human condition; to alleviate human suffering and to provide opportunities for emerging conditions that can continue to sustain life on Earth.

Science is a tool for relating to both the suffering and the richness within the world in which we live. Overcoming the limits of the implicit cultural assumptions about the nature of the world, in part by expanding the scope of awareness to include social and cultural aspects of our worldly relationships, is inherent within the scientific process. Advances in science will likely progress when scientists realize the complementary nature of the world in which we all live—as natural phenomena appearing within a social construct of reality.

"Good science" requires the presence and active involvement of "good scientists"—not only "good" in a technical sense, but as humanistic scientists with compassion for all sentient beings. The knowledge and motivation of the scientists can drive the scope of inquiries and the activities of observation, analyses, and investigation. Scientists are thus in a symbiotic relationship with the very world in which we live. Enacting such an expanded vision will require new metrics and new visions for cohabiting in the world together as a global society. A socio-cultural-ecologic vision of population health may be an aid to realizing such a process, for improving health and enhancing quality of life.

Figure 5-6. New visions for population health will likely emerge from the complexity of multiple diverse social interactions that will reframe our current situation.

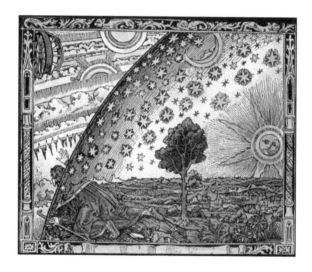

The Flammarion engraving is a wood engraving by an unknown artist. Its first documented appearance is in Camille Flammarion's 1888 book, *L'atmosphère: météorologie populaire.*

"You never change things by fighting the existing reality. To change something, build a new model that makes the existing model obsolete."[195]

Richard Buckminster Fuller

"In every age there is a turning point, a new way of seeing and asserting the coherence of the world."[194]

Jacob Bronowski

ACKNOWLEDGMENTS

The authors extend sincere appreciation to Daniel Verman, MD, Senior Counsellor in the Constanta Health Authority, Ministry of Health, for his collaboration in drafting the "Making a Healthier Community" case study based on the Constanta and Louisville Partnership that took place between 1998 and 2002.

CHAPTER 5 DISCUSSION QUESTIONS

Discussion questions are provided for team building or class exercises. Answers for all questions are provided in Appendix C.

Question Number	Question
1	What are the basic differences between the traditional medical care model and the public health or population health model? How are these differences important to a broader comprehension of health?
2	Why is consideration of the role of social determinants in health essential for assessment and planning for community/population health?
3	What are the implications of the complex interconnections of the health and social domains for policy development within a population?
4	What is the basic social-cultural-ecological construct for health? Why is it important to population health?
5	Why is the concept of positive health important as both a behavioral and a psychosocial mechanism to drive improvement in quality of life?

CHAPTER 5 SUMMARY

- Readers gained an understanding of the inherent differences between the traditional medical care model and the public or population health model.

- Insights were provided on the need for incorporating social determinants of health into the assessment and development of policies, and their relevance in assuring the health of communities.

- Insights were offered on Sir Michael Marmot's work on factors contributing to the social gradients of health and categories for social health policy development and categorization.

- A case example of a four-year (1998–2002) Healthy Communities Partnership project was discussed as it was conducted between a Constanta, Romania, and Louisville, Kentucky, collective of academic and government health and public health partners.

- The chapter gave a global perspective of the social-cultural-ecological construct and the evolving need for adoption and incorporation of this model into contemporary thinking on the advancement of population health and public health initiatives, programs and policy development.

- A model for managing population health was introduced that includes a medical care model that is not driven by measures of disease or illness. Instead measures for community health are more dependent upon societal measures.

- The potential benefits of adopting the conceptual notion of positive health (e.g., wellness) as a behavioral mechanism to drive improvement in quality of life were discussed. This concept also includes both subjective well-being and objective physical fitness.

CHAPTER 5 REFERENCES

1. Kleinman A. *Patients and healers in the context of culture: an exploration of the borderland between anthropology, medicine and psychiatry.* Vol 3: Oakland: University of California Press;1980.

2. Agar MH. *The professional stranger: an informal introduction to ethnography.* 2nd ed. San Diego, Calif.: Academic Press;1996.

3. Kelso J, Engstrøm DA. *The complementary nature.* Cambridge, Mass.: MIT Press;2006.

4. Kuhn TS. The structure of scientific revolutions, *International encyclopedia of united science,* vol. 2, no. 2. Aufl. Chicago;1970.

5. Omran AR. The epidemiologic transition: a theory of the epidemiology of population change. 1971. *Milbank Q.* 2005;83(4):731-757.

6. Verbrugge LM, Patrick DL. Seven chronic conditions: their impact on US adults' activity levels and use of medical services. *Am J Public Health.* 1995;85(2):173-182.

7. Andresen EM, Meyers AR. Health-related quality of life outcomes measures. *Arch Phys Med Rehabil.* 2000;81(12 Suppl 2):S30-45.

8. Carr SM, Lhussier M, Forster N, et al. An evidence synthesis of qualitative and quantitative research on component intervention techniques, effectiveness, cost-effectiveness, equity and acceptability of different versions of health-related lifestyle advisor role in improving health. *Health Technol Assess.* 2011;15(9):iii-iv, 1-284.

9. Neumann PJ, Goldie SJ, Weinstein MC. Preference-based measures in economic evaluation in health care. *Annu Rev Public Health.* 2000;21:587-611.

10. McGinnis JM, Williams-Russo P, Knickman JR. The case for more active policy attention to health promotion. *Health Aff (Millwood)* 2002;21(2):78-93.

11. Brownson RC, Haire-Joshu D, Luke DA. Shaping the context of health: a review of environmental and policy approaches in the prevention of chronic diseases. *Annu Rev Public Health.* 2006;27:341-370.

12. Cutler D, Miller G. The role of public health improvements in health advances: the twentieth-century United States. *Demography.* 2005;42(1):1-22.

13. Baicker K, Cutler D, Song Z. Workplace wellness programs can generate savings. *Health Aff (Millwood).* 2010;29(2):304-311.

14. Pelletier KR. A review and analysis of the clinical and cost-effectiveness studies of comprehensive health promotion and disease management programs at the worksite: 1995-1998 update (IV). *Am J Health Promot.* 1999;13(6):333-345.

15. Wakefield MA, Loken B, Hornik RC. Use of mass media campaigns to change health behaviour. *Lancet.* 2010;376(9748):1261-1271.

16. Abroms LC, Maibach EW. The effectiveness of mass communication to change public behavior. *Annu Rev Public Health.* 2008;29:219-234.

17. Lalonde M. A new perspective on the health of Canadians. In: *Canada*. MoSaS, ed. Ottawa, Ont.: Retrieved from Public Health Agency of Canada;1974.

18. Hancock T. Lalonde and beyond: looking back at "A New Perspective on the Health of Canadians." *Health Promot Int.* 1986;1(1):93-100.

19. Lalonde M. *A new perspective on the health of Canadians: a working document.* Ottawa, Ont.: Ministry of Supply and Services;1981.

20. *Healthy people. The Surgeon General's report on health promotion and disease prevention.* Washington, D.C.: U.S. Government Printing Office;1979.

21. Evans RG, Stoddart GL. Producing health, consuming health care. *Soc Sci Med.* 1990;31(12):1347.

22. Evans RG, Barer ML, Marmor TR. *Why are some people healthy and others not?: The determinants of the health of populations.* Piscataway, N.J.: Transaction Books;1994.

23. Green LW, Kreuter MW. *Health promotion planning: an educational and ecological approach.* New York, N.Y.: McGraw-Hill Humanities/Social Sciences/Languages;1999.

24. McGinnis JM, Foege WH. Actual causes of death in the United States. *JAMA.* 1993;270(18):2207-2212.

25. Mokdad AH, Marks JS, Stroup DF, Gerberding JL. Actual causes of death in the United States, 2000. *JAMA.* 2004;291(10):1238-1245.

26. Pearce N. Traditional epidemiology, modern epidemiology, and public health. *Am J Public Health.* 1996;86(5):678-683.

27. Galea S, Tracy M, Hoggatt KJ, Dimaggio C, Karpati A. Estimated deaths attributable to social factors in the United States. *Am J Public Health.*101(8):1456-1465.

28. Woolf SH. Social policy as health policy. *JAMA.* 2009;301(11):1166-1169.

29. Satcher D, Fryer GE, McCann J, Troutman A, Woolf SH, Rust G. What if we were equal? A comparison of the black-white mortality gap in 1960 and 2000. *Health Aff (Millwood).* 2005;24(2):459-464.

30. Woolf SH, Johnson RE, Phillips RL, Philipsen M. Giving everyone the health of the educated: an examination of whether social change would save more lives than medical advances. *Am J Public Health.* 2007;97(4):679-683.

31. Marmot MG, Stansfeld S, Patel C, et al. Health inequalities among British civil servants: the Whitehall II study. *Lancet.* 1991;337(8754):1387-1393.

32. Marmot M. Social differentials in mortality: the Whitehall Studies. In: Lopez A, Caselli G, Valkonen T., eds. *Adult mortality in developed countries: from description to explanation.* Oxford, England: Clarendon Press;1995:243-260.

33. Kivimaki M, Head J, Ferrie JE, et al. Why is evidence on job strain and coronary heart disease mixed? An illustration of measurement challenges in the Whitehall II study. *Psychosom Med.* 2006;68(3):398-401.

34.   Adshead F, Thorpe A. Health inequalities in England: advocacy, articulation and action. *Perspect Public Health.* 2009;129(1):37-41.

35.   De Vogli R, Macinko J, Marmot MG. Unfairness and health: evidence from the Whitehall II Study. *J Epidemiol Community Health.* 2007;61(6):513-518.

36.   World Health Organization Commission on Social Determinants of Health. Closing the gap in a generation: health equity through action on the social determinants of health. Geneva, Switzerland: World Health Organization;2008.

37.   Marmot MG. Creating healthier societies. *Bull World Health Organ.* 2004;82(5).

38.   Marmot M. Health in an unequal world: social circumstances, biology and disease. *Clin Med.* 2006;6(6):559-572.

39.   Marmot MG. Population science, prejudice and policy on alcohol. *Addiction.* 1995;90(11):1441-1443.

40.   Marmot MG, Fuhrer R, Ettner SL, Marks NF, Bumpass LL, Ryff CD. Contribution of psychosocial factors to socioeconomic differences in health. *Milbank Q.* 1998;76(3):403-448.

41.   Wilkinson RG, Marmot MG. *Social determinants of health: the solid facts.* Geneva, Switzerland: World Health Organization;2003.

42.   Wilkinson RG, Pickett KE, De Vogli R. Equality, sustainability, and quality of life. *BMJ.* 2010;341:c5816.

43.   Hancock T. Healthy communities must also be sustainable communities. *Public Health Rep.* 2000;115(2-3):151-156.

44.   Sharpe PA, Greaney ML, Lee PR, Royce SW. Assets-oriented community assessment. *Public Health Rep.* 2000;115(2-3):205-211.

45.   Raphael D. Letter from Canada: paradigms, politics and principles: an end of the millennium update from the birthplace of the Healthy Cities movement. *Health Promot Int.* 2001;16(1):99-101.

46.   Stokols D. Translating social ecological theory into guidelines for community health promotion. *Am J Health Promot.* 1996;10(4):282-298.

47.   Plsek PE, Wilson T. Complexity, leadership, and management in healthcare organisations. *BMJ.* Sep 29 2001;323(7315):746-749.

48.   Luke DA, Stamatakis KA. Systems science methods in public health: dynamics, networks, and agents. *Annu Rev Public Health.* 2012;33:357-376.

49.   Glasgow RE, Vogt TM, Boles SM. Evaluating the public health impact of health promotion interventions: the RE-AIM framework. *Am J Public Health.* 1999;89(9):1322-1327.

50.   Pearce N, Merletti F. Complexity, simplicity, and epidemiology. *International Journal of Epidemiology.* 2006;35(3):515-519.

51.   Rinpoche SM. *The Shambhala principle: discovering humanity's hidden treasure.* New York, N.Y.: Harmony Books; 2013.

52.   Wilkinson RG. *Unhealthy societies: the afflictions of inequality.* New York, N.Y.: Routledge; 1996.

53. Kawachi I, Kennedy BP. *The health of nations: why inequality is harmful to your health*. New York, N.Y.: New Press;2002.

54. Marmot MG. Status syndrome: a challenge to medicine. *JAMA*. 2006;295(11):1304-1307.

55. Kawachi I. Social capital and community effects on population and individual health. *Ann N Y Acad Sci*. 1999;896(1):120-130.

56. Kawachi I. Editorial: isn't all epidemiology social? *A J Epidemiol*. 2013;178(6):841-842.

57. Kawachi I, Kennedy BP, Lochner K, Prothrow-Stith D. Social capital, income inequality, and mortality. *Am J Public Health*. 1997;87(9):1491-1498.

58. Kennedy BP, Kawachi I, Prothrow-Stith D, Lochner K, Gupta V. Social capital, income inequality, and firearm violent crime.[erratum appears in *Soc Sci Med* 1998 Nov;47(10):1637]. *Soc Sci Med*. 1998;47(1):7-17.

59. Kennedy BP, Kawachi I, Glass R, Prothrow-Stith D. Income distribution, socioeconomic status, and self rated health in the United States: multilevel analysis. *BMJ*. 1998;317(7163):917-921.

60. Raphael D. Social determinants of health: present status, unanswered questions, and future directions. *Int J Health Serv*. 2006;36(4):651-677.

61. Baum F, Jolley G, Hicks R, Saint K, Parker S. What makes for sustainable Healthy Cities initiatives?—a review of the evidence from Noarlunga, Australia after 18 years. *Health Promot Int*. 2006;21(4):259-265.

62. AIHA. American International Health Alliance - Healthy Communitiy Partnerships in Eurasia: Constanta, Romania / Louisville, Kentucky 1998-2002. 2002; http://www.aiha.com/_content/3_What%20We%20Do/Archives/HealthcareP artnerships/ConstantaLouisville.asp. Accessed June 14, 2014.

63. Steiner RWP. *Quality of life assessments from a Healthy Communities approach to women's health In Constanta, Romania*. London, England: WONCA;2002.

64. Cole BL, Fielding JE. Health impact assessment: a tool to help policy makers understand health beyond health care. *Annu Rev Public Health*. 2007;28:393-412.

65. Veerman JL, Barendregt JJ, Mackenbach JP. Quantitative health impact assessment: current practice and future directions. *J Epidemiol Community Health*. 2005;59(5):361-370.

66. Mindell JS, Boltong A, Forde I. A review of health impact assessment frameworks. *Public Health*. 2008;122(11):1177-1187.

67. Pullen NC, Upshaw VM, Lesneski CD, Terrell A. Lessons from the MAPP demonstration sites. *J Public Health Manag Pract*. 2005;11(5):453-459.

68. Shields KM, Pruski CE. MAPP in action in San Antonio, Texas. *J Public Health Manag Pract*. 2005;11(5):407-414.

69. Kreuter MW. PATCH: its origin, basic concepts, and links to contemporary public health policy. *J Health Educ.* 1992;23(3):135-139.

70. Derose SF, Schuster MA, Fielding JE, Asch SM. Public health quality measurement: concepts and challenges. *Annu Rev Public Health.* 2002;23(1):1-21.

71. Briss PA, Zaza S, Pappaioanou M, et al. Developing an evidence-based Guide to Community Preventive Services—methods. The Task Force on Community Preventive Services. *Am J Prev Med.* 2000;18(1):35-43.

72. Zaza S, Briss PA, Harris KW. *The guide to community preventive services: what works to promote health?* New York, N.Y.: Oxford University Press;2005.

73. Guyatt GH, Feeny DH, Patrick DL. Measuring health-related quality of life. *Ann Intern Med.* 1993;118(8):622-629.

74. Haas BK. Clarification and integration of similar quality of life concepts. *Image J Nurs Sch.* 1999;31(3):215-220.

75. Patrick DL, Erickson P. *Health status and health policy.* New York, N.Y.: Oxford University Press;1993.

76. Seligman MEP. *Authentic happiness: using the new positive psychology to realize your potential for lasting fulfillment.* New York, N.Y.: Simon and Schuster;2002.

77. Kahneman D, Riis J. Living and thinking about it: two perspectives on life. In: Baylis N, Huppert FA, Keverne B, eds. *The science of well-being.* New York, N.Y.: Oxford University Press;2005:285-304.

78. Dolan P, Layard R, Metcalfe R. Measuring subjective well-being for public policy. Longon, England: Office for National Statistics;2011.

79. Preamble to the Constitution of the World Health Organization as adopted by the International Health Conference. New York, N,Y., 19-22 June, 1946; signed on 22 July 1946 by the representatives of 61 states (Official Records of the World Health Organization, no. 2, p. 100) and entered into force on 7 April 1948.

80. Centers for Disease Control and Prevention. WHO's new proposed definition. 101st Session of the WHO Executive Board, Geneva, Switzerland; January 1998. Resolution EB101.R2. Atlanta, Ga.: Centers for Disease Control and Prevention;1998.

81. Nagase M. Does a multi-dimensional concept of health include spirituality? analysis of Japan Health Science Council's discussions on WHO's 'Definition of Health'(1998). *Int J Appl Sociol.* 2012;2(6):71-77.

82. McHorney CA. Health status assessment methods for adults: past accomplishments and future challenges. *Annu Rev Public Health.* 1999;20(1):309-335.

83. Bergner M, Bobbitt RA, Kressel S, Pollard WE, Gilson BS, Morris JR. The sickness impact profile: conceptual formulation and methodology for the development of a health status measure. *Int J Health Serv.* 1976;6(3):393-415.

84.   Kaplan RM, Anderson JP. A general health policy model: update and applications. *Health Serv Res.* Jun 1988;23(2):203-235.

85.   Nelson EC, Johnson DB, Hays RD. Dartmouth CO-OP Functional Health Assessment Charts. In: Spilker B, ed. *Quality of life and pharmacoeconomics in clinical trials.* 2nd ed. Philadelphia, Pa.: Lippincott-Raven Publishers;1995:161-168.

86.   McHorney CA, Ware Jr JE, Raczek AE. The MOS 36-Item Short-Form Health Survey (SF-36): II. Psychometric and clinical tests of validity in measuring physical and mental health constructs. *Med Care.* 1993:247-263.

87.   Ware Jr JE, Sherbourne CD. The MOS 36-item short-form health survey (SF-36): I. Conceptual framework and item selection. *Med Care.* 1992:473-483.

88.   Rabin R, Charro F. EQ-5D: a measure of health status from the EuroQol Group. *Ann Med.* 2001;33(5):337-343.

89.   McDowell I, Newell C. *Measuring health: a guide to rating scales and questionnaires.* Vol. 268. New York, N.Y.: Oxford University Press;2006.

90.   Revicki DA, Kaplan RM. Relationship between psychometric and utility-based approaches to the measurement of health-related quality of life. *Qual of Life Res.* 1993;2(6):477-487.

91.   Fryback DG, Dunham NC, Palta M, et al. US norms for six generic health-related quality-of-life indexes from the National Health Measurement study. *Med Care.* 2007;45(12):1162.

92.   Gold MR, Stevenson D, Fryback DG. HALYS and QALYS and DALYS, Oh My: similarities and differences in summary measures of population Health. *Annu Rev Public Health.* 2002;23(1):115-134.

93.   Baum F. Researching public health: behind the qualitative-quantitative methodological debate. *Soc Sci Med.* 1995;40(4):459-468.

94.   Aneshensel CS, Stone JD. Stress and depression: a test of the buffering model of social support. *Arch Gen Psychiatry.* 1982;39(12):1392-1396.

95.   Stansfeld S, Head J, Marmot M. Explaining social class differences in depression and well-being. *Soc Psychiatry Psychiatr Epidemiol.* 1998;33(1):1-9.

96.   Diener E. Guidelines for national indicators of subjective well-being and ill-being. *Appl Res Qual Life.* 2006;1(2):151-157.

97.   Parrish RG. Measuring population health outcomes. *Prev Chronic Dis.* 2010;7(4):A71.

98.   Marmot M, Wilkinson R. *Social determinants of health.* New York, N.Y.: Oxford University Press;2009.

99.   Stokols D. Establishing and maintaining healthy environments. Toward a social ecology of health promotion. *Am Psychol.* Jan 1992;47(1):6-22.

100.   Engel GL. The need for a new medical model: a challenge for biomedicine. *Science.* 1977;196(4286):129-136.

101. Dahlberg, LL, Krug EG. Violence—a global public health problem. In: Krug EG, Mercy JA, Zwi AB, Lozano R, eds., *World Report on Violence and Health.* Geneva, Switzerland: World Health Organization;2002:1–56.

102. Cummins S, Curtis S, Diez-Roux AV, Macintyre S. Understanding and representing 'place' in health research: A relational approach. *Soc Sci Med.* 2007;65(9):1825-1838.

103. Muhajarine N, Labonte R, Williams A, Randall J. Person, perception, and place: what matters to health and quality of life. *Soc Indic Res.* 2008;85(1):53-80.

104. Veenhoven R. Why social policy needs subjective indicators. *Soc Indic Res.* 2002;58(1-3):33-46.

105. Green LW, Richard L, Potvin L. Ecological foundations of health promotion. *Am J Health Promot.* 1996;10(4):270-281.

106. Kartman L. Human ecology and public health. *Am J Public Health Nations Health.* 1967;57(5):737-750.

107. Capra F. *The web of life: A new scientific understanding of living systems.* New York, N.Y.: Random House Digital, Inc.;1996.

108. Plaut VC, Markus HR, Lachman ME. Place matters: consensual features and regional variation in American well-being and self. *J Pers Soc Psychol.* 2002;83(1):160.

109. Atun R. Health systems, systems thinking and innovation. *Health Policy Plan.* 2012;27(suppl 4):iv4-iv8.

110. Allee V. Reconfiguring the value network. *J Bus Strategy.* 2000;21(4):36-39.

111. Weick KE, Sutcliffe KM. *Managing the unexpected.* San Francisco, Calif.: Jossey-Bass; 2001.

112. Guastello SJ. *Managing emergent phenomena: nonlinear dynamics in work organizations.* Hillsdale, N.J.: Lawrence Erlbaum Associates, Publishers;2002.

113. Committee for the Study of the Future of Public Health, Division of Health Care Services, Institute of Medicine. *The future of public health.* Washington, D.C.: National Academy Press;1988.

114. Bartunek JM, Foster-Fishman PG, Keys CB. Using collaborative advocacy to foster intergroup cooperation: a joint insider-outsider investigation. *Human Relations.* 1996;49(6):701-733.

115. Durkheim E. *Emile Durkheim: selected writings.* New York, N.Y.: Cambridge University Press;1972.

116. Ritzer G. Sociology: a multiple paradigm science. *Am Sociol.* 1975;10(3):156-167.

117. Kindig DA. *Purchasing population health: paying for results.* Ann Arbor: University of Michigan Press;1997.

118. Kindig D, Stoddart G. What is population health? *Am J Public Health.* 2003;93(3):380-383.

119. Hanlon P, Carlisle S, Reilly D, Lyon A, Hannah M. Enabling well-being in a time of radical change: Integrative public health for the 21st century. *Public Health.* 2010;124(6):305-312.

120. Kondo N. Socioeconomic disparities and health: impacts and pathways. *J Epidemiol.* 2012;22(1):2-6.

121. Egan M, Tannahill C, Petticrew M, Thomas S. Psychosocial risk factors in home and community settings and their associations with population health and health inequalities: a systematic meta-review. *BMC Public Health.* 2008;8:239.

122. Wilkinson RG, Pickett KE. The problems of relative deprivation: why some societies do better than others. *Soc Sci Med.* 2007;65(9):1965-1978.

123. Helliwell JF, Putnam RD. The social context of well-being. *Philos Trans R Soc Lond B Biol Sci.* 2004;359(1449):1435-1446.

124. Lochner K, Kawachi I, Kennedy BP. Social capital: a guide to its measurement. *Health & Place.* 1999;5(4):259-270.

125. Kawachi I. Social capital and community effects on population and individual health. *Ann N Y Acad Sci.* 1999;896:120-130.

126. Kawachi I, Kennedy BP, Lochner K, Prothrow-Stith D. Social capital, income inequality, and mortality. *Am J Public Health.* 1997;87(9):1491-1498.

127. Hawe P, Shiell A. Social capital and health promotion: a review. *Soc Sci Med.* 2000;51(6):871-885.

128. Macintyre S, Ellaway A, Cummins S. Place effects on health: how can we conceptualise, operationalise and measure them? *Soc Sci Med.* 2002;55(1):125-139.

129. Baum F. Health for All Now! Reviving the spirit of Alma Ata in the twenty-first century: an introduction to the Alma Ata Declaration. *Soc Med.* 2007;2(1):34-41.

130. International Conference on Primary Health Care. Declaration of Alma-Ata. *WHO Chron.* 1978;32(11):428-430.

131. Irvine L, Elliott L, Wallace H, Crombie IK. A review of major influences on current public health policy in developed countries in the second half of the 20th century. *J R Soc Promot Health.* 2006;126(2):73-78.

132. World Health Organziation. Ottawa Charter for Health Promotion. 1986; http://www.who.int/hpr/NPH/docs/ottawa_charter_hp.pdf. Accessed December 22, 2009.

133. Richard L, Gauvin L, Raine K. Ecological models revisited: their uses and evolution in health promotion over two decades. *Annu Rev Public Health.* 2011;32:307-326.

134. Porter C. Ottawa to Bangkok: changing health promotion discourse. *Health Promot Int.* 2007;22(1):72-79.

135. The Jakarta Declaration on health promotion in the 21st century. *Health Millions.* 1998;24(1):29-30, 35.

136. World Health Organization. *Global strategy for health for all by the year 2000.* Geneva, Switzerland: World Health Organization;1981.

137. Hall JJ, Taylor R. Health for all beyond 2000: the demise of the Alma-Ata Declaration and primary health care in developing countries. *Med J Aust.* 2003;178(1):17-20.

138. Maciocco G, Stefanini A. From Alma-Ata to the Global Fund: the history of international health policy. *Revista brasileira de saúde materno infantil.* 2007;7(4):479-486.

139. Akin JS, Birdsall N, De Ferranti DM. *Financing health services in developing countries: an agenda for reform.* Vol 34. Washington, D.C.: World Bank Publications;1987.

140. Travis P, Bennett S, Haines A, et al. Overcoming health-systems constraints to achieve the Millennium Development Goals. *Lancet.* 2004;364(9437):900-906.

141. The Bangkok charter for health promotion in a globalized world. *Health Promot Int.* 2006;21 Suppl 1:10-14.

142. Catford J. The Bangkok Conference: steering countries to build national capacity for health promotion. *Health Promot Int.* 2005;20(1):1-6.

143. Social Exclusion Knowledge Network. *Understanding and tackling social exclusion: final report to the WHO Commission on Social Determinants of Health from the Social Exclusion Knowledge Network.* Geneva, Switzerland: WHO Commission on the Social Determinants of Health;2008.

144. Marmot M, Commission on Social Determinants of Health. Achieving health equity: from root causes to fair outcomes. *Lancet.* 2007;370(9593):1153-1163.

145. Marmot M. Achieving health equity: from root causes to fair outcomes. *Lancet.* 2007;370(9593):1153-1163.

146. Marmot M, Friel S, Bell R, Houweling TAJ, Taylor S. Closing the gap in a generation: health equity through action on the social determinants of health. *Lancet.* 2008;372(9650):1661-1669.

147. Navarro V, Muntaner C, Borrell C, et al. Politics and health outcomes. *Lancet.* 2006;368(9540):1033-1037.

148. McKeown T. *The role of medicine: dream, mirage or nemesis?* Oxford, England: Basil Blackwell Publisher Ltd.;1979.

149. Schroeder SA. We can do better—improving the health of the American people. *N Engl J Med.* 2007;357(12):1221-1228.

150. Whitehead M, Dahlgren G. *Levelling up (part 2): a discussion paper on concepts and principles for tackling social inequities in health.* Geneva, Switzerland: World Health Organization, Regional Office for Europe;2006.

151. Baum FE, Begin M, Houweling TAJ, Taylor S. Changes not for the fainthearted: reorienting health care systems toward health equity through action on the social determinants of health. *Am J Public Health.* 2009;99(11):1967-1974.

152.   Victora CG, Vaughan JP, Barros FC, Silva AC, Tomasi E. Explaining trends in inequities: evidence from Brazilian child health studies. *Lancet.* 2000;356(9235):1093-1098.

153.   Hart JT. The inverse care law. *Lancet.* 1971;297(7696):405-412.

154.   Smedley BD, Stith AY, Nelson AR. Committee on Understanding and Eliminating Racial and Ethnic Disparities in Health Care, Board on Health Sciences Policy, Institute of Medicine. *Unequal treatment: confronting racial and ethnic disparities in health care.* 2003:160-179.

155.   Isaacs SL, Schroeder SA. Class—the ignored determinant of the nation's health. *N Engl J Med.* 2004;351(11):1137-1142.

156.   Blane D, Brunner E, Wilkinson RG. *Health and social organization: towards a health policy for the twenty-first century.* New York, N.Y.: Routledge;1996.

157.   Tarlov A. Social determinants of health: the sociobiological translation. In: Blane D, Brunner E, Wilkinson R, eds. *Health and social organization: towards a health policy for the twenty-first century.* London and New York: Routledge;1996:71-93.

158.   Marmot M, Bell R. Fair society, healthy lives. *Public Health.* 2012;126, Supplement 1(0):S4-S10.

159.   Raphael D. Barriers to addressing the societal determinants of health: public health units and poverty in Ontario, Canada. *Health Promot Int.* 2003;18(4):397-405.

160.   Eakin J, Robertson A, Poland B, Coburn D, Edwards R. Towards a critical social science perspective on health promotion research. *Health Promot Int.* 1996;11(2):157-165.

161.   Whitehead M, Dahlgren G. *Levelling up, part 1: a discussion paper on concepts and principles for tackling social inequities in health.* Copenhagen, Denmark: World Health Organization, Regional Office for Europe;2006.

162.   Benach J, Malmusi D, Yasui Y, Martínez JM. A new typology of policies to tackle health inequalities and scenarios of impact based on Rose's population approach. *J Epidemiol Community Health.* 2013;67(3):286-291.

163.   Whitehead M, Popay J. Swimming upstream? Taking action on the social determinants of health inequalities. *Soc Sci Med.* 2010;71(7):1234-1236.

164.   Navarro V. What we mean by social determinants of health. *Int J Health Serv.* 2009;39(3):423-441.

165.   Wilkinson RG. The epidemiological transition: from material scarcity to social disadvantage? *Daedalus.* 1994;123(4):61-77.

166.   Lantz PM, Pritchard A.. Socioeconomic indicators that matter for population health. *Prev Chronic Dis.* 2010;7(4):(A74).

167.   Macinko J, Silver D. Improving state health policy assessment: an agenda for measurement and analysis. *Am J Public Health.* 2012;102(9):1697-1705.

168. Adler N, Stewart J, Cohen S, et al. *Reaching for a healthier life: facts on socioeconomic status and health in the U.S.* . San Francisco, Calif.: University of San Francisco. The John D. and Catherine T MacArthur Foundation Research Network on Socioeconomic Status and Health;2007.

169. Cohen S, McKay G. Social support, stress, and the buffering hypothesis: A theoretical analysis. *Handbook of psychology and health.* 1984;4:253-267.

170. Cohen S. Social relationships and health. *Am Psychol.* 2004;59(8):676.

171. Cohen S, Sherrod DR, Clark MS. Social skills and the stress-protective role of social support. *J Pers Soc Psych.* 1986;50(5):963.

172. Cohen S, Syme SL. Issues in the study and application of social support. *Social support and health.* 1985;3:3-22.

173. Campbell A, Converse PE, Rodgers WL. *The quality of American life: perceptions, evaluations, and satisfactions.* Vol 3508. New York, N.Y.: Russell Sage Foundation;1976.

174. Andrews FM, Withey SB. *Social indicators of well-being: Americans' perceptions of life quality.* New York and London: Plenum;1976.

175. Diener E, Suh EM, Lucas RE, Smith HL. Subjective well-being: three decades of progress. *Psychol bull.* 1999;125(2):276.

176. Levin LS, Ziglio E. Health promotion as an investment strategy: considerations on theory and practice. *Health Promot Int.* 1996;11(1):33-40.

177. Kickbusch I. The contribution of the World Health Organization to a new public health and health promotion. *Am J Public Health.* 2003;93(3):383-388.

178. Leon DA. Commentary: Preston and mortality trends since the mid-1970s. *Int J Epidemiol.* 2007;36(3):500-501.

179. Preston SH. The changing relation between mortality and level of economic development. *Popul Stud.* 1975;29(2):231-248.

180. Wilkinson RG, Pickett KE. Income inequality and population health: a review and explanation of the evidence. *Soc Sci Med.* Apr 2006;62(7):1768-1784.

181. Wilkinson RG. *The impact of inequality: how to make sick societies healthier.* New York, N.Y.: W.W. Norton;2005.

182. Gold R, Connell FA, Heagerty P, Bezruchka S, Davis R, Cawthon ML. Income inequality and pregnancy spacing. *Soc Sci Med.* 2004;59(6):1117-1126.

183. Hsieh C, Pugh MD. Poverty, income inequality, and violent crime: a meta-analysis of recent aggregate data studies. *Criminal Justice Review.* 1993;18(2):182-202.

184. Pickett KE, Kelly S, Brunner E, Lobstein T, Wilkinson RG. Wider income gaps, wider waistbands? An ecological study of obesity and income inequality. *J Epidemiol Community Health.* 2005;59(8):670-674.

185. Pickett KE, Wilkinson RG. Greater equality and better health. *BMJ.* 2009;339:b4320.

186.   Berkman LF, Glass T, Brissette I, Seeman TE. From social integration to health: Durkheim in the new millennium. *Soc Sci Med.* Sep 2000;51(6):843-857.

187.   Kondo N, Sembajwe G, Kawachi I, van Dam RM, Subramanian SV, Yamagata Z. Income inequality, mortality, and self rated health: meta-analysis of multilevel studies. *BMJ.* 2009;339:b4471.

188.   Rudolph L, Caplan J, Ben-Moshe K, Dillon L. *Health in All Policies: a guide for state and local governments.* Washington, D.C. and Oakland, Calif.:: American Public Health Association and Public Health Institute;2013.

189.   Public Health Agency of Canada. Crossing sectors: experiences in intersectoral action, public policy and health. Ottawa, Ont.: Public Health Agency of Canada;2007.   http://www.phac-aspc.gc.ca/publicat/2007/cro-sec/pdf/cro-sec_e.pdf. Accessed March 14, 2014.

190.   Van den Broucke S. Implementing health in all policies post Helsinki 2013: why, what, who and how. *Health Promot Int.* 2013;28(3):281-284.

191.   Kickbusch I, Buckett K. *Implementing health in all policies: Adelaide 2010.* Adelaide: Government of South Australia;2010.

192.   Tremblay MC, Richard L. Complexity: a potential paradigm for a health promotion discipline. *Health Promot Int.* 2011.

193.   Box GEP, Draper NR. *Empirical model building and response surfaces.* New York, N.Y.: John Wiley & Sons;1987.

194.   Bronowski J. *The ascent of man.* London, England: BBC Books;1973.

195.   Wikipedia contributors. Talk: Buckminster Fuller. Wikipedia, The Free Encyclopedia. April 6, 2012, 22:50 UTC Available at: http://en.wikiquote.org/wiki/Talk:Buckminster_Fuller. Accessed March 12, 2014.

SECTION II. Critical Business Aspects of the Health and Wellness of a Nation

Executive Editor,

LaQuandra S. Nesbitt, MD, MPH

Section II Overview

Critical Business Aspects of the Health and Wellness of a Nation
(Health in All Policies)

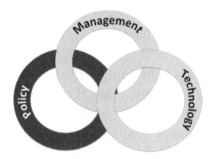

The four chapters in Section II present information on the critical business aspects of health and wellness, and the role of policy in improving population health outcomes. Oftentimes we focus on healthcare and behavior in discussions on how to improve health. For example, most would suggest increasing our physical activity/exercise and eating healthier foods as the best solution to improve obesity rates. For people to do those things, they must live in communities in which healthy food is readily available and where it is safe and easy to be active. In the case of tobacco use, smoking cessation classes are a good way to provide support to individuals who are quitting smoking; however, the most successful way to reduce the overall number of people who smoke is to increase the cost of tobacco products. While both clinical medicine and public health have embraced the impact of multidisciplinary service delivery models on health outcomes, we must now recognize the role that multisector public-private partnerships have on the population's health.

This section endeavors to present the reader with a Health in All Policies (HiAP) approach to improving population health. Each chapter provides examples of ways in which the healthcare and public health systems can work together to improve population health outcomes through service delivery and effective public policy.

Chapter 6 provides a broad overview of the concept of wellness and prevention in the context of the Patient Protection and Affordable Care Act (PPACA; also simply known as the ACA), and emphasizes the importance of such initiatives as the *Healthy People 2020* program from a population health perspective. Chapter 7 highlights the progress and challenges of chronic diseases in the United States and discusses the applications of the Chronic Care Model, and such other healthcare delivery system models as accountable care organizations, patient-centered medical homes, and clinically integrated networks. Mental health is an integral component of wellness and quality of life; Chapter 8 examines the impact of health policy, technology, and management decisions on the behavioral health system and provides examples of how behavioral health services can be more effectively delivered to improve population health outcomes. By 2030, nearly 20 percent of the U.S. population is estimated to be age 65 and over; Chapter 9 reviews the latest population health initiatives for the aging population and highlights key initiatives in chronic disease management targeting this special population.

Public health is not simply health care for poor people. It is doing the greatest good for the greatest number of people through assessment, assurance, and policy development. Although this definition is an easily accepted public health construct, many state government and local health departments are concerned about ceasing to deliver health care and accepting a new role in policy development, despite evidence suggesting that a greater impact on a population's health is achieved through effective public policy than through the provision of health services.

LaQuandra S. Nesbitt, MD, MPH
Director
Louisville Metro Department of Public Health and Wellness

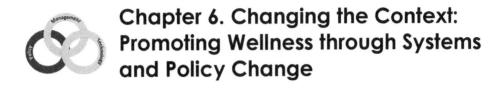

Chapter 6. Changing the Context: Promoting Wellness through Systems and Policy Change

Sarah E. Walsh, PhD, MPH

LaQuandra S. Nesbitt, MD, MPH

"No mass disorder afflicting humankind has ever been eliminated or brought under control by attempts at treating the affected individual."[1]

George W. Albee, PhD
Professor emeritus of psychology,
University of Vermont

Chapter 6 Learning Objectives

- Illustrate a model for increasing the impact of population health improvement efforts.

- Discuss the importance of shared goals for population health.

- Identify the opportunities created through recent policy changes for promoting wellness.

- Understand the importance of the *Healthy People 2020* program from a population health perspective.

- Know the infrastructure elements addressed by the 2009 HITECH Act and the 2010 Patient Protection and Affordable Care Act (ACA).

Introduction

How society manages the health of its population is evolving, and wellness strategies have become a significant factor in improving the health of communities and nations. The challenges to population health today are countered by evidence-based strategies that provide a clear focus on wellness which can improve outcomes while lowering the cost of care at both the individual and population levels. This chapter will describe one model for maximizing the impact of population health interventions—the Health Impact Pyramid—and detail several applications of that model to change the context of health and healthcare in the United States. Using the Health Impact Pyramid as our framework, we will explore recent federal policy changes that have created new opportunities to promote wellness in our communities, although additional social, economic, and technological barriers continue to impede progress. The field will continue to evolve as the next generation of workers takes up the challenge to improve population health.

Identifying the Problem

The United States spends 17.9 percent of its gross domestic product (GDP) on health care in exchange for a life expectancy of 76 years for men and 81 years for women—which most experts believe is inconsistent with this level of spending.[2]

What interventions should be introduced to achieve maximum benefit in life expectancy and quality of life?

Should the focus be technological advances in medicine designed to improve the health of the individual with a resultant improvement in the population's health status? Or should population health management and wellness be the primary objective of the healthcare system?

Should we aim to achieve equity in the social determinants of health to provide individuals the opportunity to achieve optimal health?

One could argue that all of the above are appropriate; however, with limited resources and competing political priorities, the focus should be on achieving the greatest good for the greatest number of people—the founding tenets of public health. To do so, we must understand the key factors that contribute to health outcomes—access to quality clinical care, individual health behaviors, and socioeconomic factors—and understand their relative impact.

In 2001, the Committee on Quality of Health Care in America drafted the Institute of Medicine's (IOM) landmark report, *Crossing the Quality Chasm: A New Health System for the 21st Century.* The committee established that transforming the existing healthcare system to provide care that is consistently safe, effective, patient-centered, timely, efficient, and equitable will lead to improvements in health outcomes, especially among those with one or more chronic diseases.[3] While it is reasonable to expect that improving quality in health care will improve health, achievement of this goal is based on a factor that still remains highly variable in the United States: access. Access to quality health care as defined by the IOM is "the timely use of personal health services to achieve the best health outcomes." Barriers to access include lack of insurance, limited insurance coverage or benefits, the cost of health care, limited availability of healthcare providers in a given geographic area, and a fragmented system that impedes communication between specialty and primary care providers. If the 2010 Affordable Care Act (ACA) provisions that will increase access to insurance coverage, expand primary care access points, and suspend lifetime limits on coverage are implemented successfully, these barriers will be reduced. In Massachusetts, within three years of enacting health reforms that included an individual mandate, residents were more likely to have insurance coverage and access to care than residents in neighboring states. This effect was most beneficial to disadvantaged populations, quite possibly because of the decreased need to forego care because of cost.[4]

Individual health behaviors have long been established as a significant contributor to individual health status. Obesity rates for American adults and children have grown exponentially in the past two decades.[5] At the most basic level, obesity is believed to be the result of an imbalance between caloric intake (diet) and caloric expenditure (exercise/physical activity). Physical inactivity and poor nutrition have become targets of many public health interventions designed to reduce obesity and the subsequent risk of such chronic diseases as diabetes, heart disease, arthritis, and cancer. The connection between tobacco use/smoking and many types of cancers is thoroughly documented and widely accepted by many people. Nonetheless, tobacco use rates among U.S. youth and adults remain high at 18.7 percent and 19.3 percent, respectively.[6] Unlike obesity, in which the effects on health are limited to the obese individual as a result of his or her own behaviors, tobacco smoke leads to adverse health outcomes in nonsmokers; in some instances it has been linked to increased asthma hospitalizations and ear infections in children who are exposed to secondhand smoke.[7,8] Other health behaviors like excessive alcohol intake and improper use of controlled and illegal substances have been linked to increased risks of unintentional injury, high-risk sexual behavior, and violence.[9,10] All these health behaviors can lead to increased prevalence of preventable deaths, making health behaviors an appropriate target for improving population health outcomes.

While health behaviors were historically believed to be the result of individual choice, contemporary perspectives acknowledge the role of socioeconomic factors in shaping health behaviors. Individuals without reliable transportation to a grocery store are more likely to eat the unhealthy foods available at their local corner store. Individuals with lower levels of education, low income, and inconsistent employment are more likely to smoke, abuse alcohol and other drugs, and have poor eating habits.[11] People who are in "good health" but live in enconomically deprived neighborhoods experience a higher risk of mortality than people of similar health status living in affluent neighborhoods.[12] Health-related behavior is influenced as much or more by ecological factors—the options available in one's community and the resources needed to support those behaviors —as it is by personal choice. The notion that where we live influences our health as much as how we live further supports the need for developing population health strategies that are designed to improve not only health care and health behaviors, but also the built environment.

One significant barrier to addressing social determinants of health and the development of local, state, and federal policies that aim to make it easier for individuals to engage in healthy behaviors is the ongoing debate regarding the role of government in improving health. While individual choice and freedom are fundamental American values, the authors believe that policy is a critical tool for making healthy choices available to more Americans. Promoting wellness does not require impeding individual choice, but it can and should improve Americans' knowledge and awareness of health-related issues to support making informed choices regarding their lifestyle, dietary regimens, and related social determinant factors that affect health behavior and ultimately, improve population health outcomes.

Successful Strategies

It is widely accepted that applying a purely biomedical model will have little effect on improving the health of a population. As stated previously, advances in medical care and clinical services have yielded minimal gains in life expectancy and morbidity. Moskowitz and Bodenheimer proposed a concept called "evidence-based health" that combines the practice of evidence-based medicine with community health and self-management support programs that have been proven to improve outcomes as one way to ensure that the improved health outcomes which evidenced-based guidelines are expected to yield are realized at the population level.[13] Public health officials, sociologists, and economists work to identify other factors that affect an individual's and population's holistic health; and attempts have been made to stratify these factors according to their level of impact. When resources are scarce and when demand for increased accountability and transparency regarding the use of public funds is high, the prudent practitioner of population health seeks to prioritize interventions and allocate resources to high-impact areas. As important as the interventions themselves are, the identification of appropriate population health indicators and the creation of an infrastructure to support data collection and analysis are equally important. In addition, expanding the responsibility for achieving population health improvements beyond the medical community requires the active engagement of key decision makers in sectors that influence the social determinants of health. This HiAP approach can be applied successfully only if the proper infrastructure is created and the key stakeholders understand the role they play in improving population health.

Communicating complex concepts often requires an illustrative depiction of a process, strategy, or framework. Diagrams that articulate hierarchical relationships and interactions between various domains are common in public health and can be effective tools to communuicate health improvement strategies to policy makers and other key stakeholders. To articulate the spectrum of reach and cost (low to high); their inverse relationship; and how policy change, health care, and community interventions rank along the spectrum, Grizzell developed a six-tier pyramid with the intent of influencing the distribution of funding in clinical care versus health promotion.[14] Diderichsen et al. developed an "action-oriented" framework designed to identify policy opportunities for addressing social determinants of health and achieving health equity.[15]

In an attempt to illustrate the impact of public health programs, policies, and services, Frieden developed a five-tier pyramid (Figure 6-1). This pyramid combines the interventions common in biomedical models with those often described in psychosocial models; it creates a hierarchy based on the interventions' level of impact on population health outcomes. Recognizing that the degree to which specific interventions affect population health outcomes increases as the individual effort necessary for the intervention to be successful decreases, Frieden's model illustrates the high impact of interventions that address socioeconomic factors and the relatively low population health impact of clinical interventions.[16]

Figure 6-1. The Health Impact Pyramid

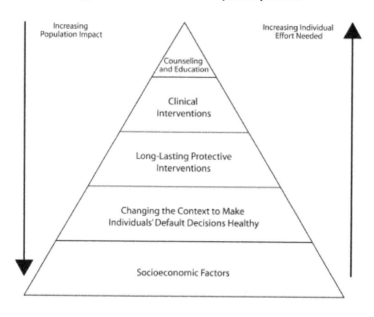

In applying the health impact pyramid as a framework, one should recognize that a diverse group of stakeholders is needed to develop and implement successful interventions across all five domains. Coalitions can be formed among a group of policymakers, as with the National Prevention Council, or between organizations that all have a shared goal of seeking to affect population-level health within a community, state, region, or nation.

Population health interventions are often perceived as targeting the population of a specific jurisdiction—city, county, state, country—however, many of the principles outlined in this chapter can be applied to subpopulations. One example is the development and implementation of comprehensive school-based health programs. School districts can change the context in which their students make health decisions by improving the nutritional value of school meals and including adequate time for physical education and activity for all grade levels. Furthermore, workplace wellness initiatives have demonstrated promise and success for improving health at the level of targeted subpopulations. While the ultimate goal should be to improve the health status of employees, intermediate targets can include decreased health care costs, decreased absenteeism, and improved productivity, resulting in improved financial performance and social responsibility for United States and multinational companies that adopt such strategies.

Convening agencies that are all part of the executive branch of government (i.e., oversight by the governor or mayor) presents few challenges relative to those faced by coalitions whose member organizations do not have a common governance structure. In addition to identifying primary goals and objective, these coalitions have to create a set of rules related to their governance structure (who leads/convenes); a process for making decisions; tracking progress by evaluating the work of the coalition; and the sharing of resources. Butterfoss and Kegler's Community Coalition Action Theory provides a framework for coalitions to move through three stages: formation, maintenance, and institutionalization.[17] This theory can assist in the elimination of commonly identified barriers to sustainability by intentionally focusing on issues related to member retention, financial resources, and establishing realistic goals and objectives. Although the direct link between multisector partnerships and population health outcomes is still not completely understood, there is evidence that these partnerships can influence behavior and systems.[18]

Common Goals

A critical success factor for multisectoral partnerships is the establishment of agreed-upon goals and objectives, and the development of metrics that evaluate the progress of the group's activities. Identifying health status indicators that correspond to the core functions of each partner organization helps to reinforce the impact of non-health-sector policies and programs on the community's health status. For example, tracking the prevalence of diabetes in a community as a key health indicator for a coalition focusing on obesity and diabetes prevention may allow the responsibility for improvement to fall squarely on the healthcare and public health systems. Given that diabetes outcomes can be a function of an individual's health literacy, measuring patterns of educational attainment in the community helps to diffuse the burden of health improvement and places some responsibility on educational entities within the community. Education is one of the social determinants of health, as discussed earlier in Chapter 5 by Steiner and Wainscott, and is one of the key socioeconomic factors that comprise the base of the Health Impact Pyramid. Similarly, viewing obesity as a function of physical activity and food intake emphasizes the role of government planning and design in creating walkable communities in which active transit is the default decision; and that of economic development to attract businesses that will make healthier food options more readily available in a given neighborhood or community.

The existence of a robust set of health indicators helps organizations track their progress in meeting population health goals for their organization and as part of a multisector partnership. Developing a set of indicators that evolves to include not just such healthcare service metrics as the percentage of population receiving age-appropriate vaccines to one that highlights the role of the social determinants of health is critical to the success of population health initiatives. In following the adage of "what's measured gets done,"[19] overtly creating time-bound metrics of performance or population status can help government and nongovernment organizations align their efforts and continually evaluate their progress. A good example of a unifying set of goals and objectives is the U.S. Department of Health and Human Services' *Healthy People* program. The current program is *Healthy People 2020*; the *Healthy People* program was launched in the 1980s as it "provides science-based 10 year national objectives for improving the health of all Americans."[20]

Originally released as the U.S. Surgeon General's report in 1979, *Healthy People* has become the decennial guide to improving population health in the United States and includes metrics related to both disease prevention and health promotion. *Healthy People 2020*, however, is the first plan to emphasize the importance of the role of socioeconomic factors in health outcomes, and to establish the social determinants of health as a topic area.[21] The topic area focuses on five key determinants: economic stability; education; social and community context; health and health care; and the neighborhood and the built environment.[22] Nonpublic health agencies that participate in multisector partnerships to improve population health will undoubtedly lead efforts to address four of the five aforementioned key determinants.

The data used to measure each objective in *Healthy People* tend to be derived from a national dataset that is not always available at the more granular levels of state, county, or city; however, states and local jurisdictions can create *Healthy People 2020* plans for their locale with benchmarks and goals specific to their population by using available data. State vital statistics and the Centers for Disease Control and Prevention's (CDC) Behavioral Risk Factors Surveillance System (BRFSS) are common sources of data; and the state and regional health information exchange (HIE) network, once established, may serve as a rich source of information for traditional health indicators. Additonal efforts should be directed toward data collection for indicators in education, economic development, neighborhood safety, and neighborhood assets. The U.S. Census and the American Community Survey may serve as good initial resources for data in these domains and can readily be linked to data from vital statistics and to a limited extent, from BRFSS.

Opportunities Created through Policy

Laws and regulations often create new opportunities to apply effective strategies for improving population health and advance our shared goals. The first decades of the twenty-first century saw game-changing federal legislative reforms that will affect many aspects of population health. When it was signed by President Barack Obama in 2010, the ACA became the most significant change to population health in a generation, with provisions that affect all facets of health care from provider education to clinical service delivery and payment to health promotion and community engagement. While the ACA created some of the largest changes, it was far from the only important policy change in recent years. During the economic downturn, Congress passed the 2009 American Recovery and Reinvestment Act (ARRA), which authorized more than $800 billion in direct spending, tax incentives, unemployment benefits, and other efforts intended to stimulate the U.S. economy. As a result of these changes, we have an improving infrastructure to support advancement of health information technologies and provider care delivery; new opportunities to advance prevention and community-based wellness; and incentives to change the way health care services are delivered. Each of these factors is discussed in more detail in the following sections.

Infrastructure

As described in the preceding section, *Healthy People 2020* creates a shared national agenda for public health improvement. But these goals are meaningless without the information needed to track our progress towards them. As Donald Berwick famously noted, "Some is not a number. Soon is not a time."[23] National data collection efforts like the American Community Survey, the Health Effectiveness Data and Information Set, the National Health Interview Survey, and the Behavioral Risk Factor Surveillance System provide the data needed to evaluate our progress. The Data.gov website was launched in 2009 as part of President Obama's Open Government Initiative.[24] This website provides increased access to a host of federal datasets to support innovation and evaluation. As has been noted throughout this text, the technological innovations that emerge from this work will be a centerpiece of the population health ecosystem.

The quality of available data has been improved by federal efforts. A provision of the ACA established national standards for data collection and reporting, coordinating the way information on race, ethnicity, sex, language, and disability status is gathered to improve comparability. This same provision established a commitment to identify a similar set of questions for tracking demographic information on sexual orientation and gender identity. These efforts will provide new insights on health status within the lesbian, gay, bisexual, and transgender (LGBT) community, a segment of the population that has been largely ignored by most studies.

For the health care sector, another significant provision of the ARRA was a section known as the Health Information Technology for Economic and Clinical Health or HITECH Act. The HITECH Act was designed to expand the use of health IT—specifically, electronic health records (EHRs), a key technological innovation in recent years.

The HITECH Act defined criteria and standards for the meaningful use of EHRs, which initiated the proliferation of health information exchanges (both private and public) in which data could be safely shared between EHR systems to improve coordination of care. The meaningful use criteria and standards are being defined by the Office of the National Coordinator for Health Information Technology (ONC-HIT) in three phases that started in 2011. As of mid-2013, Stages 1 and 2 were defined by the HIT Policy and Standards Committees but subsequently revised:

> Under the revised schedule, Stage 2 would be extended through 2016 and Stage 3 would begin in 2017 for those providers that have completed at least two years in Stage 2," explained acting national coordinator Jacob Reider, MD, and Rod Tagalicod, director of the CMS office of health standards and services.

> CMS plans to release proposed rulemaking for Stage 3 in the fall of 2014 and corresponding ONC proposed rulemaking for the 2017 edition of the ONC Standards and Certification Criteria will also be released in the fall of 2014, which will outline further details for this proposed new timeline.[25]

Eligible providers and eligible hospitals who have adopted EHRs according to the standards have been rewarded with incentive payments to encourage meaningful use. After Phase III is implemented, however, the current regulations call for providers and hospitals who do not adopt an EHR system by the specified deadline (originally set for 2016) will forfeit up to 3 percent of Medicare payments.

At the individual level, EHRs will help patients obtain better coordinated care from their various providers. Health information exchange is critical with EHRs as an underlying technology. In Chapter 12, Yasnoff will introduce and discuss the concept of health record banks (HRBs) as another option for helping achieve the goals of care coordination. Should a patient become ill on vacation, for example, HRBs will permit a new provider to immediately access a patient's medical history from the patient's primary care provider. This is good news for individual patients, but the benefits grow exponentially when applied at the population health level. HRBs will create better access to aggregate data and allow for improved population health management. Our existing Internet, telecommunications, and banking infrastructure can be used to facilitate HRB development and operation. HRBs meet the requirements for making comprehensive, aggregated electronic patient information available when and where needed, while fully protecting individual privacy and making information available for health care and population health research.

Prevention and Community-based Wellness

Beyond the data, recent legislation has increased our understanding of best practices for improving population health. In 2001, the *Guide to Community Preventive Services*—also known as the *Community Guide*—was first published. The *Community Guide* was created to highlight the effectiveness of various health promotion interventions.[26] Based on the available literature, the *Community Guide* identifies interventions that have been proven effective; those for which additional evidence is needed; and those that are known to be ineffective and should be avoided. The *Community Guide* has an easily navigated website that provides useful synopses of the scientific literature; however, in some respects it reflects the "old way." For example, the evidence-based recommendations to increase breast cancer screening include client reminders and one-on-one education[27]—approaches typical of the high-effort, low-impact tip of Frieden's Health Impact Pyramid. While the *Community Guide* also recommends more "upstream" strategies, like reducing structural barriers and costs, it does not really address root causes.

More recently, another provision of the ACA established the National Prevention Council, which does reflect the importance of social determinants of health and the role of multisector partnerships in improving population health. The National Prevention Council comprises senior leaders from various agencies within the executive branch of the federal government. Building upon the work of the *Community Guide*, the National Prevention Council released our nation's first National Prevention Strategy in 2011.[28] Reflecting the importance of the social determinants of health, the National Prevention Strategy (Figure 6-2) focuses on four strategic directions:

- Healthy and safe community environments
- Clinical and community preventive services

- Empowered people

- Elimination of health disparities

Figure 6-2. National Prevention Strategy, America's Plan for Better Health and Wellness[28]

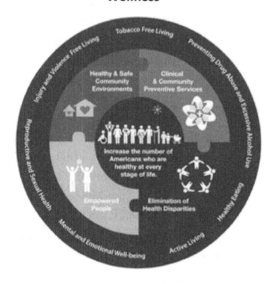

The National Prevention Strategy outlines specific recommendations for improving health within the context of each strategic direction and across sectors. These recommendations underscore the importance of partners inside and outside the healthcare sector, with explicit roles for the federal government, state and local policymakers, private industry, schools and universities, nonprofit organizations, families, and individuals. The recommendations outlined in the National Prevention Strategy are focused on the base layers of Frieden's Health Impact Pyramid: promoting protective interventions, changing the context for health behavior and recognizing the importance of socioeconomic factors. One example of a non-health-sector agency developing policy that will impact population health outcomes is the U.S. Department of Agriculture's role in developing dietary guidelines and creating requirements for food products made available to participants in free and reduced-price school meal programs as well as the Women, Infant, and Children Supplemental Nutrition Program (WIC).

The role of the Centers for Disease Control and Prevention (CDC) in improving population health continues to evolve from its original role in communicable disease prevention to include comprehensive approaches to the key threats to the health of the U.S. population. ARRA included $650 million in funding to the CDC to support community-based prevention, an effort that became known as Communities Putting Prevention to Work (CPPW). The CPPW initiative funded 50 communities to implement strategies to increase physical activity, improve nutrition, and decrease obesity and tobacco use in efforts to prevent chronic disease. While many local and national efforts have attempted to address these issues, the CPPW initiative looked beyond individuals to their environments. Funded communities worked to change the context to encourage healthy behaviors for all residents by reducing exposure to tobacco advertising, increasing access to fresh produce and healthy foods, encouraging active transportation by creating safe spaces for pedestrians and cyclists, and other evidence-based approaches.

This model of environmental change to prevent chronic disease became the foundation of another federal grants initiative. In 2010, the ACA established the Community Transformation Grants program to address the root causes of chronic disease and poor health. The Community Transformation Grants program identified three priority areas: tobacco-free living; active living and healthy eating; and quality clinical and preventive services. In the first two years of the program, more than 100 communities were funded to engage partners and create healthier environments.

In addition to the work that the CPPW initative and Community Transformation Grant recipients are doing to promote healthier lifestyles, many states and communities have adopted policies to change the context of health behavior. One example of changing the context is a smoke-free workplace policy. Smoke-free environments are the only way to fully protect nonsmokers from the serious health risks associated with secondhand smoke.[29] At the time of this printing, according to the CDC, 26 states plus the District of Columbia have adopted comprehensive smoke-free laws covering all workplaces, including bars and restaurants.[30]

Policy can also be used to change the context of behaviors related to healthy foods and nutrition. The ACA included a provision to require chain restaurants with 20 or more locations to provide nutrition information for the items on their menus. Research has shown that people will order foods with fewer calories and reduce the number of calories they consume when presented with nutrition information.[31] At the time of this text's publication, the Food and Drug Administration (FDA) was still developing the regulations for this provision of the ACA. Despite the delays with the federal policy, state and local jurisdictions have already implemented nutrition labeling regulations. Because of existing city and state laws, as well as the impending federal regulation, many establishments have incorporated caloric content into their menus, thereby providing consumers with the opportunity to make informed decisions.

Advocates and policy makers have looked beyond calorie content to improve the nutritional content of the foods available in their communities. In 2003, the FDA began requiring food manufacturers to list the *trans* fat content on package nutrition labels. Consumption of *trans* fats is associated with an increased risk of coronary heart disease and other adverse health outcomes. While some communities have encouraged restaurants to voluntarily reduce or eliminate *trans* fats in their foods, others have enacted policies to ban them entirely. Research suggests that *trans* fat bans are an effective strategy for reducing the *trans fat* content of meals purchased at fast-food establishments.[32]

Health Care Delivery: Access and Integration

Recent legislative and policy changes have improved our population health infrastructure and created opportunities for community-based interventions, but that is not all that has changed. Policy has also changed the way health care is delivered.

Establishing such community-based support systems as patient navigation programs can bridge the divide between the community and the healthcare system. Health care in the United States is a confusing and complicated system for population health students to understand. It presents even more challenges for the general public. Beginning with Harold Freeman's work in Harlem in the 1990s to the present day, a growing body of evidence has emerged in support of patient navigation.[33] Patient navigators are laypersons who are knowledgeable about the health system and who can help patients make and keep appointments, get their questions answered, and identify resources to lower the barriers to care. Patient navigator programs have been shown to improve patient outcomes and even reduce mortality. In light of this, President Bush signed the Patient Navigator and Outreach and Chronic Disease Prevention Act of 2005, which authorized a federal grants program to support patient navigator programs. The 2005 Act allocated funding through 2010, at which time the ACA reauthorized the act for five more years.

One of the most widely recognized changes to the healthcare system created by the ACA is increasing consumer access to care by requiring nearly all Americans to have health insurance or pay a fine. This provision is sometimes called the individual mandate. As the previous sections emphasized, this mandate was far from the only major change stemming from the ACA—but it was one of great significance for health care consumers in the United States. The requirement that most people have health insurance did not exist in isolation. Through a phased implementation process, the law will also increase the number of people eligible for Medicaid (in states that elected this provision); provide incentives to small businesses to provide health insurance for their employees; modify the way insurance companies can charge for their coverage to help curb costs; create insurance exchanges in which individuals and small businesses can shop for coverage, and other efforts to increase coverage.

The ACA prohibited insurance companies from denying coverage to individuals with preexisting conditions, eliminated copays for certain preventive services, and reduced instances of gender rating (in which women are charged higher rates for coverage than men). The ACA is not, however, the first time that the federal government has regulated insurance companies to improve access to care for individuals. The Paul Wellstone and Pete Domenici Mental Health Parity and Addiction Equity Act of 2008 required group health plans to treat behavioral health and medical benefits similarly in their pricing structures. Under this law, copays and treatment limitations could not be any more restrictive for behavioral health services than for other types of health care.

When the ACA was passed in 2010, it expanded the provisions of the Mental Health Parity and Addiction Equity Act. Under the ACA, benefits for mental health and substance use disorders are included as essential health benefits for all plans. It also expanded the requirements of the 2008 law beyond large group plans to small group and individual health insurance plans. It is hoped that the increased access to behavioral health services created through parity legislation will help lower the high numbers of people with mental illness who do not get treatment.

Case Study: Health Impact Pyramid Application

Throughout this chapter, we have highlighted several important policy changes from recent years. In many cases, these laws and regulations have created opportunities through incentives, grant programs, and other mechanisms to change the context of population health improvement. Communities cannot capitalize on these opportunities without buy-in from network leadership. Working across sectors, decision makers and administrators can leverage these opportunities to implement change at the local level. One example of this type of network leadership comes from Louisville, Kentucky.

In Louisville, the city has applied the lessons of Frieden's Health Impact Pyramid to identify interventions that would maximize the impact on population health. The city formed a leadership team comprising representatives from public health,

Case Study: Health Impact Pyramid Application

education, parks and recreation, zoning and licensing, economic development, public transit, public works, housing authority, public safety, community services, and human resources. This multisector leadership team has worked to lower the prevalence of tobacco use in the jurisdiction. While the county passed an ordinance in 2008 preventing the use of tobacco products in workplaces, many public venues such as parks continue to be prime locations for high rates of secondhand smoke exposure. In working through the leadership team, the departments of public health, parks and recreation, and public safety were able to develop a pilot program to reduce exposure to secondhand tobacco smoke at high-volume pools and spraygrounds throughout the community. In addition, Louisville is a recipient of a Community Transformation Grant. Funding from this grant will support the leadership team and the community coalition in implementing policies that will ensure that at least 30 percent of publicly owned and operated multi-unit housing will be smoke-free. The public housing initiative has spurred interest from the private rental housing community as well, and the city is in the process of developing goals for privately owned and operated smoke-free housing. Also, with the support of the leadership team, the county's public school system implemented a policy in July 2013 requiring all campuses to be 100 percent smoke-free.

Policy Implications

In the beginning of the twenty-first century, new policies significantly changed the healthcare system in the United States and are enabling new opportunities to improve population health. These reform laws are serving as the beginning of a new approach to promoting health and wellness in the United States.

The nation needs to look beyond the health sector and engage a broad array of partners in health improvement. The community models tested through the demonstration grants awarded by the Communities Putting Prevention to Work and Community Transformation Grants initiatives have yielded policy implications for other communities. The social determinants of health tell us that our environments, the economy, and our education system all have a profound influence over community health status, as discussed in Chapter 5 by Steiner and Wainscott. A HiAP approach means that population health professionals must engage partners across sectors to consider the health implications of their proposed policies. Transportation planners should consider the impact of new road designs on traffic congestion, but a HiAP approach means they should also look at air quality, pedestrian safety, and active transport. School administrators should design their curricula to prepare students for college or the workforce, but a HiAP approach means they should also prepare students to lead a healthy lifestyle. Local governments should recruit businesses to expand their community's economy, but a HiAP approach means they must also consider strategies to keep the workforce healthy and able to work.

Conclusion

Throughout this text, three central themes have emerged as critical contructs in population health improvement: network leadership, HiAP, and technological innovation. Promoting wellness is no exception to this trend and highlights the intersections among these themes.

Frieden's Health Impact Pyramid provides a framework for identifying effective policy solutions to promote population health. It tells us that the strategies that have the largest impact on population health are those which require the least effort on the part of the individual—strategies that address socioeconomic factors; change the context to make the healthy choice the easy or default choice; and long-lasting protective interventions. Clinical interventions, counseling, and education require significant effort from individuals in order to succeed and are therefore less effective at the population level.

Recent federal policy changes reflect this framework and have directly or indirectly addressed the base levels of the Health Impact Pyramid. In several cases, the policy changes created opportunities to promote wellness by supporting technological innovation. By incentivizing the use of EHRs and improving the quality of health data and information available to innovators, policy drives technological innovation. In other cases, the policy changes created opportunities for network leadership to come together to promote wellness at the state and local levels. By creating funding opportunities for cross-sectoral efforts to change community context, federal policy motivates collaboration among local leaders. In turn, these new innovations and engaged leaders drive novel interventions to advance wellness.

When resources are limited, population health practitioners should continue to explore the ways engaged leaders, public policy, and technology can be leveraged to maximize the effectiveness of public health interventions and promote wellness.

CHAPTER 6 DISCUSSION QUESTIONS

Discussion questions are provided for team building or class exercises. Answers for all questions are provided in Appendix C.

Question Number	Question
1	List an example of an intervention for each tier of the Health Impact Pyramid. How much individual effort is necessary for the intervention to succeed?
2	What are the five key determinants of health addressed by *Healthy People 2020*? How is this version different from previous editions of the *Healthy People* series?
3	How did the American Recovery and Reinvestment Act support technological innovation for population health improvement?
4	A provision of the ACA will require chain restaurants to post nutritional information about their menu items. In which tier of the Health Impact Pyramid does this intervention fit? Why?
5	What health information technology infrastructure elements were addressed in the chapter from the 2009 HITECH Act and the 2010 ACA?

CHAPTER 6 SUMMARY

- When resources are scarce, it is prudent to prioritize interventions and allocate resources to high-impact areas.

- The population health impact of a given intervention increases as the individual effort needed for the effort to be successful decreases.

- Shared goals and metrics are a critical factor for success in multisector partnerships.

- Recent federal policy changes have improved infrastructure, created new opportunities to advance prevention and community-based wellness, and incentivized changes in the way health care services are delivered.

- Leveraging policy changes, connecting leaders, and supporting technology and innovation are key tools for promoting wellness.

CHAPTER 6 REFERENCES

1.   Albee GW. Psychopathology, prevention and the just society. *J Prim Prev.* 1983;4(1):5-40.

2.   World Health Organization. World Health Organization Country Profiles: United States of America. http://www.who.int/countries/usa/en/. Accessed April 17, 2013.

3.   Institute of Medicine, Committee on Quality of Health Care in America. *Crossing the quality chasm: a new health system for the 21st century.* Washington, D.C.: National Academies Press;2001.

4.   Pande AH, Ross-Degnan D, Zaslavsky AM, Salomon JA. Effects of healthcare reforms on coverage, access, and disparities: quasi-experimental analysis of evidence from Massachusetts. *Am J Prev Med.* 2011;41(1):1-8.

5.   US Department of Health and Human Services, Centers for Disease Control and Prevention. Behavioral Risk Factor Surveillance System. http://apps.nccd.cdc.gov/brfss/. Accessed April 23, 2013.

6.   U.S. Surgeon General. *Preventing tobacco use among youth and young adults: A Report of the Surgeon General.* Atlanta, Ga.: U.S. Department of Health and Human Services, Centers for Disease Control and Prevention, National Center for Chronic Disease Prevention and Health Promotion, Office on Smoking and Health;2012.

7.   Hawkins SS, Berkman L. Increased tobacco exposure in older children and its effect on asthma and ear infections. *J Adolesc Health.* 2011;48(5):647-650.

8.   Gerald LB, Gerald JK, Gibson L, Patel K, Zhang S, McClure LA. Changes in environmental tobacco smoke exposure and asthma morbidity among urban school children. *Chest.* 2009;135(4):911-916.

9.   World Health Organization. *Alcohol and injury in emergency departments: summary of the report from the WHO Collaborative Study on Alcohol and Injuries.* Geneva, Switzerland: World Health Organization;2007.

10.   Heiligenberg M, Wermeling PR, van Rooijen MS, et al. Recreational drug use during sex and sexually transmitted infections among clients of a city sexually transmitted infections clinic in Amsterdam, the Netherlands. *Sex Transm Dis.* 2012;39(7):518-527.

11.   Mezuk B, Rafferty JA, Kershaw KN, et al. Reconsidering the role of social disadvantage in physical and mental health: stressful life events, health behaviors, race, and depression. *Am J Epidemiol.* 2010;172(11):1238-1249.

12.   Doubeni CA, Schootman M, Major JM, et al. Health status, neighborhood socioeconomic context, and premature mortality in the United States: The National Institutes of Health-AARP Diet and Health Study. *Am J Public Health.* Apr 2012;102(4):680-688.

13.   Moskowitz D, Bodenheimer T. Moving from evidence-based medicine to evidence-based health. *J Gen Inten Med.* Jun 2011;26(6):658-660.

14. Grizzell J. Think Health Agenda instead of Health Care Agenda: High Reach / Low Cost Health Agenda Programming. April 23, 2013; http://www.csupomona.edu/~jvgrizzell/healthagenda/intervention_pyramid.htm. Accessed December 25, 2013.

15. Commission on Social Determinants of Health. *A conceptual framework for action on the social determinants of health. DRAFT.* Geneva, Switzerland: World Health Organization;2007.

16. Frieden TR. A framework for public health action: the health impact pyramid. *Am J Public Health.* 2010;100(4):590-595.

17. Butterfoss FD, Kegler MC. Toward a comprehensive understanding of community coalitions moving from practice to theory. In: DiClemente RJ, Crosby RA, Kegler, MC, eds. *Emerging theories in health promotion practice and research: strategies for improving public health.* San Francisco, Calif.: Jossey-Bass;2002:157-193.

18. Woulfe J, Oliver TR, Zahner SJ, Siemering KQ. Multisector partnerships in population health improvement. *Prev Chronic Dis.* Nov 2010;7(6):A119.

19. Ibid.

20. US Centers for Disease Control and Prevention. *Healthy People 2020.* http://www.cdc.gov/nchs/healthy_people/hp2020.htm. Accessed August 1, 2013.

21. Koh HK, Piotrowski JJ, Kumanyika S, Fielding JE. Healthy people: a 2020 vision for the social determinants approach. *Health Educ Behav.* Dec 2011;38(6):551-557.

22. US Department of Health and Human Services. *Healthy People 2020 Objectives.* http://www.healthypeople.gov/2020/topicsobjectives2020/overview.aspx?topicid=39. Accessed April 29, 2013.

23. Berwick D. Talk presented at Institute for Healthcare Improvement annual meeting. Orlando, Florida, December 14, 2004.

24. US Government. About Data.gov. http://www.data.gov/about. Accessed April 14, 2013.

25. Sullivan T. CMS, ONC extend meaningful use. *HealthcareIT News.* December 2013. http://wwwhealthcareitnews.com/news/cms-onc-propose-mu-delay. Accessed June 9, 2014.

26. Truman BI, Smith-Akin CK, Hinman AR, et al. Developing the Guide to Community Preventive Services--overview and rationale. The Task Force on Community Preventive Services. *Am J Prev Med.* Jan 2000;18(1 Suppl):18-26.

27. Community Preventive Services Task Force. Cancer prevention and control: client-oriented interventions to increase breast, cervical, and colorectal screening. http://www.thecommunityguide.org/cancer/screening/client-oriented/index.html. Accessed April 14, 2013.

28. National Prevention Council. *National prevention strategy.* Washington, D.C.: U.S. Department of Health and Human Services, Office of the Surgeon General;2011.

29. US Department of Health and Human Services. *The health consequences of involuntary exposure to tobacco smoke: a report of the Surgeon General.* U.S. Department of Health and Human Services, Centers for Disease Control and Prevetion, Coordinating Center for Health Promotion, National Center for Chronic Disease Prevention and Health Promotion, Office on Smoking and Health;2006.

30. Tynan M, Babb S, MacNeil A, Griffin M. State smoke-free laws for worksites, restaurants, and bars--United States, 2000-2010. *MMWR Morb Mortal Wkly Rep.* 2011;60(15):472-475.

31. Roberto CA, Larsen PD, Agnew H, Baik J, Brownell KD. Evaluating the impact of menu labeling on food choices and intake. *Am J Public Health.* 2010;100(2):312-318.

32. Angell SY, Cobb LK, Curtis CJ, Konty KJ, Silver LD. Change in trans fatty acid content of fast-food purchases associated with New York City's restaurant regulation: a pre-post study. *Ann Intern Med.* 2012;157(2):81-86.

33. Freeman HP. Patient navigation: a community centered approach to reducing cancer mortality. *J Cancer Educ.* Spring 2006;21(1 Suppl):S11-14.

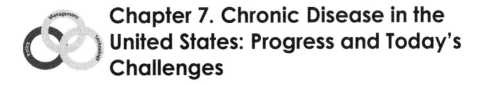

Chapter 7. Chronic Disease in the United States: Progress and Today's Challenges

Renee Vannucci Girdler, MD, FAAFP

James G. O'Brien, MD, FRCPI

"It is better to look ahead and prepare than to look back and regret."[1]

Jackie Joyner-Kersee
Retired American Olympic gold medalist

Chapter 7 Learning Objectives

- Understand the current and future impact of chronic disease on population health.

- Discuss application of the Chronic Care Model through public health and medical care efforts in the management of chronic disease.

- Describe how recent health and social policy reforms and technology are affecting the trends in chronic disease outcomes in the United States.

- Understand the current healthcare delivery system models, which include accountable care organizations, patient-centered medical homes, and clinically integrated networks, as organizational structures serving patient populations dealing with chronic disease.

- Gain new insights about twenty-first-century health information technology innovation opportunities to help mitigate chronic disease.

Introduction

During the twenty-first century, Americans can expect to live longer but with the expense of living with one or more chronic conditions. While medical technology is advancing rapidly, there have been numerous unintended consequences from its implementation in efforts to reduce medical errors and combat the prevalence of chronic disease.

In addition, the delivery and financing of care in response to the rapid increase of chronic disease is occurring at a much slower rate. New models of care that focus on disease prevention and chronic disease management have been needed, and health policy and regulatory reforms of the past decade have resulted in a paradigm shift in how care is delivered across the spectrum of care settings. This chapter will describe how expansion of the chronic care model, Accountable Care Organizations (ACOs), the Patient Centered Medical Home (PCMH), and Clinically Integrated Networks (CINs) are making positive strides to address the needs for improved care coordination and access to care for patients with chronic diseases; and how advances in such health information technologies as patient-based portals and electronic health records (EHRs) affect outcomes for patients with chronic disease.

Demographics: A Century of Change (1900–2000)

Over the last hundred years, the world's population has experienced increased longevity along with the accompanying burden of continued prevalence of chronic illness. Declines in fertility rates and increases in life expectancy contribute to the aging of the world's population, in contrast to the high fertility and mortality a century ago.[2] This change, combined with the number of aging Baby Boomers, will result in an increase in the number of persons over the age of 65 in the next 20 years.[3] By 2040, the number of people in the United States over 65 will double and those over 85 will triple.[4] This figure represents an increase in those over 65 from 35 million in 2000 to an estimated 79.7 million in 2040.[3] Due to higher mortality in the 1900s, fewer people survived to old age and the population-level needs for long-term medical care were not as great as they are today. Life expectancy at birth in the United States (U.S.) is now 76 years for men and 81 years for women, and projected to increase to 77 years for men and 82 years for women by 2020.[5] Women live longer than men and hence acquire more chronic conditions. As people age, they are more likely to develop a chronic condition requiring treatment and management. The effects of aging are felt not only by the elderly but also by their families. Approximately 50 percent of caregivers are employed full-time outside the home, and one-third have minor children at home who require nurturing and support.[3] The oldest members of the 77 million Baby Boomer generation became eligible for retirement in 2008. With the size of the American family generally getting smaller, there are fewer adult children to help care for elderly parents. Also, these children often live farther away from their parents than they did a generation ago. In addition, there are more women, the traditional caregivers, in the workforce.

The leading causes of death have transitioned in the twenty-first century from acute illness or such infectious diseases as pneumonia and tuberculosis accompanied by poor sanitation, overcrowding, and lack of medical care, to chronic conditions and degenerative diseases. By the mid-twentieth century, the focus of care became treatment of such noninfectious acute diseases as heart attacks and stroke. By the end of the twentieth century, more people survived these acute events and were living longer with such chronic diseases as diabetes and hypertension.[3]

Even human immunodeficiency virus (HIV) infection has become a chronic condition that requires comprehensive care rather than a short-term death sentence. Nearly 50 percent of deaths in the United States in 2010 were due to heart disease and cancer, which represent the two leading causes of death according to the Centers for Disease Control and Prevention (CDC).[6] These trends are coupled with the broader acceleration of change occurring throughout society as the result of technological advances affecting various aspects of life. Consequently, the U.S. healthcare system urgently needs to move away from an emphasis on acute episodic care toward planned and longitudinal models of care. In the early twenty-first century, the focus on patients with chronic illness and especially those with multiple chronic conditions has become a high priority.

Prevalence of Chronic Disease/Multimorbidity

Such chronic diseases as diabetes, hypertension, and asthma take a toll on patients, their families, and the medical care system in addition to being a primary concern of the global healthcare system in light of burgeoning costs and stress on clinical resources. On the other hand, such technological advances as the increased adoption of electronic health records (EHRs) and the growth of Big Data[7] have given physicians, provider organizations, and government agencies better tools to collect and track information on the trends and prevalence of chronic diseases. Improved data collection thus provides insights that were not readily accessible at the population level even a decade ago.

The co-occurrence of multiple chronic conditions (MCC) within one person is referred to as multimorbidity.[8] In 2005, 133 million Americans, or 45 percent of the population, were living with at least one chronic condition. By 2020, that number is expected to increase to 157 million, or 48.3 percent of the population, with 81 million having more than one chronic condition, or MCC as illustrated in Figure 7-1.[9,10]

Figure 7-1. Number of People with Chronic Conditions[9]

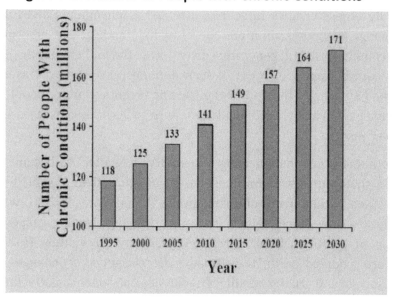

Source: ACP *Effective Clinical Practice*

The sharp increase in the prevalence of chronic conditions is attributed to the aging of the general population; the fact that people are living longer with chronic conditions; and a rise in such disease-specific risk factors as obesity and lack of physical activity along with lifestyle factors. Eighty percent of people over 65 in the United States have at least one chronic disease, and 50 percent have at least two chronic conditions.[2] As the number of people with chronic conditions increases, health care costs, including long-term and home-health care expenditures, are also expected to increase. Furthermore, the number of children who are overweight and who develop diabetes in their lifetime is increasing.

The health care needs of patients with MCC are complex, requiring numerous health care providers and caregivers to be involved in their care. This complexity often results in care that is fragmented and difficult to coordinate, and leads to more frequent hospitalizations, polypharmacy, and adverse drug events.[3] The use of such technological innovations as telehealth interventions, coupled with dedicated care management programs, has demonstrated opportunities to improve outcomes and reduce health care expenditures associated with such chronic diseases as heart disease, diabetes, and chronic obstructive pulmonary disease (COPD).[4]

Poor quality of life, disability, activity limitations, and increased psychological distress are more prevalent in those with MCC.[5,6] Chronic diseases affect the elderly segment of the patient population disproportionately and are major causes of disability and death, accounting for 60 percent of deaths and 47 percent of the global burden of disease.[7]

Costs

"More than 75 percent of health care costs are due to chronic conditions."[15] DeVol et al. reported in 2007 that the impact of seven chronic diseases on the economy is $1.3 trillion annually, with a projected increase to $4.2 trillion dollars by 2030.[16] Almost all Medicare dollars and approximately 80 percent of Medicaid dollars are spent on care for frail elders and those with multiple chronic conditions. Two-thirds of Medicare expenditures are for patients with five or more chronic conditions, who on average see fourteen different physicians a year.[12] As the number of providers a patient has to engage with increases, the patient is more likely to have difficulty understanding and remembering instructions about their care. Seventy-five percent of hospital days, office visits, home health visits, and prescription drugs are attributed to those with chronic conditions.[3] These facts foreshadow what we can expect as the population ages.

According to a recent cost of diabetes study by the American Diabetes Association (ADA), more than 2 million adults in the United States, or 9.3 percent of the adult population, received the diagnosis of diabetes in 2012.[17] Diabetes is the leading cause of such multiple chronic complications as renal failure, lower limb amputations, and blindness, as well as a major contributor to heart disease and stroke. The risk of death from diabetes is approximately twice that of people of similar age without diabetes and is the seventh leading cause of death in the United States.[18] The ADA estimates the total cost of diagnosed diabetes, including direct medical costs and reduced productivity, at $245 billion in 2012—which was a 41 percent increase in costs compared to 2007.[17] Medical expenses more than double for a person with diabetes compared to someone without the disease.[19] The prevalence of diabetes in the United States is projected to increase significantly over the next several decades, with an estimated one in three adults expected to be diagnosed with diabetes by 2050, based on current trends and projections.

Obesity and sedentary lifestyles increase the risk of developing diabetes, impede its successful treatment, and are prevalent conditions throughout the United States. As such, weight loss and improved physical fitness for adults with type 2 diabetes mellitus has been shown to result in significant improvement in health-related quality of life.[19,20] Limited health literacy[21] and lower socioeconomic status[20] are prevalent among patients with diabetes and are also associated with poorer health outcomes. Such lifestyle interventions as the National Diabetes Prevention Program have demonstrated promise with the greatest impact in older adults; the program was shown to be effective in all racial and ethnic groups.[22]

In addition, problems with medication use occur daily and add substantial costs to the healthcare system, due to poor patient compliance, inappropriate dosing, and under- and overtreatment, as well as medication-induced functional impairment. The morbidity and mortality costs associated with medication-related problems actually exceed the amount spent on the medications themselves.[23] Conversely, comprehensive medication management for patients with complex chronic conditions has been well documented to result in safe, appropriate, and effective medication use,[24] which yields significant return on investment (ROI) in efforts to reduce health care medication expenditures.

The average ROI on comprehensive medication management ranges from 3:1 to12:1 with an average of 5:1. This figure reflects a decrease in hospital admissions, physician visits, and emergency room admissions as well as reduction in unnecessary and inappropriate medications.[25,26]

Dementia imposes a substantial financial burden on society with increasing prevalence in the future, when 14.7 percent of those over 70 will be affected. The yearly monetary cost per person is $31,000–$56,000 depending on the method of calculation.[27] In contrast to other chronic diseases, Alzheimer's has virtually no effective treatments that modify the course of the disease. Currently, available therapies only slow the rate of decline in a subset of patients at best. Alzheimer's imposes the greatest burden on caregivers with the debilitating progress of the disease: increasing physical dependence, troublesome behaviors, and finally death.

The cumulative consequences of diabetes and other chronic conditions are demonstrated by their impact on population health, reduced social engagement, and costs to society as substantial individual- and population-level challenges. These trends illustrate the need for a Health in All Policies (HiAP) approach to the analysis of and actions taken on relevant social and health policies that may affect a patient's abilities to gain access to affordable high-quality medical care and social services; and to improve opportunities for managing and reducing the prevalence of these chronic conditions.

The costs of care are skyrocketing, particularly for those requiring frequent and ongoing care; and these costs have a direct impact on the budget of many families. Health insurance in America has been an increasing financial burden on families over the last two decades. The most common cause of bankruptcy is now related to health care expenses. In the United States, there are over 40 million uninsured people and a significant number of others are underinsured. With the implementation of the health insurance mandate under the 2010 Affordable Care Act (ACA), a June 2013 *Health Affairs* article discussed five scenarios related to the expansion of Medicaid coverage. Based on the analysis of states opting in or out and expanded subsidies or partial expansion of the program, there would still be a range of 24.3 million to 51.7 million persons who are uninsured by 2016.[28]

While the cost of acute health care services continues to rise and efforts are made to control those costs, virtually no investment has been made in prevention or wellness care until the last few years. There is as of 2014 increased funding through the ACA for new incentives to support workplace wellness programs, community transformation programs, and pilot programs to test the effectiveness of providing individual wellness plans to members of at-risk populations who utilize community health centers. The impact of such new initiatives as these will take time to emerge, but today the United States still has a disease care system that cannot respond to the chronic disease crisis in an affordable manner. Such safety net resources as the trust fund for Medicare, are likely to be depleted within the next decade without radical change, further exacerbating the current healthcare cost crisis.[29]

Palliative Care

Because chronic disease by its nature is incurable, the pursuit of curative approaches is futile; therefore palliation should be axiomatic in a treatment plan. Palliative care should not be thought of as less intense than curative care, or construed as abandonment or giving up.

In fact, palliative care may be more intense and comprehensive, but its purpose differs from that of curative care in that its endpoint is not cure but symptom relief, reduction of complications, improvement in quality of life, and prolongation of life. Whereas curative care may involve only one intervention, palliative care typically requires an interdisciplinary approach. In terms of chronic care management within palliative care, it is evident that there is tremendous variation in health care use and cost. Quality outcomes and costs do not seem to correlate with the quantity of care provided during this phase of life as measured and seen at the individual patient or population level. The greatest expense incurred by Medicare patients is typically realized during the last six months of life. This evidence can be found in the *Dartmouth Atlas of Health Care 2006*.[30]

Many individuals in the last six months of life have frequent expensive visits to the hospital that often provide very little benefit and perhaps increase discomfort for some. Some of these conditions—dementia, for example, now acknowledged as a terminal disease—are frequently a major challenge to hospital care. New models of care are urgently required with better patient-centeredness, along with family and community involvement and better coordination across all aspects of health care.

Current System Preparedness

Physicians contacted in a 2001 survey said that they did not believe their training adequately prepared them to treat patients with chronic conditions. They did not feel prepared to coordinate in-home and community services; educate patients with chronic conditions; manage the psychological and social aspects of chronic care; provide effective nutritional guidance; and manage chronic pain.[31]

Physicians felt less satisfied in caring for patients with chronic illness due to inadequate training, difficulty with coordination of care, and inadequate payment systems for patients with chronic illnesses. Likewise, patients were most concerned about inability to pay health care expenses; becoming a burden to family and friends; and losing their independence.[31] These issues are supported by the fact that out-of-pocket spending is much higher for patients with chronic conditions, despite their having some type of insurance. Our system has not been prepared to treat patients with MCC; moreover, the patient's role in developing a management plan has been undervalued. The healthcare system must continue to adapt to change with the provision of new models of care that integrate the medical, behavioral, and social aspects of care, and further strengthen the patient-centeredness of care.

Care Model Transformation

Chronic Care Model

The Institute of Medicine's 2001 report, *Crossing the Quality Chasm: A New Health System for the 21st Century*, identified an increased prevalence in chronic conditions as one of the major reasons for inadequate quality of care.[32] Over a decade later, and despite the need for less fragmented and better integrated, patient-centered, and continuous care, physicians and caregivers still face the challenge of dealing with the needs of patients with chronic illnesses. Financing the increased costs of chronic diseases is only one part of the equation. Changes must come in care delivery as well. One strategy for promoting change is the Chronic Care Model (CCM), developed from research in the early 1990s by Wagner and colleagues.[33] This evidence-based model focuses on the delivery of planned, proactive, population-based care rather than acute episodic care for patients with chronic diseases. The six components of this model are illustrated in Figure 7.2. They include: 1) self-management support; 2) delivery system design; 3) decision support; 4) clinical information systems; 5) community resources; and 6) organization of the health system.

Figure 7.2. Chronic Care Model[33]

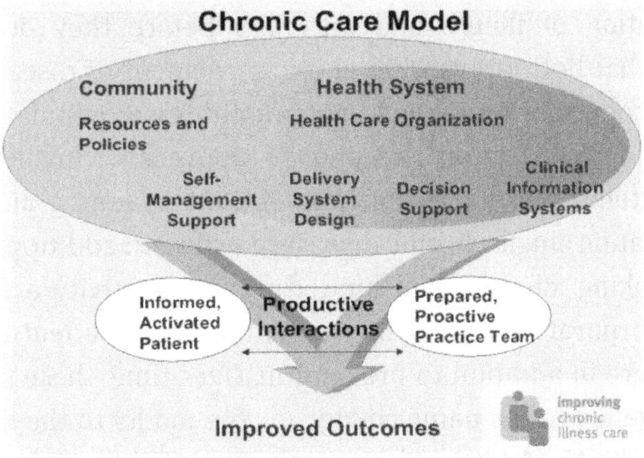

Source: ACP *Effective Clinical Practice*

To achieve the objective of improving patient outcomes, the CCM utilizes registries and electronic health records to identify gaps in care (examples of clinical information systems); multidisciplinary teams (such as the formal engagement of community health teams per Section 3502 of the ACA); effective use of community resources; evidence-based guidelines (decision support); and self-management support.[34] Each element of the CCM enables greater productivity across the healthcare delivery system and opportunities to improve care at the community's population level.

Published evidence supports the positive effect of the CCM on patient outcomes and quality of care in primary care practices, community health centers, and such integrated health care settings as Kaiser Permanente.[35-38] For example, patients in the congestive heart failure collaborative had fewer emergency department visits, spent fewer days in the hospital, and used recommended therapies more often.[39] Most of the literature reflects highly motivated, larger practice organizations that focus on patients with a single chronic condition. Likewise, many of the interventions of the CCM are poorly reimbursed or not reimbursed at all—such that many health plans and Medicaid agencies have turned to disease management programs to improve the care of patients with chronic illness. Financial incentives and payment for quality of care may be needed to extend this model of care to smaller practices.

In 2003, Barr and colleagues[40] proposed the Expanded Chronic Care Model (ECCM) to incorporate prevention and population health promotion into the existing CCM. Three additional components of the model include building healthy public policy, creating supportive environments, and strengthening community action.[40] This expanded model integrates prevention, social determinants of health, and enhanced community participation. The focus is changed from hospital-based illness and disability to a community-based focus on the prevention of illness and disability before they occur. The CCM is broadened so that both prevention and management of disease are addressed, and health outcomes for individuals, communities and populations are targeted. This comprehensive interdisciplinary approach involving community engagement attempts to focus on interventions spanning an MCC population rather than treating single chronic diseases in silos. In addition, such root causes of MCC as smoking, obesity, and limited physical activity are addressed. This model has incorporated high-quality care, including patient-centeredness and timeliness of care in addition to prevention. Over time, these proposed changes to the CCM have led to the name change for the model to the Expanded Chronic Care Model or ECCM. Additional research is needed to evaluate these changes on multimorbid patients and caregiver burden from a cost-effectiveness perspective.

One example of a CCM in an academic medicine setting comes from our work at the University of Louisville in the Department of Family and Geriatric Medicine, where we participated in a national collaborative over a multiyear period to improve outcomes for patients with chronic conditions.

Case Study: Academic CCM Project Application

The Department of Family and Geriatric Medicine (DFGM) at the University of Louisville School of Medicine, along with 22 other medical schools and teaching hospitals, participated in the Association of American Medical Colleges' (AAMC) Academic Chronic Care Collaborative from 2005 to 2007, based on the Chronic Care Model and focused on diabetes care. This project was supported by the Robert Wood Johnson Foundation, and tested system changes in academic medical centers to determine the effect on chronic conditions.

The goal of the AAMC collaborative was to improve the care of patients with chronic illness and the education of the health care teams providing the care in academic settings. The department was able to show that this multidisciplinary approach to diabetes care had the greatest effect on improving such key process measures as the rate of diabetic foot exams, retinal screening, and the setting of self-management goals. These measures were most dependent on the team's providing the service to the patient. Such clinical measures as controlling blood pressure and glycosylated hemoglobin (HbA1c) levels were not as significantly affected.[41] This finding was attributed to the fact that these measures required changes in patient behavior, and barriers to access or adherence were not understood or addressed. Therefore, a chronic care coordinator was added to the healthcare team and charged with identifying all patients with diabetes, scheduling planned visits, group visits, and any other preventive services needed. Other self-management support provided to diabetic patients included a licensed clinical social worker, registered dietitians, and a certified diabetes educator, who were available at planned visits. In addition, listings of community resources were provided to every diabetic patient. Despite significant improvement in outcomes, the majority of patients were not at goal for glycemic control (HbA1c < 7%), lipid control (LDL< 100), and blood pressure control (BP < 130/80), as outlined in *Healthy People 2020* national objectives. Between July 2010 and December 2012, patients showed the following improvements toward the aforementioned target objectives:

- 19 percent improvement in glycemic control (26%–45%),

- 28 percent improvement in lipid control (18%–46%), and

- 7 percent improvement in blood pressure control (25%–32%).

The *Healthy People 2020* goals for these parameters are 59 percent, 58 percent, and 57 percent respectively.[22] The DFGM sponsors a peer intervention called the Living Well Workshop, a community-based program utilizing peer facilitators and a structured protocol to teach self-management skills to patients with a chronic disease. This program is modeled after the Chronic Disease Self-Management Program (CDSMP) from Stanford School of Medicine, which has shown such improved outcomes as decreased emergency room and outpatient visits,

Case Study: Academic CCM Project Application

decreased health distress, fatigue, disability, fewer limitations on social role activities, and improved self-efficacy, in addition to lower costs associated with chronic diseases.[42] The CDSMP has been adopted by the Administration on Aging for use in senior centers and churches across the nation.[43] To further demonstrate improvement in diabetes biomarkers; self-management behaviors related to diet, physical activity, and medication adherence; and diabetes-related quality of life, a peer intervention that is more individualized and links the peers and patients in their communities is under development. Peer advocates will be trained in diabetes self-management, motivational interviewing, and nutrition support in diabetes, physical activity, and medication adherence.

Efforts like the Living Well Workshop and participation in the AAMC Collaborative demonstrate a commitment to supporting a population-level focus on addressing the challenges associated with chronic conditions.

Patient-Centered Medical Homes

The CCM and the IOM medical home concept have been incorporated into the Joint Principles of the Patient-Centered Medical Home (PCMH),[44] which include:

- *Personal physician*: each patient has a personal physician who provides continuous and comprehensive care;

- *Physician-directed medical practice*: the personal physician is responsible for all of the patient's health care needs or arranges for that care;

- *Coordinated/integrated care*: care is facilitated across the complex healthcare system and community by registries and information technology;

- *Quality and safety*: incorporation of care plans, evidence-based medicine, continuous quality improvement, patient-centered care, and patient participation in quality improvement activities;

- *Enhanced access*: open access, expanded hours, and new options for communication between patients and their team is offered;

- *Payment*: recognizes the value provided to patients who have a patient-centered medical home.

The PCMH concept combines primary care attributes with new models of health care delivery and payment reform. This model is viewed as a promising strategy to improve healthcare quality, improve patient satisfaction, and decrease cost.

Accountable Care Organizations and Clinically Integrated Networks

As public- and private-payer accountable care organization (ACOs) models have evolved over the past five years, three design principles for ACOs emerged from the work of Elliot Fisher, Mark McClellan, and colleagues as summarized in a 2009 *Health Affairs* article.[45] These principles are:

- *Accountability*: instituting and maintaining local organizational accountability for the continuum of patients' care and placing physicians in leadership both organizationally and clinically;

- *Performance measurement*: comprehensive measures of outcomes, quality, and cost;

- *Payment reform*: increased value represented by improved health and outcomes and reduced cost of care.

Part of the need for ACOs was from lessons learned in the managed care era; hence the focus on payment reforms, the call for greater physician leadership, and greater insight into health outcomes with clinical quality measures applied at the level of the population served by each ACO. Improving chronic disease management is central to the focus of ACOs and is tied to the strategies for lowering health care expenditures at the population level.

One of the underlying tenets for establishing ACOs is to have a clinical integration program. As described earlier in Chapter 2, clinical integration programs (or clinically integrated networks [CINs]) are also growing across the country as models separate from ACOs.

These models of care exist in regional markets and can play an integral focus on improving the management of chronic conditions. In their 2011 work entitled, *Clinical Integration. A Roadmap to Accountable Care*, Bruce Flareau, Ken Yale, and colleagues summarized requirements for CINs as follows:[46]

- Physician leadership: physicians lead the development of quality, cost, and access initiatives;

- Care coordination: primary and specialty care participation in coordinating care;

- Clinical protocols: used for a wide range of diseases and conditions;

- Clinician responsibility: ensure compliance with clinical protocols;

- Infrastructure: have appropriate systems and processes to meet the goals and objectives, as well as training;

- IT integration: use of appropriate information technology and clinical decision support;

- Performance: monitoring and improvement of physician performance; and

- Outcomes: measurable outcomes that demonstrate improved quality.

These three models (ACOs, PCMHs, and CINs) are part of the changing care delivery structure in the U.S. healthcare system. As these models continue to evolve along with the infusion of new health information technologies, opportunities to improve chronic disease care and management will improve. Research on the effectiveness of each model in meeting the care delivery needs for different segments of the population and in rural versus urban areas will be important to help assess best practices for diffusion and application throughout the industry in future years.

Promising Practices

The nature of any chronic disease, due to its seriousness and complexity, requires not only a skilled health care provider but also a system that allows for and supports self-management. Patients make the majority of their disease management decisions outside the presence of health professionals. Dwindling clinical resources for management support, provider time, and increasing numbers of people with chronic diseases mandate the innovative creation of care models providing greater flexibility, convenience, and support access for these populations.

The incorporation of health literacy into the Care Model (formerly CCM) has been proposed recently to assist a patient's self-management skills, decision making, and engagement in their own health care. Far too often patients do not understand medical instructions and lack information about their medical conditions. One national health literacy survey revealed that only 12 percent of Americans can complete tasks needed to navigate the health system.[47] Specific interventions from the 2010 Agency for Healthcare Research and Quality (AHRQ) Health Literacy Universal Precautions Toolkit have been incorporated into the Care Model.[48] Patient feedback; utilization of the teach-back method in patient interactions; shared decision making between providers and patients; user-friendly patient portals in the electronic health record; and addressing the social and cultural vulnerabilities of health are all examples of incorporating the Health Literate Care Model proposed by Koh et al. in 2013 into the existing Care Model.[49] These components are in line with *Healthy People 2020* objectives, which include improvement in shared decision making and interactions between providers and patients and increasing the use of personalized health information.[50] Advances in technology with EHRs and patient portals create new options for access and communication, and promote self-management through provision of clinical summaries and written care plans. Smartphone applications are currently being utilized as a means of delivering behavioral health interventions. For example, studies are under way to determine whether patients with type 1 diabetes mellitus who use electronic self-help tools and receive feedback show improvement in glycemic control.

There is a growing body of evidence that peer interventions improve clinical outcomes.[51-54] The World Health Organization (WHO) recognized peer support as a promising approach to diabetes management in 2007.[55] The ACA includes community health workers among the integral components of the national health workforce.[53] The success of the intervention is based on a nonhierarchical, reciprocal relationship through shared life experiences. One of the objectives of the ACA is to reduce health disparities in the United States through prevention and early detection; health care access and coordination; insurance coverage and continuity; and diversity and cultural competency among health care providers.[56]

Community health workers are one example of patient navigators, who offer a promising solution in targeting healthcare disparities through facilitation of health care access and improving quality for underserved populations. Patient navigators have a role in these areas through advocacy and care coordination such that access to preventive screening, community services, Medicaid and PCMHs are all improved. By addressing disparities associated with diversity and culture, patient navigators engage patients to improve trust and strengthen patient-provider communications. While there are different models of peer interaction, including professional-led group visits with peer exchange, face-to-face group self-management programs, peer coaches (mentors or advocates), community health workers, support groups, telephone-based peer support and Web-based peer support;[52] community health workers and peer advocates are similar in that they both have knowledge of the community and can bridge gaps between patients and their health care providers.[54] Peer advocates, however, share the firsthand experience of living with or being a caretaker for someone with a chronic disease. When properly matched, they share other experiences and life challenges with their mentees. As a result, peer advocates are uniquely qualified to provide the four key functions of peer support: assistance in daily management; social and emotional support; linkages to clinical care and community resources; and ongoing support over time.[57]

Unintended Consequences

As the industry has been and is still shifting to pay-for-performance and a value-driven care system, the benefits of performance measurement (PM) systems have been documented. For instance, PCMHs have shown improvements in processes of care and clinical outcomes for patients with diabetes mellitus (DM), asthma, congestive heart failure (CHF), COPD, and depression. Team-based care and chronic disease management are embedded in the PCMH model.

The Veterans Health Administration (VA) conducted a study in 2009 to identify unintended negative consequences of PM systems for patients. These include: (1) inappropriate clinical care; (2) distraction of providers from patient concerns; and (3) compromised patient education and autonomy.[58] PM systems may encourage polypharmacy to meet medication guidelines while less time is spent on addressing educational needs and issues that are important to the patient.

While ACOs aim to reduce costs and improve quality of care, concern exists that vulnerable populations, the clinically at-risk and the socially disadvantaged, may not have access to an ACO.[59] All groups, not just the privileged, should have access to this new health care delivery model. Providers may often try to avoid caring for high-cost or high-need patients, since they make it more difficult to achieve quality performance measures. Furthermore, socially disadvantaged populations often live in areas where participation in an ACO occurs at the community or healthcare organization level. Many of these organizations may lack the capability and infrastructure to form an ACO or lie outside a geographic area to be integrated in an ACO, all of which creates additional barriers for disadvantaged populations.

Future policy regarding the design of ACOs should focus on access to all populations, evaluation of both the patient and caregiver experience, and carefully designing financial rewards for those who care for challenging populations.

Policy Implications

Despite advances in understanding the leading causes of chronic diseases, additional information is needed to prevent and decrease the effects of chronic diseases in the future. Chronic disease programs should be evidence-based, comprehensive, and applicable to all populations in society. In addition to improving coordination of care, there must be a corresponding emphasis on preventive care.

Incentives that pay for improvement in health care should continue to focus on chronic disease management, as seen in the clinical quality measures for the Centers for Medicare and Medicaid Services (CMS) Shared Savings Program (i.e., Medicare ACOs) that require performance evaluation on measures for diabetes, depression, hypertension, coronary artery disease, and heart failure.[60] Future directions for policy innovation to support the ongoing battle against chronic disease should address health disparities related to diversity and cultural competence, care coordination and barriers to access, health literacy in the electronic health record, and patient-centered care that focuses on patient engagement.

Research involving the complexities of social policies from the HiAP perspective should also be encouraged because environmental, housing, and labor all have policy implications that, if neglected, can affect the prevalence and patient self-management of chronic disease either positively or negatively. Medical organizations in conjunction with public health agencies must work collaboratively to address population health management focused on prevention as well as care management.

Conclusion

The U.S. healthcare system is facing the greatest challenge in its history, namely coping with and responding to the burden of chronic disease and its attendant demands. This conclusion is not conjecture, as we are aware of the growth of the population already in the pipeline, which is quite lengthy—starting with childhood obesity and type 2 diabetes mellitus and progressing in the adult years to multimorbidities with disabilities and reduced quality of life.

Our system of health care has prioritized acute care over chronic care with little investment in prevention. The system has been poorly coordinated at all levels for decades, but there are signs of hope and promise for improvement, with the focus of such new care delivery models as PCMHs, ACOs, and CINs that focus on meeting this essential need for better care coordination. Chronic disease treatment is really palliative in nature rather than curative, especially in end-of-life stages of care. Interventions at this stage incur such massive expenses as cardiac stents or bypass surgery, joint replacements, or dialysis, which might have been prevented with minimal expense at an earlier stage.

There is now widespread acknowledgment that the current system is unable to respond adequately to this challenge. It has given rise to a variety of programs to manage chronic disease, as seen through the 2010 enactment of the ACA and programs that have been spawned from this legislation. Expanding care teams to include peer advisors and a patient-centric approach to disease management will help to improve outcomes for those with chronic diseases as the nation moves forward in the twenty-first century.

ACKNOWLEDGMENTS

The authors wish to thank Jeri R. Reid, MD, and Demetra Antimisiaris, PharmD, CGP, FASP, both associate professors in the Department of Family and Geriatric Medicine at the University of Louisville School of Medicine, for providing content research support to the development of this chapter.

CHAPTER 7 DISCUSSION QUESTIONS

Discussion questions are provided for team building or class exercises. Answers for all questions are provided in Appendix C.

Question Number	Question
1	List the components of the Chronic Care Model. How is the Expanded Chronic Care Model different?
2	How can such technology as electronic health records, disease registries, and Web-based portals affect chronic disease outcomes?
3	A provision of the Affordable Care Act is to reduce health disparities in the United States. How might patient navigators offer a solution in targeting healthcare disparities?
4	What percentage of healthcare costs are expended on chronic disease?
5	What percentage of the population is predicted to have type 2 diabetes mellitus by 2050?

CHAPTER 7 SUMMARY

- The cumulative consequences of chronic diseases are demonstrated by the impact on health, social aspects, and costs to society; and pose a substantial challenge to individual patients and public health.

- New models of care that focus on disease prevention, chronic disease management, and health outcomes for individuals, communities, and populations offer promising solutions for the future.

- The nature of any chronic disease requires not only a skilled healthcare provider but also a system that allows for and supports self-management.

- Advances in technology with the electronic health record, smartphone applications, and patient portals create new options for access and communication.

CHAPTER 7 REFERENCES

1. Luby L. Be Inspired by Great Women in History. *365 Barrington.* March 6, 2011. http://365barrington.com/2011/03/06/340-be-inspired-by-great-women-in-history/. Accessed June 15, 2014.

2. Kinsells K, Velkoff V. US Census Bureau, Series P95/01-1. *An aging world: 2001.* Washington, D.C.: Government Printing Office;2001.

3. Robert Wood Johnson Foundation. Partnership for Solutions. *Chronic care: making the case for on-going care.* Princeton, N.J.: Robert Wood Johnson Foundation;2010.

4. Administration on Aging. *A profile of older Americans: 2012.* Washington, D.C.: Administration on Aging; 2012.

5. US Census Bureau. *State and national population projections: 2012.* Washington, D.C.: US Census Bureau; 2012.

6. Centers for Disease Control and Prevention. QuickStats: number of deaths from 10 leading causes—National Vital Statistics System, United States, 2010. *Morb Mortal Wkly Rep.* 2010;62:155.

7. Barr P. Analyze this: health systems get help with big data. *Hosp Health Netw.* 2013;87(6):16.

8. Marengoni A et al. Aging with multimorbidity: a systematic review of the literature. *Ageing Res Rev.* 2011;10(4):430-439.

9. Wu SY, Green A. Projection of chronic illness prevalence and cost inflation. *ACP Effective Clinical Practice.* Santa Monica, Calif.: RAND Corp; 2000.

10. [No authors listed.] Tackling the burden of chronic diseases in the USA. *Lancet.* 2009;373(9659):195.

11. National Center for Chronic Disease Prevention and Health Promotion. Chronic disease notes and reports: special focus. *Healthy Aging.* 1999;12(3).

12. Vogeli C et al. Multiple chronic conditions: prevalence, health consequences, and implications for quality, care management, and costs. *J Gen Intern Med.* 2007;22((Suppl 3)):391-395.

13. Baker LC, Johnson SJ, Macaulay D, Birnbaum H. Integrated telehealth and care management program for Medicare beneficiaries with chronic disease linked to savings. *Health Aff (Millwood).* 2011;30(9):1689-1697.

14. World Health Organization. *Global strategy on diet, physical activity, and health.* Geneva, Switzerland: World Health Organization;2004.

15. U.S. Centers for Disease Control and Prevention. *The power to prevent, the call to control. At a glance* 2009; http://www.cdc.gov/chronicdisease/resources/publications/AAG/chronic.htm . Accessed July 17, 2013.

16.   Devol R, Bedroussian A. *An unhealthy America: the economic burden of chronic disease.* Santa Monica, Calif.: Milken Institute;2007.

17.   Yang W, Dall TM, Halder P, Gallo P, Hogan PF. Economic costs of diabetes in the U.S. in 2012. *Diabetes Care.* 2013;36(4):1033-46.

18.   US Centers for Disease Control and Prevention. National diabetes fact sheet: national estimates and general information on diabetes and pre-diabetes in the United States;2011. http://www.cdc.gov/diabetes/pubs/factsheet11.htm. Accessed August 1, 2013.

19.   Polonsky WH, Anderson BJ, Lohrer PA, Welch G, Jacobson AM, Aponte JE. Assessment of diabetes-related distress. *Diabetes Care.* 1995;18(6):754-760.

20.   Williamson DA, Rejeski J, Lang W, Van Dorsten B, Fabricatore AN, Toledo K. Impact of a weight management program on health-related quality of life in overweight adults with type 2 diabetes. *Arch Intern Med.* 2009;169(2):163-171.

21.   Kim S, Love F, Quistberg DA, Shea JA. Association of health literacy with self-management behavior in patients with diabetes. *Diabetes Care.* 2004;27(12):2980-2982.

22.   US Centers for Disease Control and Prevention. *Healthy People 2020.* http://www.cdc.gov/nchs/healthy_people/hp2020.htm. Accessed August 1, 2013.

23.   Johnson JA, Bootman JL. Drug-related morbidity and mortality and the economic impact of pharmaceutical care. *Am J Health Syst Pharm.* 1997;54(5):554-558.

24.   Roughead EE, Barratt JD, Ramsay E, et al. The effectiveness of collaborative medicine reviews in delaying time to next hospitalization for patients with heart failure in the practice setting: results of a cohort study. *Circ Heart Fail.* 2009;2(5):424-428.

25.   Cipolle R, Strand, L., Morley, P. *Pharmaceutical care practice: the clinician's guide.* New York, NY: McGraw-Hill;2004.

26.   Isetts BJ, Schondelmeyer SW, Artz MB, et al. Clinical and economic outcomes of medication therapy management services: the Minnesota experience. *J Am Pharm Assoc.* 2008;48(2):203-211.

27.   Hurd MD, Martorell P, Delavande A, Mullen KJ, Langa KM. Monetary costs of dementia in the United States. *N Engl J Med.* 2013;368(14):1326-1334.

28.   Price CC, Eibner C. For states that opt out of Medicaid expansion: 3.6 million fewer insured and $8.4 billion less in federal payments. *Health Aff (Millwood).* 2013;32(6):1030-1036.

29.   Medicare Trustees. Letter of Transmittal: Board of Trustees of the Federal Hospital Insurance and Federal Supplementary Medical Insurance Trust Funds. Washington, D.C.: Medicare Trustees;2006.

30.   Dartmouth Medical School, Center for Evaluation of Clinical Science. Variations among states in the management of severe chronic illness. Part One: Care during the last six months of life. In: *The care of patients with severe chronic illness: an online report on the Medicare program. The Dartmouth Atlas of Health Care 2006.* Lebanon, N.H.: Trustees of Dartmouth College;2006.

31.   Mathematica Policy Research I. *National public engagement campaign on chronic illness–physician survey.* Princeton, N.J.: Mathematica Policy Research, Inc.;2001.

32.   Institute of Medicine. Underlying reasons for inadequate quality of care. In: *Crossing the Quality Chasm: A New Health System for the 21st Century.* Washington, D.C.: National Academies Press;2001:25-33.

33.   MacColl Institute for Healthcare Innovation. Improving chronic illness care: the chronic care model. http://www.improvingchroniccare.org/index.php?p=Chronic+Care+Model&s=124. Accessed August 1, 2013.

34.   Martinez J, Ro M, Villa NW, Powell W, Knickman JR. Transforming the delivery of care in the post-health reform era: what role will community health workers play? *Am J Public Health.* 2011;101(12):e1-5.

35.   Wagner EH, Grothaus LC, Sandhu N, et al. Chronic care clinics for diabetes in primary care: a system-wide randomized trial. *Diabetes Care.* 2001;24(4):695-700.

36.   Nutting PA, Dickinson WP, Dickinson LM, et al. Use of chronic care model elements is associated with higher-quality care for diabetes. *Ann Fam Med.* 2007;5(1):14-20.

37.   Landon BE, Hicks LS, O'Malley AJ, et al. Improving the management of chronic disease at community health centers. *N Engl J Med.* 2007;356(9):921-934.

38.   Sadur CN, Moline N, Costa M, et al. Diabetes management in a health maintenance organization: efficacy of care management using cluster visits. *Diabetes Care.* 1999;22(12):2011-2017.

39.   Asch SM, Baker DW, Keesey JW, et al. Does the collaborative model improve care for chronic heart failure? *Med Care.* 2005;43(7):667-675.

40.   Barr VJ, Robinson S, Marin-Link B, et al. The expanded Chronic Care Model: an integration of concepts and strategies from population health promotion and the Chronic Care Model. *Hosp Q.* 2003;7(1):73-82.

41.   Girdler RV. Chronic disease management delivery of planned care by the family physician and a multidisciplinary team. *KAFP Journal.* 2009;64:8-11.

42.   Lorig KR, Ritter P, Stewart AL, et al. Chronic disease self-management program: 2-year health status and health care utilization outcomes. *Med Care.* 2001;39(11):1217-1223.

43.   Hudson Scholle S, Torda P, Peikes D, Han E, Genevro J. *Engaging patients and families in the medical home.* Rockville, Md.: Agency for Healthcare Research and Quality;2010.

44.   American Academy of Pediatrics, Implementation. NCfMH. Joint principles of the Patient-Centered Medical Home. 2007; http://www.medicalhomeinfo.org/downloads/pdfs/JointStatement.pdf. Accessed September 25, 2013.

45.   Fisher ES, McClellan MB, Bertko J, et al. Fostering accountable health care: moving forward in medicare. *Health Aff (Millwood).* 2009;28(2):w219-231.

46. Flareau B, Yale K, Bohn JM, C. K. History and case for action. *Clinical integration: a roadmap to accountable care*. Virginia Beach, Va: Convurgent Publishing;2011.

47. Kutner M, Greenberg E, Y. J, Paulsen C. *The health literacy of America's adults: results from the 2003 national assessment of adult literacy* Washington, D.C.: National Center for Educational Statistics;2006. NCES 2006-483.

48. DeWalt DA, Callahan L, Hawk VH, Broucksou KA, Hink A, Rudd R. Health Literacy universal precautions toolkit (Internet). Rockville, Md.: Agency for Healthcare Research and Quality;2010.

49. Koh HK, Brach C, Harris LM, Parchman ML. A proposed 'health literate care model' would constitute a systems approach to improving patients' engagement in care. *Health Aff (Millwood).* 2013;32(2):357-67.

50. US Department of Health and Human Services. *Healthy People 2020 Objectives.* http://www.healthypeople.gov/2020/topicsobjectives2020/overview.aspx?topicid=39. Accessed April 29, 2013.

51. Fisher EB, Boothroyd RI, Coufal MM, et al. Peer support for self-management of diabetes improved outcomes in international settings. *Health Aff (Millwood).* 2012;31(1):130-139.

52. Heisler M. Different models to mobilize peer support to improve diabetes self-management and clinical outcomes: evidence, logistics, evaluation considerations and needs for future research. *Fam Pract.* 2010;27(Suppl 1):i23-32.

53. Ramirez AG, Turner BJ. The role of peer patients in chronic disease management. *Ann Intern Med.* 2010;153(8):544-545.

54. Natale-Pereira A, Enard KR, Nevarez L, Jones LA. The role of patient navigators in eliminating health disparities. *Cancer.* 2011;117(15 Suppl):3543-3552.

55. World Health Organization. *Peer support programmes in diabetes: report of a WHO consultation 5–7 November 2007.* Geneva, Switzerland: World Health Organization;2008.

56. Dohan D, Schrag D. Using navigators to improve care of underserved patients: current practices and approaches. *Cancer.* 2005;104(4):848-855.

57. Peers for Progress. What is peer support? http://pcmhforprogress.org/learn-about-peer-support/what-is-peer-support. Accessed July 17, 2013.

58. Powell AA, White KM, Partin MR, et al. Unintended consequences of implementing a national performance measurement system into local practice. *J Gen Intern Med.* 2012;27(4):405-412.

59. Lewis VA, Larson BK, McClurg AB, Boswell RG, Fisher ES. The promise and peril of accountable care for vulnerable populations: a framework for overcoming obstacles. *Health Aff (Millwood).* 2012;31(8):1777-1785.

60. RTI International. *Accountable care organization 2012 program analysis. Quality performance standards. Narrative measure specifications. Final report.* Baltimore, Md.: Centers for Medicare and Medicaid Services;2011.

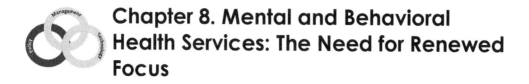

Chapter 8. Mental and Behavioral Health Services: The Need for Renewed Focus

Catherine Batscha, DNP, PMHCNS-BC, PMHNP-BC
Anthony Zipple, ScD, MBA
Scott Hedges, MD
Sandra Wilkniss, PhD

"There is no health without mental health."

United Nations Secretary-General Ban Ki Moon
Message on World Mental Health Day
October 10, 2011

Chapter 8 Learning Objectives

After reading this chapter the student will be able to:

- Discuss personal, family, and societal impacts of common behavioral health issues in the United States.

- Understand issues in the integration of evidence-based care for psychiatric and medical illnesses in the context of current legislation.

- Identify trends in technology that affect behavioral health treatment.

- Discuss issues affecting parity and policy development in the behavioral health arena.

Introduction

As Secretary General Moon's comment suggests, mental health is an integral component of wellness and quality of life. The Institute for Health Metrics and Evaluation of the University of Washington ranks depression as the third cause of disability in most regions worldwide. Anxiety disorders are in the top ten causes of disability, and schizophrenia and bipolar disorder rank in the top twenty world-wide.[1] The impact of behavioral health disorders on the ability of people to lead productive lives and realize goals makes the understanding of behavioral health issues imperative. There are numerous segments of the population in need of behavioral health support. One example is the nation's servicemen, servicewomen, and veterans who have a recognized need for mental health services to assist them and their families with the mental health and emotional effects of serving in combat situations and extended military deployments.[2,3]

Mental health is a true public health issue, and public health professionals must be increasingly aware of both the range of problems that can necessitate mental health treatment and the range of treatments to which mental health problems respond. *The New Freedom Commission Report* begins with a vision of a:

> future when everyone with a mental illness will recover, . . . when mental illnesses can be prevented or cured, . . . when mental illnesses are detected early, . . . when everyone with a mental illness at any stage of life has access to effective treatment and supports—essentials for living, working, learning, and participating fully in the community.[4]

This chapter will discuss five areas that relate to leadership and/or policy in the delivery of effective mental health services. First, we will discuss the impact of mental health on individuals, families, and the community. Second, evidence-based services that have the potential to improve treatment outcomes in people with mental illnesses are discussed. Third, we will discuss the 2010 Affordable Care Act (ACA) and its implications for behavioral health. Fourth is a review of technology and behavioral health applications. Finally, the chapter closes with a discussion of policy in the United States and its effects on behavioral health practice.

Impact of Behavioral Health

Behavioral Health Overview

The National Institute of Mental Health (NIMH) estimates that 26 percent of adults in the United States (U.S.) suffer from a diagnosable mental disorder in a given year.[5] Fourteen percent of people in the United States have a moderate or serious mental illness, and comorbidities are common among people with serious mental illness.[6] Mental illnesses account for 25 percent of all years lost to disability and premature mortality in the United States.[7] The Centers for Disease Control and Prevention (CDC) lists mental and emotional problems as the fifth self-reported cause of disability in the United States, with the cost of associated care increasing.[8] Behavioral health disorders are also common in children. Approximately 15 percent, or eight million U.S. children between four and 17 years of age, have diagnosable mental illnesses or emotional disturbances; and 5 percent of U.S. children take medications for treatment of these disorders.[9,10]

The prevalence of behavioral health disorders and their likelihood to cause disability combine to create significant costs to society. In 2009 there were over 2 million people receiving supplemental security income (SSI) benefits in the United States for a diagnosis of a mental disorder.[10] Currently, 69 percent of people receiving SSI, and over 30 percent of people receiving social security disability insurance (SSDI), have a diagnosed mental disorder.[11] In the United States, the direct costs of behavioral health disorders exceed 150 billion dollars annually. Lost wages associated with these disorders cost an additional 190 billion dollars. The indirect costs of mental illness bring the costs to a staggering half trillion dollars a year.[12] Mental illnesses were responsible for 20 percent of Medicare expenditures and 23 percent of Medicaid expenditures in the United States in 2010.[13]

These conditions and disorders are also costly to society because of increased mortality in people experiencing them. Suicide was the tenth leading cause of death in 2010, accounting for over 38,000 deaths (or 1.6 percent of total deaths) in the United States.[14] Suicide was also one of eight causes of death that increased significantly in its rate of occurrence between 2009 and 2010.[14] Suicide has received significant attention in recent years as the United States struggles with a rate of suicide among active-duty military and veterans that doubled between 2004 and 2008, and which far exceeds the suicide rate in the general population.[15] The rate of suicide in the general population has been increasing since 2008 as well, with the worldwide economic downturn suggested as a cause.[16]

Substance abuse and addiction also cause mortality as well as disability. Misuse of synthetic opiates has emerged as a leading cause of mortality, with 350,000 emergency room visits in 2009 as a result of synthetic opiate abuse and a death rate from synthetic opiates that increased fourfold between 1999 and 2009.[17] Attempts to reduce deaths from synthetic opiates by restricting access to prescriptions without increasing treatment options have had the unintended consequence of driving up the rates of death from heroin.[18]

Behavioral Health and Physical Illness

As noted earlier, serious mental illnesses cause significant behavioral health and disability burden. It is important to point out that people with mental illnesses consume a higher percentage of health care costs than the general public, and are more likely to have comorbid medical illnesses. Individuals with serious mental illness have a 25-year shorter life expectancy than the general population.[19] This figure means that the life expectancy of someone in the United States living with a serious mental illness is closer to that of a person in the Republic of Cameroon or Ghana than that of a citizen of the United States.

Individuals with serious mental illness are at high risk of cardiovascular disease, metabolic disorders, and lifestyle-related conditions resulting from tobacco use, poor nutrition, and a sedentary lifestyle.[20] Approximately two-thirds of the shortened life expectancy can be attributed to these common, often preventable, treatable conditions. Such chronic illnesses as diabetes or hyperlipidemia are less likely to be treated in people with mental illness than in the general public.[21] A 2013 study shows that a majority of primary care providers may be unaware of the consensus guidelines for metabolic monitoring of people receiving antipsychotic medications.[22] This lack of awareness is of particular concern, given the increasing use of second-generation antipsychotics for treatment of disorders other than psychosis, and in pediatric populations.

It is well established that the presence of a comorbid mental illness also increases the likelihood of adverse outcomes in physical illness. Depression is a common comorbidity that is frequently encountered in primary care settings. The presence of depression can affect outcomes in medical illness either through inflammatory effects; an association with behaviors that might lead to the development of disease; or its impact on the likelihood of adherence to treatment. Comorbid depression affects outcomes in diabetes, congestive heart failure, arthritis, asthma, and COPD; and is associated with higher utilization of health care services and higher health care costs.[23]

Human Costs

The human costs borne by individuals affected by serious mental illness are even more concerning than the significant financial costs. People with mental illness are almost three times more likely to be impoverished than people without mental illness and the distance from poverty level is greater.[11] Twenty-six percent of individuals who are homeless have serious mental illnesses,[24] and 46 percent have comorbid mental illness and substance abuse.[25] The number of people with mental illnesses who are incarcerated have led some advocates to suggest that jails and prisons are increasingly replacing conventional behavioral health treatment facilities.[26] Fifty-six percent of people in state prisons, 45 percent of federal prisoners, and 64 percent of people in local jails have mental illnesses, with costs of incarceration reaching 15 billion dollars annually. Seventy percent of incarcerated people with mental illness have been imprisoned for nonviolent offenses. The majority of prisoners with mental illnesses and substance abuse do not receive treatment.[25]

It is clear that there are significant stressors for the families of people with mental illnesses. The social costs of caring for a family member with a serious mental illness are extensive and well documented. Shortages of appropriate services often force families to shoulder a disproportionate amount of the burden of providing ongoing support for loved ones struggling with a mental illness.[27] The shift away from hospital-based care is associated with financial strain from lost income; reduced quality of life; stress-related illnesses, depression; and even excess mortality in family members.[28] Unrelieved symptoms of a mental illness increase the number of days missed from work by caregivers.[29] If a mental illness is chronic, the family's perception of its burden increases.[30] Family members have identified several important issues for family caregivers: services that extend beyond control of symptoms; an increased focus on collaboration between service users, family, and clinicians; and development of policies with input from all stakeholders.[31]

It is ironic that the impact of serious mental illness in the United States continues to be so great, given the strides in identifying effective behavioral health interventions during the last generation. A growing array of evidence-based practices demonstrated to reduce the effects of mental illness and help people live full and complete lives in spite of their diagnosis is now available to providers. A sample of these interventions is included as follows:

- *Assertive community treatment (ACT):* ACT teams are interprofessional teams, including psychiatrists and nurses on each team, which provide community-based intensive psychiatric and rehabilitative services to people with serious mental illness. Teams are available to provide services on a 24-hour basis and focus on avoidance of hospitalization and attainment of rehabilitation goals.[32] ACT dramatically decreases hospitalization rates and crises among people with severe mental illness, particularly those who have frequent hospitalizations.[33-35]

- *Supported employment:* Supported employment has evolved from programs in which people worked in a setting with others with disabilities (sheltered workshop) to a service in which people are helped to find competitive employment in an area of their choosing and provided with the individualized support necessary to maintain employment. This model of services is called Individual Placement and Support (IPS). IPS services have demonstrated that up to 65 percent of individuals with serious mental illness who would like to be employed can work at least part time.[36,37]

- *Cognitive behavioral therapy (CBT):* Cognitive behavioral therapy was developed by Aaron Beck in the 1950s; it focuses on the interactions among thoughts, emotions, and behaviors, and interventions that are effective in relieving distress in one of these areas. CBT has been shown to be extraordinarily effective in the treatment of affective disorders, anxiety, and most recently, in the treatment of psychosis.[38-40]

- *Integrated dual disorders treatment (IDDT):* IDDT is an intervention model based on the premise that treating either substance abuse or mental illness in someone who has co-occurring diagnoses is less effective than treating both simultaneously. Assertive outreach is used to engage people in treatment in this model, in which services for addiction and mental illness are provided by the same clinical team. IDDT is effective in treating both mental illness and substance abuse in the 20 percent to 40 percent of individuals with serious mental illness who have significant co-occurring disorders.[41]

- *Pharmacological interventions:* Medications remain an evidence-based treatment for people with serious mental illness. Antipsychotic medications have become increasingly well tolerated as side effect profiles have changed with the advent of the so-called atypical antipsychotics. On the other hand, concerns about metabolic syndrome have emerged as a disadvantage of this class of medications, which makes it prudent to employ such adjunctive interventions as CBT for psychosis that may reduce the need for medication. Interventions that encourage active involvement in decisions about medication and understanding on the part of clinicians about factors that promote or hinder adherence are essential to the effective use of medications.[42]

- *Recovery-focused services:* Recovery and empowerment are increasingly viewed as essential parts of an individual's journey toward wellness and attainment of life goals even in the face of continuing symptoms. Recovery-focused services, including direct peer support services, illustrate a dramatic and productive shift in the dominant treatment paradigm for significant mental illness.[43] Recovery has become the guiding structure for standards of care.

- *Intensive child and adolescent services:* Services that are community-based can reduce hospitalization, dropouts from and costs of services, and can increase patients' levels of functioning.[44]

In short, severe mental illness and related behavioral health disorders create significant individual, familial, and community burdens. The financial, quality-of-life, and public safety implications would logically make mental illness a public health priority. Despite increased ability to reduce the burden of serious mental illness through successful treatment, however, there may actually be *decreasing* levels of societal commitment to effective intervention. For example, state spending on behavioral health services in the United States has been reduced by more than $1.6 billion between FY2009 and FY2012.[45] Fewer than 25 percent of people with serious mental illness receive any vocational services, with a fraction having access to supported employment services, which have been shown to significantly reduce the use of medical and behavioral health services while improving employment outcomes.[46] The most recent state-by-state report card from the National Alliance on Mental Illness (NAMI) gives the United States an average grade of "D" in terms of quality and availability of services.[47] Given the rates of severe mental illness, treatment reimbursement rates for services and treatments in the United States are quite low, with psychiatrists having the lowest median income among physicians.[48] In part this low rate of reimbursement is because insurance plans have tended to treat mental illnesses as different from physical illnesses. Billing codes for behavioral health care have traditionally been reimbursed at a lower rate than codes used in primary care.[49] In addition, 98 percent of consumers with employer insurance plans had behavioral health benefit limits.[50] The Paul Wellstone and Pete Domenici Mental Health Parity and Addiction Equity Act enacted in 2008 prohibits arbitrary limits on behavioral health; however, the definition of "arbitrary" remains somewhat controversial. Behavioral health providers, like most health providers in the United States, have been relatively slow to leverage the opportunities available through improved electronic technology.[51] To achieve truly integrated care and provide evidence-based treatment will require some adjustments to the way services are conceptualized and funded.

Violence and Mental Illness

A widespread societal perception is that people with mental illnesses are highly likely to be violent; this perception may be fueled by media reports.[52] In the aftermath of the 2009 Fort Hood mass murder of 13 military personnel; the 2011 shooting rampage in Tucson, Arizona; the 2012 elementary school shooting in Newtown, Connecticut, by a person with a mental illness; and the 2013 killing of 12 people at the Washington Navy Yard (headquarters of U.S. Naval Operations) in Washington, D.C., by a man who had called police to report distress from hearing voices, there is a renewed focus on the connection between violence and mental illness and ways to reduce the risk of violence in society.

This focus on mental illness as a cause of violent behavior is stigmatizing and overlooks two important issues. First, mass shootings are a rare though tragic occurrence. In 2012 mass shootings accounted for 0.003 percent of all shooting deaths.[53] To focus on mental illness as a risk factor for large-scale shootings detracts from the magnitude of the problem of gun violence in our society and lends itself to such simplistic solutions as the proposed reporting to authorities of all persons admitted for psychiatric hospitalization in Connecticut. Second, the likelihood of suicide in someone with a mental illness far outweighs the likelihood of homicide.[53] Identification of and engagement in effective treatment for patients with acute cases of mental illness and who have been determined to be a danger to themselves or others is a highly useful first step in preventing future gun violence.

Americans dramatically overestimate the risk of violence associated with mental illness. In Pescosolido et al.'s survey of 1,444 Americans, using standardized vignettes to assess views of mental illness and treatment approaches, the survey respondents estimated the risks of violence associated with mental illness to be much higher than the actual risk.[54]

Assessing the absolute nature of any link between mental illness and violence is difficult because of the variety of conditions that can be considered a mental illness and the many intervening variables that affect the expression of violence. Evidence from literature; however, provides some supportive findings:

- Individuals with serious mental illness are far more likely to be victims of violence or crime than they are to be perpetrators.[55]

- People with severe mental illnesses such as schizophrenia, bipolar disorder, or psychosis, are 2½ times more likely to be attacked, raped, or mugged than the general population.[56]

- Only a small portion of crime is attributable to people with mental illnesses.[57]

- We do know that people with untreated mental illness or mental illness with untreated substance abuse disorders are more likely to commit crimes or engage in violence than the general population or a person with mental illness who is receiving treatment.[58]

- People with mental illness who have no symptoms of substance abuse do not present higher risks than their neighbors. As Steadman et al. report, "There was no significant difference between the prevalence of violence by patients without symptoms of substance abuse and the prevalence of violence by others living in the same neighborhoods who were also without symptoms of substance abuse."[59]

- *The MacArthur Violence Risk Assessment Study*[60] echoes Steadman et al.'s findings and stands out as the most sophisticated attempt to date to disentangle these complex interrelationships. In this study of 1,136 subjects, the prevalence of violence among those with a major mental disorder who did not abuse substances was indistinguishable from that of their neighborhood controls. However, the presence of both a mental illness and an untreated substance abuse problem doubled the risk.

- Current estimates are that about 10 percent of all homicides are committed by people with severe mental illness, *almost all of whom are undiagnosed or untreated.*[61-63] Ten percent is higher than the expected rate of 6 percent, based on the number of Americans with serious mental illnesses, but still constitutes a small percentage of total homicides in the United States. Virtually all these homicides are attributable to individuals outside service provider systems of care.

- In a recent study of homicide defendants, 47 percent met diagnostic criteria for substance abuse; however, only eight percent of defendants with a diagnosis had received treatment within the preceding three months— offering limited opportunities for prevention.[64]

The conflicting evidence and the fact that intervening variables like co-occurring substance abuse or absence of treatment dramatically affect the actual incidence of violence make it difficult to assess the absolute relationship between mental illness and violence. A diagnosis of a mood disorder or psychosis should be considered a *risk factor* for violence rather than a *direct cause.* In other words, the presence of a mental illness is, under certain circumstances, a predictor of violence in the same way that gender (men are more likely to commit these acts) and a variety of socioeconomic variables (race, education, income level) are also risk factors for violence. A mental illness does not in itself *cause* an increase in violence, but when combined with other factors the presence of a mental illness may increase risk. Some of the most examined interrelated factors are failure to diagnose and treat the illness, and untreated substance abuse. The irony is that during this time of increased public concern over the risk of violence in people with mental illness, funding for mental health services has been slashed by the states.[45]

Organizing Behavioral Health Services: Implications of the ACA

The ACA was originally scheduled to provide access to coverage for an estimated 32 million Americans who are uninsured in 2014.[65] The ACA essential benefits packages will increase services available to individuals, including provisions requiring a benefit for treatment of mental health and substance use disorder services, prescription drugs, rehabilitation, and prevention and wellness services. An estimated 10 percent to 20 percent increase in counselors for mental health and addictions services will be needed to provide services.[66]

Primary care providers will receive additional incentives and grants to coordinate care with behavioral health and addiction services, including the co-location of behavioral health providers. Mental health screenings will be linked with required annual physical and wellness examinations. The ACA will increase Medicare payments for preventive health care and health promotion. With a high comorbidity rate, people with serious mental illnesses are at greater risk of many preventable diseases. The outcome of increased access to preventive health and coordinated care will contribute to the prevention of or reduction in obesity, tobacco use, diabetes, and heart disease; and ultimately improve the health of people with severe mental illnesses.

In addition, the ACA will fund new federal initiatives to develop innovative interventions through service research. This landmark health reform expands coverage for psychiatric hospitals to allow Medicaid coverage of private inpatient psychiatric facilities. New school-based health center grants that offer mental health and addiction services will be available. Community-based service options for individuals with a mental health and/or substance use condition will also be expanded.

The ACA will move reimbursement for providers to a cost-based reimbursement system based on prospective payments. Prospective payments are based on a provider fee for each encounter regardless of the amount of time required. Just as the new 2013 Current Procedural Terminology (CPT) code sets offer opportunities for psychiatrists and other psychiatric prescribers to change revenue streams by allowing them to use Evaluation and Management (E/M) codes, the prospective payment system offers opportunities for potential revenue increases as well. Community mental health centers will have many new opportunities to provide and expand treatment options, particularly in the areas of chemical dependency treatment and the expansion of men's services.

The federal rules for accountable care organizations (ACOs) will have a profound impact on the behavioral health industry. An ACO is a legal entity made up of an integrated group of providers and hospitals that are collectively accountable for the costs of health care for a specific population of patients. This accountability includes the achievement of predetermined quality standards as well. Similar to the HMOs of the 1990s, ACOs are positioned to have a prominent effect on healthcare systems, requiring behavioral health providers to position themselves strategically to take advantage of the expanded ACOs' impact. In this context, ACOs provide a pathway for patient access to behavioral health providers. Successful behavioral health providers, hospitals, and primary care providers will be fully merged in this new era of health care networks.

Many ACOs across the country include patient-centered medical homes (PCMHs) supported by specialists, including those in behavioral health. The ACO strategy revolves around the premise that providers and hospitals that are integrated and working together will have a greater impact on improving the health and well-being of their patients with less duplication of services. When ACOs achieve identified quality and clinical outcomes, their participants share the savings. One of the objectives is to create an environment in which an ACO has an incentive to provide high-quality care; produce positive clinical outcomes; and promote prevention by inspiring healthy patient behavior.

ACOs can receive global payments for services based on a blended payment model that includes: (1) fee-for-service [50 percent]; (2) a care management fee [20 percent]; and (3) performance incentives based on clinical measures [30 percent].[67] Shared savings based on increasing quality and reducing costs are split contractually among the provider, the payer, and the employer/government.

The Centers for Medicare and Medicaid Services (CMS) does not prohibit behavioral health and substance use care organizations from being included as part of an ACO. CMS does, however, prohibit behavioral health organizations from forming their own ACOs or from creating health homes (defined below) led by behavioral healthcare entities. The objective is to encourage behavioral health providers to partner and integrate with community partners to reduce the historic separation of these providers.

Patients with depression and associated mood disorders have the highest medical costs, even when compared with such other risk factors as obesity, high blood sugar, and high blood pressure.[68] A recent study examining health insurance claims determined that members with depression had 48 percent higher health care expenditures.[69] Additional studies indicate that depression costs billions in lost productivity in the workplace and significant related disability costs.[70] Furthermore, researchers agree that the costs associated with mood disorders and mental health issues are greatly underreported and underestimated. The presence of depression also increases costs and produces poorer outcomes in people with chronic medical illness. Approximately 74 percent of all health care costs result from four health conditions: cardiovascular disease, cancer, diabetes, and obesity; 80 percent of cardiovascular disease and diabetes cases are preventable, and 90 percent of obesity cases can be prevented.[71] The collaboration between medical providers and behavioral health providers to help patients stay engaged with their wellness plans has profound implications for medical cost savings. Such emerging techniques as motivational interviewing are easily adapted in either behavioral or primary care settings for promoting positive health behavior changes.

The industry transformation occurring with the increased adoption of primary care-focused medical home models has been documented extensively in the healthcare industry literature. Proposed in 2007 by the American Academy of Family Physicians (AAFP), the American Academy of Pediatrics (AAP), the American College of Physicians (ACP), and the American Osteopathic Association (AOA), the PCMH model aims to provide comprehensive, coordinated, and continuous care for all populations from children to seniors. It requires a team-based physician-led approach that seeks to enhance the role of primary care and organize care around the patient.

Contrasting with the PCMH model is the health home model. There are important differences between the two and opportunities for collaboration in both models (Table 8-1). Health homes are a population-based integrated care model targeting consumers with chronic conditions, which coordinate medical and behavioral health care services with community and social supports. While health homes and medical homes were born of the same concept, health care reform legislation established health homes as a new state Medicaid option for service delivery specifically for enrollees with chronic conditions. To encourage states to take up the new option, the ACA authorized a temporary 90 percent federal match rate (FMAP or Federal Medical Assistance Percentage) for health home services specified in the law.

Table 8-1. Differences between Health Homes and Patient-Centered Medical Homes[72]

Category	Health Homes	Patient-Centered Medical Homes
Populations served	Individuals with approved chronic conditions	All populations served
Staffing	May include primary care practices, community mental health centers, federally qualified health centers, health home agencies, ACT teams, and others	Are typically defined as physician-led primary care practices, but may also employ mid-level practitioners
Payers	Currently a Medicaid-only construct	In existence for multiple payers: Medicaid, commercial insurance, and others
Care focus	Strong focus on behavioral health (including substance abuse treatment), social support, and other services (including nutrition, home health, coordinating activities, and others)	Focused on the delivery of traditional medical care: referral and lab tracking, guideline adherence, electronic prescribing, provider-patient communication, and others
Technology	Use of IT for coordination across continuum of care, including such in-home solutions as remote monitoring in patient homes	Use of IT for traditional care delivery

Health homes are designed to be person-centered systems of care that facilitate access to and coordination of the full array of primary and acute health care services; behavioral health care; and long-term community-based services and supports with the option of being led by professionals other than physicians. On November 16, 2010, CMS issued guidance to the states, outlining the requirements, choices, funding opportunities, and expectations for states interested in adopting the health home option through a state plan amendment (SPA). CMS encourages states with existing or planned PCMH initiatives to compare those programs to the definition of health homes under the ACA, and to design their health homes to complement those initiatives.

The ACA guidelines for eligible participation in health homes include:[73]

- Persons with two chronic conditions;
- Those with one chronic condition and risk of a second;
- Those with one "serious and persistent" mental health condition.

Both children and adults who meet these criteria are eligible for health home services; individuals who are dually eligible for Medicaid and Medicare cannot be excluded. States can target health home services to those with particular chronic conditions or to those with higher numbers or severity of chronic or mental health conditions. In addition, because the Medicaid "comparability" requirement is waived, states can offer health home services in a different amount, duration, and scope than services provided to individuals not in the health home population.

In many states the health home model builds on the medical home model, expanding the linkages and breadth of services to support the needs of those with chronic illnesses. The goal of the Medicaid home health model is to improve clinical outcomes and overall healthcare quality for persons with long-term conditions, as well as reduce per-capita healthcare expenditures by delivering more effective coordinated care. Unlike the PCMH model, states have flexibility to determine eligible health home providers. The provider may be a designated professional entity such as a health clinic or home health agency, or a team of health professionals that may include mental health workers, dietitians, nurses, and pharmacists.

Health home services that are eligible for the 90 percent FMAP include: comprehensive care management; care coordination and health promotion, comprehensive transitional care from inpatient to other settings, including appropriate follow-up; individual and family support; referral to community and social support services if relevant; and the use of health information technology (health IT) to link services.

CMS guidance establishes standards for health homes to ensure they have the capacity for a "whole-person" approach to care that identifies needed clinical and nonclinical services and supports, and provides or makes linkages to all such care. Health homes will provide quality-driven, cost-effective, and culturally appropriate person- and family-centered health home services. As part of this whole-person approach, the states will be required by CMS to coordinate with the Substance Abuse and Mental Health Services Administration (SAMHSA) in designing their approaches to health homes.

In addition to the development of a care plan for each individual that integrates and coordinates all needed clinical and nonclinical services and supports, health homes must use health IT to link services; facilitate communication between and among providers, the individual, and caregivers; and provide feedback to practices. Health homes must establish a continuous quality improvement program, and collect and report data that support evaluation.

Being able to integrate behavioral health services into primary care services has the potential to reduce the fragmentation of health care services in the United States. The integration of treatment of some disorders, such as depression, into primary care has already begun and been shown to be an efficient and cost-effective way of delivering behavioral health services.[74] The integration of treatment for such serious mental illnesses as schizophrenia into primary care seems less certain to be successful. The literature demonstrates that people with serious mental illness are less likely than the general public to be treated with the standard of care for diagnosed comorbidities.[75,76] In this case, even access has not always translated into treatment. It may be that using behavioral health services as an entry into primary care may be effective as a way to increase access for people who have serious mental illnesses.[77] The experience of providers who have implemented a model integrating primary care services with behavioral health centers indicates recurrent difficulties with recruitment and retention of providers; obtaining space necessary for integrated services; state-specific difficulties in licensing and billing; finding EHRs that are adequate to meet both primary and behavioral health requirements; and difficulties in keeping consumers engaged in treatment.[78]

The following case study of a joint collaborative venture between the University of Louisville Pediatrics Program and Seven Counties Services Child and Families division provides an example of integrating behavioral health services with primary care services in an academic medical center setting.

Case Study: Integrated Primary and Behavioral Health Care for Children

The University of Louisville Pediatrics Program (U of L) and Seven Counties Services Child and Families Division (SCS) began an innovative community partnership to provide integrated child health services in one location. Pediatricians routinely treat children for physical illnesses who also have significant mental health issues. Early psychosocial stressors are shown to have lifelong adverse effects, so prevention and early intervention are crucial to successful health care outcomes with children. Conversely, children treated for behavioral illnesses in a solely psychiatric setting often experience undiagnosed and untreated physical illnesses.

The concept of the integrated clinic was to use collocated providers to bring complementary expertise to the child and family. Specifically, community mental health providers are expert in case management, behavioral health treatment, and navigation of the social service environment. These services are viewed by pediatric practices as time-consuming, costly, and difficult work that interferes with pediatric primary care services. Collocation also allowed families who might present to a pediatrician with a behavioral health issue to be linked to behavioral health providers more simply and to bypass any stigma that might be perceived in going to a psychiatric provider. Likewise, as children in behavioral health are prescribed medications that may impact weight and metabolism, follow-up is simplified in a collocated pediatric practice.

This program evolved over a three-year period, as staff from both groups addressed the issues of different funding streams, legal limitations to integrating primary care, and knowledge gaps between professions. The model that emerged was one in which a social worker from SCS provides screening, assessment, and ongoing treatment of behavioral health issues, as well as providing social work consultation and case management services at the pediatric site. With this new partnership, children and their families receive both physical and behavioral health care services at their primary care location.

As of 2013, this partnership has served over 700 children with co-occurring diagnoses, with an average patient satisfaction rating of 4.75 on a 5-point scale. Physician satisfaction with the service has averaged 4.9 on a 5-point scale. Over 95 percent of children seen have been able to be maintained in a community setting, with concomitant cost savings. Partnerships with the University of Louisville's Kent School of Social Work and Department of Pediatrics have provided students with the opportunity to learn clinical practice in an integrated-care setting.

In our changing health care environment, this program sees integrated primary and behavioral health care as a model that is efficient and cost-effective; that generates better health care outcomes and is more convenient for consumers.

Case Study: Integrated Primary and Behavioral Health Care for Children

The program intends to use lessons learned from its implementation to expand to other locations.

A second example that demonstrates the integration of behavioral health and primary care services is the Phoenix Health Center for the Homeless in Louisville, Kentucky. A case study of this progressive collaboration is provided at the end of this chapter and involves services focused on improving community support for the indigent and medically underserved segment of the Louisville population.

Behavioral Health and Information Technology

Information technology has increased the ability to accumulate, store, retrieve, and analyze data at a rate that has the potential to revolutionize health care by making data relevant to an individual patient's treatment available to a provider almost immediately. Despite its potential, however, information technology has been slow to be adopted in the arena of behavioral health. Historically, the cost of equipment has been part of the reason that providers have not implemented electronic health records (EHRs); but the development of EHR systems and ongoing support required to keep these systems functioning, upgrade them, and ensure compliance with new regulations is a larger obstacle to effective use. The Health Information Technology for Economic and Clinical Health act (HITECH) established the Meaningful Use of EHRs program (Meaningful Use) providing substantial financial incentives ($19 billion) for implementation of EHRs by eligible providers and eligible hospitals, as well as penalties for those who do not adopt these systems. The Meaningful Use program was established as a three-stage program and scheduled for full implementation by 2016.

While the HITECH program has benefited many providers in transitioning to more comprehensive use of health care technology, behavioral health care providers and organizations were notable exclusions from the program's eligible providers and hospitals. This exclusion complicates integration of the medical record—an essential component of coordinated care—in the behavioral health world. Structuring the system so that behavioral health providers can effectively obtain and use technology to improve access and outcomes will require capital investment and leadership—which is essential to ensuring the ability of behavioral health care providers and long-term care providers (another excluded entity) to operate effectively in the evolving health care landscape. Some policy makers are working to change this (e.g., Senator Whitehouse's bill), but they face an uphill battle. Exciting developments in technology that have the potential to increase access to and treatment for individuals requiring behavioral health treatment become less available because of the inability of behavioral health providers to obtain funds that might be used to implement them.

Big Data is increasingly being discussed in health care as a way of facilitating a clinician's ability to implement evidence-based care in an individualized manner. The ability to generate data has become progressively less expensive. For example, sequencing an individual's DNA costs about $1000 currently.[79] This lowered cost has exciting implications for research into the biology and treatment of mental illness because of its ability to help us to understand disorders with multiple contributory genetic and environmental factors. Using an individual's genotype to determine effective treatment of a disorder has already begun. Cheek swabs can be used in an outpatient setting to collect DNA to predict an individual's response to antipsychotic, antidepressant, or stimulant medications. This personalized medicine may be used to maximize effectiveness and minimize side effects for people with behavioral health disorders.[80] Development of large data sets has been proposed as a way of connecting people with needed treatment, an issue with controversial implications for individuals with serious mental illness. The Healthcare Information and Management Systems Society Policy Summit in 2013 discussed the potential uses of data to "monitor those who should be on medications" for psychiatric illnesses.[81] Other projects are working to flag in real time soldiers and veterans at risk of suicide based on communication patterns in social media and mobile communications.[82] In many ways the complexity of the brain and disorders affecting it is particularly suited for Big Data analytics because of the amount of data that would be generated in any attempt to understand functioning on the level of the neuron. On the other hand, the potential to discover information that would be distressing or embarrassing to a person is a concern in medicine and even more of a concern in behavioral health. A widespread approach to data accumulation and analysis for purposes of monitoring treatment may well be perceived as unwelcome, unhelpful, and intrusive by the very people that it is intended to assist. The task is to build a framework in which the potential benefits of data in helping to identify and engage people in treatment can be used while avoiding invasions of privacy and coercion.

Technology has more pragmatic and smaller-scale applications that also have the potential to improve health care delivery. The use of EHRs in treatment of behavioral health disorders has potential benefits in both behavioral health and primary care settings. As the treatment of such illnesses as depression and anxiety are integrated into primary care settings, tools that assist clinicians in the differential diagnosis of common mental health disorders are essential to providing optimal care. The PHQ-9 is a standardized 9-question self-rating scale that indicates the severity of depressive symptoms.[83] If a patient completes a form online before an appointment or enters responses directly into a computer in the waiting room, the scale can become part of the medical record that is immediately available to the clinician scheduled to see the person. This method allows, for example, the flagging of indications of risk of suicide, which sets in motion a process that leads to a behavioral health evaluation.[84] Stigma is identified as a reason that people do not seek treatment or continue treatment for behavioral health problems.[85,86] Patients may actually prefer disclosing such sensitive information as suicidality to a computer rather than a clinician,[87] and this method relieves the clinic of the necessity to reenter data from a paper-and-pencil form. Technology may provide a mechanism for people who might not otherwise seek treatment for a problem to investigate solutions.

Primary care providers must also be able to identify people who may not be appropriate for treatment in a primary care setting. A certain number of people who present to primary care as depressed do not have unipolar depression but rather bipolar disorder. Treatment of these individuals with antidepressants has the potential to precipitate manic episodes, disrupting lives, and potentially necessitating hospitalization. The use of computerized rating scales may prevent misdiagnosis in this population.[88]

One of the greatest potential advantages of EHRs in behavioral health is their ability to provide decision support to clinicians. For patients on certain medications, such as antipsychotics, clinicians could be prompted to perform screening exams for such issues as metabolic disorders or tardive dyskinesia at predetermined intervals. This focus can be sharpened to provide support specific to certain medications. For instance, in a patient receiving clozapine for schizophrenia, a drop in neutrophils (a potentially serious side effect of clozapine) could initiate notification of the clinician prescribing the drug.

Technology has health-related uses outside the clinic or hospital. New in-home technology applications have the potential to increase the use of mental health services to influence health-related behaviors in people with psychiatric diagnoses. For example, RiverBend Behavioral Health Services in Massachusetts reported decreased use of emergency department services for mental health reasons and urgent visits to primary care and behavioral health clinics in people who used the Health Buddy®—a two-way device that enables communication between provider and patient around a list of personalized health-related questions. The Health Buddy®, developed by Bosch, has monitoring, educational, and coaching applications for behavioral health issues and common comorbid medical diagnoses.[89]

Applications (apps) used on smartphones or tablets can be used to provide immediate information, daily coaching, or networking opportunities for people with behavioral health needs.[90] Mobilyze, an app being developed by Northwestern University, can be used by individuals to track activities and mood using GPS, accelerometers, and data entered into the phone. If a pattern suggesting depression is noted, the person is prompted by an automated text to take such appropriate actions as calling a support person or increasing activity.[91] Another smartphone app, MoodKit, is available for five dollars and leads a person through thought tracking, mood monitoring, or engagement in activities using a cognitive therapy framework.[92]

Because only 63 percent of people with schizophrenia own smartphones, this population is harder to reach. However, smartphone applications are acceptable to individuals with schizophrenia and their clinicians for use in monitoring medication adherence, mood regulation, sleep, social functioning and symptom management.[93] Smartphones have also been used to alert clinicians to early signs of relapse in schizophrenia.[94] An app in development for bipolar disorder, MoodRhythm, may help to track moods and recognize early signs of mania and depression through patient-generated logs as well as analysis of volume and rate of speech.[95] Such apps may be preferable to paper-and-pencil mood logs due to their ease of use. Web-based technologies have been used to reduce alcohol consumption;[96] prevent posttraumatic stress disorder (PTSD);[97] as a nonstigmatizing way to obtain help for problem gambling;[98] to decrease symptoms in anxiety disorders;[99] and for problem solving in nonclinical samples.[100]

The use of technology to deliver part of an intervention to someone engaged in more traditional mental health treatment settings can also be effective. Computer-assisted cognitive behavior therapy (CBT) makes it possible to increase the number of people that can receive this evidence-based treatment, either by integrating the use of computers into treatment or using computerized

CBT programs as a form of self-help. Computerized CBT programs for treatment of depression, anxiety, and PTSD in adults and children include:

- Good Days Ahead (http://www.mindstreet.com/)

- Beating the Blues (http://www.beatingtheblues.co.uk/)

- The Climate Clinic (http://www.climateclinic.tv/)

- Fear Fighter (http://www.fearfighter.com/)

- Camp Cope-A-Lot (http://cope-a-lot.com/)

Exposure treatments for PTSD are evolving with virtual reality simulation being used as a way in which veterans can experience realistic combat simulations. Exposure treatments can have a high dropout rate because of the realistic and anxiety-provoking nature of the simulation; however, they also have the potential to be more helpful than the usual forms of treatment.[101,102]

Expanding specialty services to areas of the country that lack provider capacity to serve the local community is a way in which technology may be used to improve access to care. Project ECHO, a private-public partnership developed at the University of New Mexico, is now partnering with General Electric and the Robert Wood Johnson Foundation to develop and test an innovative telehealth mental health clinic. Project ECHO was developed as a model of remote medical education and interactive supervision and mentoring. Through Project ECHO, experts at academic medical centers can share specialized knowledge with local clinicians, bringing evidence-based medicine to everyday medical practice. The new mental health clinic model uses telehealth education and supervision to expand treatment capacity and integration of mental health and substance abuse treatment with primary care services.[103]

The potential clinical gains of computerized decision support, access to lab reports and imaging, and cloud-based storage of records must be balanced against the necessity to protect patient information. This mandate is even greater in behavioral health, in which medical records routinely contain information that is even more sensitive than that found in primary care records and can be even more damaging if a breach occurs. In a system with a single integrated medical record, psychiatric clinicians have concerns that certain information not be made available. Labeling psychotherapy notes as such and further restricting their access is one way to prevent disclosure without a separate release. It is imperative that such parts of the record as medication lists, which must be available to all treating clinicians, are in fact part of the common record. Failure to share essential information, even if intentions are to protect patient privacy, hinder efforts at care coordination[104] and render computerized decision support useless. System managers should also consider that separating primary care and behavioral health records too completely may have the unintended effect of preserving stigma by making it seem that psychiatric information is so shameful that it should not be shared even for purposes of improving care.

Behavioral Health Policy Implications

Federal investment in behavioral health intervention is in a critical period. Two major new federal laws and one significant U.S. Supreme Court decision have shifted the course of behavioral health policy. Still, efforts to capitalize on this momentum are at risk of waning. Enactment of the Paul Wellstone and Pete Domenici Mental Health Parity and Addiction Equity Act of 2008 (MHPAEA), and the ACA along with the 1999 *Olmstead* decision were the culmination of long and hard-fought battles to elevate the visibility and importance of the nation's behavioral health needs to the level of our health care needs. Building on this new plateau, is where federal, state and local efforts must focus to repair the "shambles" of a system, as described by former President George W. Bush's New Freedom Commission.[4] Repair efforts must include robust implementation of the provisions of these laws, and a legislative agenda that shores up the failing behavioral health care infrastructure and plugs policy gaps that impede the advancement of behavioral health care along with the rest of the health care sector.

Implementing Current Law

The intent of current law is to place health insurance coverage of mental health and substance use treatment on a par with coverage for medical and surgical care. Parity of coverage is a major lever in ensuring access to affordable care for those previously underserved. The MHPAEA instituted a major change in coverage parity, and the ACA memorialized and expanded on this policy.

In June 1999, the United States Supreme Court held in *Olmstead v. L.C.* that unjustifiably segregating a person with a mental disability is in violation of the Americans with Disabilities Act and constitutes discrimination. As a result, public entities must provide community-based services to persons with mental disabilities when services are appropriate, desired by the individual, and can be reasonably accommodated, taking into account the resources available to the public entity and the needs of others who are receiving disability services from the entity.[105]

In 2009, the Department of Justice Civil Rights Division launched an aggressive effort to enforce the *Olmstead* decision. In a one-year period the division facilitated resolution on or investigated over 1,400 cases. More affordable housing and effective supports are needed to sustain community-based living for people with serious behavioral health disorders—those who are often institutionalized in nursing homes or similar settings.

The MHPAEA, enacted in 2008, requires that when group health insurance plans (those with more than 50 insured employees) cover mental health and substance use disorder benefits, that coverage can be no more restrictive than that provided for medical-surgical benefits. These plans cannot impose more restrictive financial arrangements (e.g., copayment and coinsurance) or treatment limitations (such as the number of outpatient visits or inpatient days) on mental health or substance use disorder benefits than those imposed on medical or surgical benefits covered by the plan. The ACA health reform law built on MHPAEA to extend parity protections to non-grandfathered health plans in the individual and small-group markets, effectively extending protections to most plan options.

The requirements of the MHPAEA have been in effect for most plans since January 2010, and the expansion provided for in the ACA was scheduled to go into effect on January 1, 2014. However, the Department of Health and Human Services (HHS) and the Treasury have yet to promulgate final regulations for implementing parity provisions, serving to delay full implementation. In the meantime, class-action lawsuits have been filed in California and New York to push insurers to adhere to federal and state laws governing parity. Timely regulation in this space is needed to ensure that behavioral health delivery system reforms do not fall behind.

The ACA provides one of the largest expansions of mental health and substance use disorder insurance coverage in decades. The ACA provides for numerous opportunities to improve behavioral health care access and quality via new financing arrangements and delivery system reforms. Under the law all new small-group and individual-market plans will be required to cover ten essential health benefit categories, including mental health and substance use disorder services, and will be required to cover them at parity with medical and surgical benefits. Currently approximately 30 percent of individuals with substance use disorders and 20 percent of people with mental illness have no coverage through individual plans. Many more people have inadequate coverage. The largest impact will likely be through expansion of coverage to approximately 32 million previously uninsured Americans[65] through private insurance options, the new health insurance marketplaces (also called exchanges) with premium subsidies for low-income individuals, and Medicaid expansion to all individuals (including childless adults) under 138 percent of the federal poverty level.

How states will implement coverage expansion remains in flux. In the summer of 2012, the U.S. Supreme Court held that states have the option to expand Medicaid to those newly eligible under the law, effectively widening access to millions of eligible Americans. By 2013, just about half the states were implementing Medicaid expansion, and roughly half planned to establish their own exchanges. However, with a large federal investment in funding Medicaid coverage for the newly eligible (100 percent initially and slowly tapering to 90 percent,compared with an average of 50 percent federal matching funding for Medicaid programs), the expansion remained an attractive option, and more states began to take it up over time. As of March 2014, 27 states plus the District of Columbia are expanding Medicaid coverage; 19 others do not plan to move forward with expansion; and the remaining five states are still debating the option.[106]

In addition, the ACA includes many provisions that directly impact behavioral health safety net services, workforce, research, education, and person-centered community-based delivery system models. For example, it includes programs that facilitate the integration of primary and behavioral health care, such as grants to school-based health centers (construction and operations); grants to co-located primary and specialty care in community-based mental health settings; and CDC-funded community transformation grants. The ACA also includes major workforce provisions with particular emphasis on vulnerable populations and underserved areas, such as expanding community health centers (construction and operations); behavioral health specialty workforce loan repayment and scholarship programs; expansion of the National Health Service Corps; behavioral health training programs for primary care providers; and grants to community-based teaching health centers.[107] The tenor of the ACA is one that is person-centered and prevention-focused, and that emphasizes value-based care. To that end, the focus on cost-effective evidence-based practice and early identification and intervention are paramount.

With the MHPAEA, the ACA, and *Olmstead* perceived as the law of the land, the bulk of policy work in the area of behavioral health will be in assuring optimal implementation of the laws. Some opportunities and challenges exist, such as:

Parity: As mentioned earlier, final regulations on mental health and substance abuse coverage parity are vital to ensuring not only full implementation of MHPAEA, but also to prepare adequately for the delivery system reforms ramping up to full speed in 2014. For example, as health homes, ACOs, and other shared savings programs emphasizing a team-based, multidisciplinary approach spread, parity requirements will shape access to high-quality evidence-based care. This improved access will stimulate growth in the behavioral health workforce; foster effective coordination of care in team-based approaches; and, improve outcomes. President Obama called for final regulations to be released following the 2012 Newtown, Connecticut shootings, but the final rule is still awaited.

Infrastructure: Many prominent health care leaders have observed the fragmentation and utter lack of infrastructure upon which to build a modern behavioral health system (e.g., the Institute of Medicine, the Surgeon General, and former President George W. Bush's New Freedom Commission). SAMHSA could serve as the lead federal entity responsible for setting up and executing a behavioral health modernization plan. SAMHSÅ has not been empowered to do so, however.

SAMHSA was last reauthorized by Congress in 2000 as part of the Children's Health Act (PL 106-310) and has been level-funded ever since. Most of its authorizations expired in 2003. Some legislation has provided authorization and funding for additional programming through SAMHSA. These include the Sober Truth on Preventing Underage Drinking Act of 2005, also called the STOP Act, which requires SAMHSA to collaborate with other federal agencies to prevent alcohol use by minors; the Garrett Lee Smith Memorial Act of 2004, which authorizes SAMHSA to support youth suicide prevention activities in states and on college campuses; and the No Child Left Behind Act of 2002, which enables SAMHSA to consult with the Secretary of the Department of Education on the soliciting and awarding of grants through this program. A major reauthorization is needed, however, to address such issues as ensuring equitable investment in our communities via SAMHSA block grants; increased performance measurement and accountability of SAMHSA-funded programs; bolstering SAMHSA's role in expanding and diversifying the behavioral health provider workforce; and building on SAMHSA's role in primary prevention and the recent partnership with the Health Resources and Services Administration (HRSA) in behavioral health and primary care integration efforts. Reauthorizing and adequately funding SAMHSA and investing in the limited cross-agency partnerships between SAMHSA, CMS, HHS's Assistant Secretary for Planning and Evaluation, and HRSA could serve as a catalyst for integrating the highly fragmented system on federal and state levels. At this point, reauthorization is not immediately forthcoming, due in part to conflicting philosophical and political views in Congress.

One example of the value of a SAMHSA, CMS, and HRSA partnership would be its co-ownership of the promotion and adoption of primary and behavioral health care integration nationwide through a number of different initiatives. These include a provision in the ACA that allows states to establish health homes through their Medicaid programs; new Medicaid waiver authority given to the states to redesign the behavioral health aspects of their Medicaid programs; a demonstration program for integrating primary care and behavioral health care integration grants nationwide; and the establishment of the SAMHSA–HRSA Center for Integrated Health Solutions to support this purpose.

Current Legislative Efforts and New Opportunities

The most recent legislative vehicle that showed promise for improvements to the behavioral health system, particularly for children and youth, was the gun control legislation debated in Congress soon after the shootings in Newtown, Connecticut. The mental health legislation, called the Mental Health Awareness and Improvement Act, was offered as an amendment by Senators Harkin and Alexander, chair and ranking member of the Committee of Jurisdiction over Discretionary Health Programs. The legislation would provide for grant funding to develop schoolwide mental health programs and promote partnerships between schools and clinical mental health services. It provides for suicide prevention and mental health awareness training and early intervention to help students with mental health or substance abuse problems; reauthorizes suicide prevention programs; and commissions a study of obstacles to mental health access and substance abuse treatments specifically for children. Due to irreconcilable political differences over the underlying bill, this legislation died in the Senate.

A second amendment to the gun control bill with major implications for access to behavioral health care is the Excellence in Mental Health Act, a bill sponsored by Senator Stabenow that provides for the creation of Federally Qualified Behavioral Health Centers. This model recognizes the unique role behavioral health providers can play in community mental health by expanding the Federally Qualified Health Center model to those behavioral health providers who can demonstrate the capacity for integrated health care.

These are examples of the most promising infrastructural changes currently considered in Congress. In addition, through appropriations legislation, many of the behavioral health workforce improvement provisions in the ACA (noted above) still require funding, which has been stalled in the debate over whether the ACA will survive.

With unprecedented emphasis on comparative effectiveness research as a means to identify cost-effective health care options, an ACA provision, there is much hope for widespread adoption of evidence-based practices in behavioral health. Already, depression screening in youth, which has been ranked highly by the U.S. Preventive Services Task Force, is being required in the Medicaid screening program for youth (Early Periodic Screening, Diagnostic, and Treatment Program) and elsewhere. The ACA also includes clear goals for developing and meaningfully using quality metrics across disciplines via the Patient-Centered Outcomes Research Institute (PCORI). Funding opportunities for innovative delivery system reform ideas via the Center for Medicare and Medicaid Innovation can expedite innovations in identification and the rapid translation and promotion of routine use of evidence-based practices in behavioral health care.

Finally, delivery system reforms will depend upon high-quality behavioral health care. Reports on the early development of new models for reducing hospital readmissions, effective care coordination in Medicare shared-savings models, and managing complex populations, all point to successful management of the behavioral health needs of patients as a key ingredient to success.

Conclusion

This overview of behavioral health issues in this country makes clear the complexities inherent in understanding the current state of these services in the United States. Despite the significant cost of behavioral health disorders and the promise of evidence-based treatments, funding for treatment has been dramatically decreased over the past decades and the concept of parity has not been fully implemented by insurance providers. The delivery of comprehensive health services to people with serious mental illness has been fragmented; consequently these individuals have substantially higher mortality from treatable chronic diseases than the general public. Behavioral health providers must prepare to use both technology and the expanded opportunities for integrating primary and behavioral health care that are components of the ACA in order to optimize outcomes for this underserved population.

Case Study: Phoenix Health Center: Collaborative Primary Health Care Integration

History

What is now the Phoenix Health Center for the Homeless began with a collaborative effort between Family Health Centers, Seven Counties Services, the Coalition for the Homeless, the City of Louisville, and the St. John Center. A federal Healthcare for the Homeless grant was awarded in 1987 to begin operation of the clinic. The grant provided funding for a nurse practitioner, a medical assistant, a part-time physician from Family Health Centers, and a three-member social service outreach team from Seven Counties to serve the homeless. In its first year of operation, this center provided services to 1,822 patients. In achieving its goal of providing much-needed services to the homeless, Phoenix Health is also helping to decrease the number of unnecessary emergency room visits by this population.

The current Phoenix Health Center services include: primary health care; basic dental services; mental health counseling and treatment; laboratory services; substance abuse assessment and access to treatment; and outreach and case management for disabled adults and families who have children with special needs. There is no charge to patients for the above services including medications.

Phoenix Health is located within Louisville's downtown hospital district. This location is ideal, as it is near the highest density areas of Louisville's homeless population and is also in close proximity to the hospitals. For homeless clients with basic health needs, hospital personnel can effectively refer and direct them to the Phoenix Health location.

Primary funding for Phoenix Health is provided through three federal grants: the Health Resources and Services Administration's Bureau of Primary Health Care; the Department of Housing and Urban Development (HUD); and the Substance Abuse and Mental Health Services Administration (SAMHSA). Local foundation grants have also been used to sustain services and purchase equipment. The program is largely dependent upon federal funds for program expenses. Most clinics for the indigent and medically underserved depend on Medicaid as a primary source of financial support, however, only 3 percent of the patients who use the health center have Medicaid, and only 1 percent have Medicare; 96 percent have no insurance and no ability to pay for health care services.

Collaboration

In order to address the mental health and substance abuse needs of this population, Family Health Centers, a federally qualified health center, elected to collaborate with Seven Counties Services, the region's community mental health center and safety net provider of mental health services.

Seven Counties provides an onsite psychiatric nurse practitioner as well as a mobile

Case Study: Phoenix Health Center: Collaborative Primary Health Care Integration

unit of four case managers called the Homeless Outreach Team. Seven Counties' participation as a partner has enabled Phoenix Health's clients to gain access to much-needed mental health services, but it has also helped open new avenues for community supports that have helped clients obtain permanent housing.

After a client achieves housing, they are no longer eligible for services through Phoenix Health. Seven Counties' case managers are also responsible for transitioning these clients to physical health services at Family Health Centers and other mental health services available through Seven Counties.

This collaboration has enabled Phoenix Health to operate a truly integrated health care center, serving both physical and mental health care needs as they are identified.

Integrated Staffing Model

Phoenix Health's revised staffing model includes:

1. One part-time physician – Family Health Centers
2. Three full-time nurse practitioners – Family Health Centers
3. Three medical assistants – Family Health Centers
4. One dentist – Family Health Centers
5. Two social workers – Family Health Centers
6. Three front-office staff – Family Health Centers
7. One prescribing psychiatric nurse practitioner – Seven Counties
8. Four mental health case managers – Seven Counties
9. One mental health coordinator – Family Health Centers

Service Process

Phoenix Health does not accept appointments. Each morning homeless clients arrive for physical health care services. As they are waiting to be seen, the mental health coordinator conducts screenings to determine who may require a visit with the psychiatric nurse practitioner. In addition, those clients who are seen by a primary care physician may be immediately referred to the psychiatric nurse practitioner. Many times the doctor may call "down the hall" for an immediate psychiatric evaluation or consultation. Conversely, if the psychiatric nurse practitioner discovers any physical health requirement during the psychiatric session, a primary care physician will be called for immediate care.

After the mental health care visit or screening, Phoenix Health clients may be referred to Seven Counties' case management services, the Homeless Outreach Team. These case managers will work with clients to determine whether they are eligible for any benefits, including Social Security or disability. They may also begin the process of seeking housing. Temporary housing is sometimes offered through

Case Study: Phoenix Health Center: Collaborative Primary Health Care Integration

Extended Care Housing, which allows for up to nine months of housing while the status of disability applications is pending. Again, once benefits are established and the client is no longer homeless, the Homeless Outreach Team will work to connect the client to ongoing services through the Family Health Center and Seven Counties Services.

Outcomes

The Phoenix Health Center has approximately 5,000 persons per year receiving services, which translates to over 15,000 visits. Nearly 20 percent of Phoenix Health's clients utilize mental health services. This seamless integration of physical and mental health care enables clients to receive much-needed mental health services quickly and easily. These services not only address mental health needs but also provide community supports that enable these clients to establish Social Security benefits and other insurance while seeking housing.

Finally, through this collaborative approach to health care, Phoenix Health is helping to prevent unnecessary and expensive emergency room visits by providing high-quality physical and mental health care. After receiving care at Phoenix Health, the likelihood of these clients showing up in emergency rooms decreases dramatically.

CHAPTER 8 DISCUSSION QUESTIONS

Discussion questions are provided for team building or class exercises. Answers for all questions are provided in Appendix C.

Question Number	Question
1	Why has parity taken so long to be identified as an issue and why is it still not fully realized?
2	What role does stigma play in behavioral health's receiving so little attention in the public health arena? Discuss the role of professional training in perpetuating or dispelling stigma.
3	What are potential ways to organize health care delivery to maximize outcomes in behavioral health disorders?
4	Will current efforts at healthcare reform (the ACA for example) result in access for all to appropriate and effective behavioral health services? If not, what else can we do?
5	Behavioral health services have historically not been addressed in the public health arena. Given the effect of comorbid behavioral health conditions on outcomes in illness, does it make sense to continue this separation? If not, what behavioral health conditions would you identify as priorities for public health?

CHAPTER 8 SUMMARY

- Behavioral health disorders are common and costly, and they complicate effective treatment of medical illnesses with which they are comorbid.

- Stigma associated with mental illness can color the public perception of people with mental illness, and prevent people from seeking needed mental health services.

- Lack of parity and years of cuts to mental health funding have limited access to affordable evidence-based treatment for serious mental illnesses.

- Technology can expand access to service and extend the capacity of specialty providers; however, the ineligibility of behavioral health providers for incentives hinders adoption of new technologies.

- The country is in an exciting period of transition as the Affordable Care Act and the Mental Health Parity and Addiction Equity Act increase mental health coverage and integrate screening for common behavioral health disorders into primary care.

CHAPTER 8 REFERENCES

1. Institute for Health Metrics and Evaluation (IHME). *The global burden of disease: generating evidence, guiding policy.* Seattle, Wash.: IHME;2013. http://www.healthmetricsandevaluation.org/gbd/publications/policy-report/global-burden-disease-generating-evidence-guiding-policy. Accessed December 23, 2013.

2. Bonner L. Community mental health services for young adults challenged. *News Observer.* December 22, 2012. http://www.newsobserver.com/2012/12/22/2561984/community-mental-health-services.html. Accessed December 23, 2013.

3. Executive Order—Improving access to mental health services for veterans, service members, and military families [press release]. Washington, D.C.: The White House. August 12, 2012.

4. The President's New Freedom Commission on Mental Health. *Achieving the promise: transforming mental health care in America.* Final Report. Rockville, Md.: SAMHSA;2003.

5. National Institute of Mental Health. The numbers count: mental disorders in America. http://www.nimh.nih.gov/health/publications/the-numbers-count-mental-disorders-in-america/index.shtml#Intro. Accessed December 23, 2013.

6. Kessler RC, Chiu WT, Demler O, Walters EE. Prevalence, severity, and comorbidity of 12-month DSM-IV disorders in the National Comorbidity Survey Replication. *Arch Gen Psychiatry.* 2005;62(6):617-627.

7. United States Department of Health and Human Services (HHS). *Healthy People 2020*: Mental Health. Washington, D.C.: HHS;2010. http://www.healthypeople.gov/2020/LHI/mentalHealth.aspx?tab=determinants. Accessed December 23, 2013.

8. Olin GL, Rhoades JA. *The five most costly medical conditions, 1997 and 2002: estimates for the US civilian noninstitutionalized population.* Medical Expenditure Panel Survey. Rockville, Md.:Agency for Healthcare Research and Quality;2005.

9. Simpson G, Cohen RA, Pastor PN, Reuben CA. *Use of mental health services in the past 12 months by children aged 4-17 years: United States, 2005-2006.* US Department of Health and Human Services. Atlanta, Ga.: Centers for Disease Control and Prevention, National Center for Health Statistics;2008.

10. Social Security Administration. SSI Annual Statistical Report 2009. Washington, D.C.: Social Security Administration;2010.

11. Vick B, Jones K, Mitra S. Poverty and severe psychiatric disorder in the US: evidence from the medical expenditure panel survey. *J Ment Health Policy Econ.* 2012;15(2):83-96.

12. Rampell C. The half-trillion-dollar depression. *New York Times Magazine.* July 2, 2013. http://www.nytimes.com/2013/07/02/magazine/the-half-trillion-dollar-depression.html. Accessed June 10, 2014.

2

2

13. Morgan L. The chronic condition multiplier effect on cost. *Open Minds Circle.com* September 24, 2013. http://www.openminds.com/market-intelligence/executive-briefings/092413-chronic-conditions.htm. Accessed June 10, 2014.

14. Murphy SL, Xu J, Kochanek KD. Deaths: preliminary data for 2010. *Natl Vital Stat Rep.* 2012;60(4):1-69.

15. Logan J, Skopp NA, Karch D, Reger MA, Gahm GA. Characteristics of suicides among US army active duty personnel in 17 US states from 2005 to 2007. *Am J Public Health.* 2012;102(S1):S40-S44.

16. Reeves A, Stuckler D, McKee M, Gunnell D, Chang S-S, Basu S. Increase in state suicide rates in the USA during economic recession. *Lancet.* 2012;380(9856):1813-1814.

17. Calcaterra S, Glanz J, Binswanger IA. National trends in pharmaceutical opioid related overdose deaths compared to other substance related overdose deaths: 1999–2009. *Drug and Alcohol Depend.* 2013;131(3):263-270.

18. Cheves J. Kentucky drug deaths decline slightly in 2012, but heroin deaths up sharply. *Lexington Herald Leader.* July 26, 2013. http://www.kentucky.com/2013/07/26/2734183/kentucky-drug-deaths-decline-slightly.html. Accessed June 10, 2014.

19. Parks J, Svendsen D, Singer P, Foti M, eds. Morbidity and mortality in people with serious mental illness. Alexandria, Va.: National Association of State Mental Health Program Directors;2006. http://www.dsamh.utah.gov/docs/mortality-morbidity_nasmhpd.pdf. Accessed December 23, 2013.

20. Hert M, Schreurs V, Vancampfort D, Winkel R. Metabolic syndrome in people with schizophrenia: a review. *World Psychiatry.* 2009;8(1):15-22.

21. Nasrallah HA, Meyer JM, Goff DC, et al. Low rates of treatment for hypertension, dyslipidemia and diabetes in schizophrenia: data from the CATIE schizophrenia trial sample at baseline. *Schizophr Res.* 2006;86(1):15-22.

22. Mangurian C, Giwa F, Shumway M, et al. Primary care providers' views on metabolic monitoring of outpatients taking antipsychotic medication. *Psychiatr Serv.* 2013;64(6):597-599.

23. Katon WJ. Epidemiology and treatment of depression in patients with chronic medical illness. *Dialogues Clin Neurosci.* 2011;13(1):7.

24. National Coalition for the Homeless (NCH). Mental Illness and homelessness. Washington, D.C.: NCH;2009. http://www.nationalhomeless.org/factsheets/Mental_Illness.html. Accessed December 23, 2013.

25. National Alliance on Mental Illness (NAMI)Virginia. Fact sheet: mental illness and the criminal justice system. Richmond: NAMI Virginia;2008. http://namivirginia.org/assets/pdfs/MIandCriminalJusticeSystem.pdf. Accessed December 23, 2013.

26. Torrey EF, Kennard AD, Eslinger D, Lamb R, Pavle J, Center TA. *More mentally ill persons are in jails and prisons than hospitals: A survey of the states.* Arlington, Va.: Treatment Advocacy Center;2010.

27. Awad AG, Voruganti LN. The burden of schizophrenia on caregivers. *Pharmacoeconomics.* 2008;26(2):149-162.

28. Viana MC, Gruber MJ, Shahly V, et al. Family burden related to mental and physical disorders in the world: results from the WHO World Mental Health (WMH) surveys. *Revista Bras Psiquiatr.* 2013;35:115-125.

29. Rabinowitz J, Berardo CG, Bugarski-Kirola D, Marder S. Association of prominent positive and prominent negative symptoms and functional health, well-being, healthcare-related quality of life and family burden: a CATIE analysis. *Schizophr Res.* 2013;150(2-3):339-342.

30. Koutra K, Basta M, Roumeliotaki T, et al. 1365–Family functioning, expressed emotion and family burden in relatives of first-episode and chronic patients with schizophrenia and bipolar disorder: preliminary findings. *Eur Psychiatry.* 2013;28(Supp 1):1.

31. Wallcraft J, Amering M, Freidin J, et al. Partnerships for better mental health worldwide: WPA recommendations on best practices in working with service users and family carers. *World Psychiatry.* 2011;10(3):229-236.

32. National Alliance on Mental Illness. Assertive community treatment: investment yields outcomes. September 2007. http://www.nami.org/Template.cfm?Section=act-ta_center&template=ContentManagement/ContentDisplay.cfm&ContentID=52382. Accessed December 23, 2013.

33. Burns T, Catty J, Dash M, Roberts C, Lockwood A, Marshall M. Use of intensive case management to reduce time in hospital in people with severe mental illness: systematic review and meta-regression. *BMJ.* 2007;335(7615):336.

34. Dieterich M, Irving CB, Park B, Marshall M. Intensive case management for severe mental illness. *Cochrane Database Syst Rev.* 2010(10):CD007906.

35. Latimer E. Economic considerations associated with assertive community treatment and supported employment for people with severe mental illness. *J Psychiatry Neurosci.* 2005;30(5):355-359.

36. Bond GR, Drake RE, Becker DR. An update on randomized controlled trials of evidence-based supported employment. *Psychiatr Rehabil J.* 2008;31(4):280.

37. Campbell K, Bond GR, Drake RE. Who benefits from supported employment: a meta-analytic study. *Schizophr Bull.* 2011;37(2):370-380.

38. Butler AC, Chapman JE, Forman EM, Beck AT. The empirical status of cognitive-behavioral therapy: a review of meta-analyses. *Clin Psychol Rev.* 2006;26(1):17-31.

39. Kingdon D, Dimech A. Cognitive and behavioural therapies: the state of the art. *Psychiatry.* 2008;7(5):217-220.

40. Rector NA, Beck AT. Cognitive behavioral therapy for schizophrenia: an empirical review. *J Nerv Ment Dis.* 2001;189(5):278-287.

41. Drake RE, Mercer-McFadden C, Mueser KT, McHugo GJ, Bond GR. Review of integrated mental health and substance abuse treatment for patients with dual disorders. *Schizophr Bull.* 1998;24(4):589-608.

42. Weiden PJ. Understanding and addressing adherence issues in schizophrenia: from theory to practice. *J Clin Psychiatry. Supplement.* 2007;68(14):14-19.

43. Hogan MF. New Freedom Commission report: The president's New Freedom Commission: recommendations to transform mental health care in America. *Psychiatr Serv.* 2003;54(11):1467-1474.

44. McDonald KM, Sundaram V, Bravata DM, et al. Closing the quality gap: a critical analysis of quality improvement strategies (Vol. 7: Care Coordination). Rockville, Md.: Agency for Healthcare Research and Quality;2007.

45. Honberg R, Kimball A, Diehl S, Usher L, Fitzpatrick M. State mental health cuts: the continuing crisis. National Alliance for the Mentally Ill (NAMI). November 2011. http://www.nami.org/ContentManagement/ContentDisplay.cfm?ContentFileID =147763. Accessed December 23, 2013.

46. National Alliance on Mental Illness (NAMI). Treatment and services: supported employment. http://www.nami.org/Content/NavigationMenu/Inform_Yourself/About_Ment al_Illness/About_Treatments_and_Supports/Supported_Employment1.htm;200 3. Accessed December 23, 2013.

47. National Alliance on Mental Illness (NAMI). Grading the states. 2009; http://www.nami.org/Content/NavigationMenu/Grading_the_States_2009/Gra ding_the_States_20091.htm. Accessed December 23, 2013.

48. McLaughlin J. 200 Statistics on physician compensation. *Becker's ASC Review.* February 6, 2013. http://www.beckershospitalreview.com/compensation-issues/200-statistics-on-physician-compensation-2014.html. Accessed June 10, 2014.

49. American Academy of Child and Adolescent Psychiatry Committee on Health Care Access and Economics Task Force on Mental Health. Improving mental health services in primary care: Reducing administrative and financial barriers to access and collaboration. *Pediatrics.* 2009;123(4):1248-1251.

50. W.K. Kellogg Foundation. Mental health parity state of the states November 2002 update,April 2003. http://www.wkkf.org/resource-directory/resource/2003/07/mental-health-parity-state-of-the-states-november-2002-update. Accessed December 23, 2013.

51. Navia B. Bridging the gap between behavioral health and EHRs in New Jersey. *Health IT Buzz.* May 17, 2013. http://www.healthit.gov/buzz-blog/electronic-health-and-medical-records/bridging-gap-behavioral-health-ehrs-jersey/. Accessed December 23, 2013.

52. Corrigan PW, Powell KJ, Michaels PJ. The effects of news stories on the stigma of mental illness. *J Nerv Ment Dis.* 2013;201(3):179-182.

53. Gold LH. Gun violence: psychiatry, risk assessment, and social policy. *J Am Acad Psychiatry Law.* September 1, 2013 2013;41(3):337-343.

54. Pescosolido BA, Monahan J, Link BG, Stueve A, Kikuzawa S. The public's view of the competence, dangerousness, and need for legal coercion of persons with mental health problems. *Am J Public Health.* 1999;89(9):1339-1345.

55. Hiroeh U, Appleby L, Mortensen PB, Dunn G. Death by homicide, suicide, and other unnatural causes in people with mental illness: a population-based study. *Lancet.* 2001;358(9299):2110-2112.

56. Hiday VA, Swartz MS, Swanson JW, Borum R, Wagner R. Criminal victimization of persons with severe mental illness. *Psychiatr Serv.* 1999;50(1):62-68.

57. Mulvey EP. Assessing the evidence of a link between mental illness and violence. In: American Psychiatric Association, *Violent behavior and mental illness: a compendium of articles from psychiatric services and hospital and community psychiatry.* Arlington, Va,: American Psychiatric Publishing;1997:14.

58. Elbogen EB, Johnson SC. The intricate link between violence and mental disorder: results from the National Epidemiologic Survey on Alcohol and Related Conditions. *Arch Gen Psychiatry.* 2009;66(2):152-161.

59. Steadman HJ, Mulvey EP, Monahan J, et al. Violence by people discharged from acute psychiatric inpatient facilities and by others in the same neighborhoods. *Arch Gen Psychiatry.* 1998;55(5):393.

60. Appelbaum PS, Robbins PC, Monahan J. Violence and delusions: data from the MacArthur violence risk assessment study. *Am J Psychiatry.* 2000;157(4):566-572.

61. Grunberg F, Klinger B, Grumet B. Homicide and deinstitutionalization of the mentally ill. *Am J Psychiatry.* 1977;134(6):685.

62. Matejkowski JC, Cullen SW, Solomon PL. Characteristics of persons with severe mental illness who have been incarcerated for murder. *J Am Acad Psychiatry Law.* 2008;36(1):74-86.

63. Wilcox DE. The relationship of mental illness to homicide. *Am J Forensic Psychiatry.* 1985;8(6):3-15.

64. Martone CA, Mulvey EP, Yang S, Nemoianu A, Shugarman R, Soliman L. Psychiatric characteristics of homicide defendants. *Am J Psychiatry.* 2013;170(9):994-1002.

65. DeParle NA. The Affordable Care Act helps America's uninsured. *The White House Blog.* Sept. 16, 2010. http://www.whitehouse.gov/blog/2010/09/16/affordable-care-act-helps-america-s-uninsured. Accessed December 23, 2013.

66. SAMHSA predicts 10% to 20% more mental health and addiction professionals needed by 2018. *Open Minds Weekly News Wire.* June 10, 2013. http://www.openminds.com/market-intelligence/news/061013mhcd1.htm. Accessed June 10, 2014.

67. Grier P. Health care reform bill 101: who will pay for reform? *Christian Science Monitor.* March 21, 2010.

http://www.csmonitor.com/USA/Politics/2010/0321/Health-care-reform-bill-101-Who-will-pay-for-reform. Accessed December 23, 2013.

68. Katon WJ. Clinical and health services relationships between major depression, depressive symptoms, and general medical illness. *Biol Psychiatry.* 2003;54(3):216-226.

69. Goetzel RZ, Pei X, Tabrizi MJ, et al. Ten modifiable health risk factors are linked to more than one-fifth of employer-employee health care spending. *Health Aff (Millwood).* 2012;31(11):2474-2484.

70. Horwitz JR, Kelly BD, DiNardo JE. Wellness incentives in the workplace: cost savings through cost shifting to unhealthy workers. *Health Aff (Millwood).* 2013;32(3):468-476.

71. US Centers for Disease Control and Prevention. The power to prevent, the call to control: At a glance 2009. December 2009. http://www.cdc.gov/chronicdisease/resources/publications/aag/chronic.htm. Accessed December 24, 2013.

72. Smith A. Overview of the Medicaid health home care coordination benefit. National Council webinar, June 7, 2011.

73. Centers for Medicare and Medicaid Services. Health Homes. 2013. http://medicaid.gov/Medicaid-CHIP-Program-Information/By-Topics/Long-Term-Services-and-Support/Integrating-Care/Health-Homes/Health-Homes.html. Accessed December 24, 2013.

74. Katon W, Russo J, Lin EB, et al. Cost-effectiveness of a multicondition collaborative care intervention: A randomized controlled trial. *Arch Gen Psychiatry.* 2012;69(5):506-514.

75. Hennekens CH, Hennekens AR, Hollar D, Casey DE. Schizophrenia and increased risks of cardiovascular disease. *Am Heart J.* 2005;150(6):1115-1121.

76. Kurdyak P, Vigod S, Calzavara A, Wodchis WP. High mortality and low access to care following incident acute myocardial infarction in individuals with schizophrenia. *Schizophr Res.* 2012;142(1–3):52-57.

77. Kim J, Higgins T, Gerolamo A, Esposito D, Hamblin A. Early lessons from Pennsylvania's SMI Innovations project for integrating physical and behavioral health in Medicaid. Hamilton, N.J.: Center for Health Care Strategies, Inc.;2012.

78. Scharf DM, Eberhart NK, Schmidt N, et al. Integrating primary care into community behavioral health settings: programs and early implementation experiences. *Psychiatr Serv.* 2013;64(7):660-665.

79. Insel T. Director's blog: An emerging era of big data. February 15, 2012. www.nimh.nih.gov/about/director/2012/an-emerging-era-of-big-data.shtml. Accessed December 24, 2013.

80. Genesight Technology. http://assurexhealth.com/products/. Accessed December 24, 2013.

81. Maheu M. BIG DATA discussion at HIMSS Policy Summit 2013 mentions mental health. September 26, 2013. http://telehealth.org/blog/big-data-discussion-at-

himss-policy-summit-2013-mentions-mental-health/. Accessed December 24, 2013.

82. Durkheim Project. The Durkheim Project will analyze opt-in data from veterans' social media and mobile content-seeking real-time predictive analytics for suicide risk Durkheim Project press release, July 2, 2013. http://www.durkheimproject.org/news/durkheim-project-will-analyze-opt-in-data/. Accessed December 24, 2013.

83. Kroenke K, Spitzer RL, Williams JB. The PHQ-9. *J Gen Intern Med.* 2001;16(9):606-613.

84. Lawrence ST, Willig JH, Crane HM, et al. Routine, self-administered, touch-screen, computer-based suicidal ideation assessment linked to automated response team notification in an HIV primary care setting. *Clin Infect Dis.* 2010;50(8):1165-1173.

85. Conner KO, Copeland VC, Grote NK, et al. Mental health treatment seeking among older adults with depression: the impact of stigma and race. *Am J Geriatr Psychiatry.* 2010;18(6):531-543.

86. Judge A, Estroff S, Perkins D, Penn D. Recognizing and responding to early psychosis: A qualitative analysis of individual narratives. *Psychiatr Serv.* 2008;59(1):96-99.

87. Kobak KA, Reynolds WM, Greist JH. Computerized and clinician assessment of depression and anxiety: respondent evaluation and satisfaction. *J Pers Assess.* 1994;63(1):173-180.

88. Gill J CY, Grimes A., Klinkman M. S. Using electronic health record-based tools to screen for bipolar disorder in primary care patients with depression. *J Am Board Fam Med.* 2012;25(3):283-290.

89. Riverbend Community Mental Health, Concord, N.H. Health Buddy 2013 Program of Significance by National Council for Behavioral Health. [press release];2013. http://riverbendcmhc.org/press-release/health-buddy-2013-program-of-significance-by-national-council-for-behavioral-health/. Accessed December 24, 2013.

90. CoCentrix. Health IT can enhance mental healthcare through smartphone apps. http://cocentrix.com/health-it-mental-healthcare-smartphone-apps/?doing_wp_cron=1380763033.4598519802093505859375.Accessed December 24, 2013.

91. Kerr D. Can a smartphone sense depression. 2012. http://news.cnet.com/8301-1023_3-57373705-93/can-a-smartphone-sense-depression/. Accessed December 24, 2013.

92. Broida R. MoodKit: Can an app improve your mood? *CNET.* May 2011. http://reviews.cnet.com/8301-19512_7-20066426-233.html. Accessed December 24, 2013.

93.   Ben-Zeev D, Kaiser SM, Brenner CJ, Begale M, Duffecy J, Mohr DC. Development and usability testing of FOCUS: a smartphone system for self-management of schizophrenia. *Psychiatr Rehabil J.* 2013;36(4):289-96.

94.   Ainsworth J, Palmier-Claus JE, Machin M, et al. A comparison of two delivery modalities of a mobile phone-based assessment for serious mental illness: native smartphone application vs text-messaging only implementations. *J Med Internet Res.* 2013;15(4):e60.

95.   Steele B. Smartphone app for bipolar patients wins $100K prize. *Cornell Chronicle.* July 3, 2013. http://news.cornell.edu/stories/2013/07/smartphone-app-bipolar-patients-wins-100k-prize. Accessed December 23, 2013.

96.   Schulz DN, Candel MJ, Kremers SP, Reinwand DA, Jander A, de Vries H. Effects of a web-based tailored intervention to reduce alcohol consumption in adults: randomized controlled trial. *J Med Internet Res.* 2013;15(9):e206.

97.   Mouthaan J, Sijbrandij M, de Vries GJ, et al. Internet-based early intervention to prevent posttraumatic stress disorder in injury patients: randomized controlled trial. *J Med Internet Res.* 2013;15(8):e165.

98.   Rodda S, Lubman DI, Dowling NA, Bough A, Jackson AC. Web-based counseling for problem gambling: exploring motivations and recommendations. *J Med Internet Res.* 2013;15(5):e99.

99.   Klein B, Meyer D, Austin DW, Kyrios M. Anxiety online: a virtual clinic: preliminary outcomes following completion of five fully automated treatment programs for anxiety disorders and symptoms. *J Med Internet Res.* 2011;13(4):e89.

100.   Gaffney H, Mansell W, Edwards R, Wright J. Manage Your Life Online (MYLO): A Pilot Trial of a Conversational Computer-Based Intervention for Problem Solving in a Student Sample. *Behav Cogn Psychother.* 2013:1-16.

101.   McLay RN, Wood DP, Webb-Murphy JA, et al. A randomized, controlled trial of virtual reality-graded exposure therapy for post-traumatic stress disorder in active duty service members with combat-related post-traumatic stress disorder. *Cyberpsychol Behav Soc Netw.* 2011;14(4):223-229.

102.   Rizzo A, Parsons TD, Lange B, et al. Virtual reality goes to war: a brief review of the future of military behavioral healthcare. *J Clin Psychol Med Settings.* Jun 2011;18(2):176-187.

103.   Hall SD. Project ECHO expansion to help rural docs provide mental health services. *Fierce HealthIT.* June 19, 2013. http://www.fiercehealthit.com/story/project-echo-expansion-help-rural-docs-provide-mental-health-services/2013-06-19. Accessed December 23, 2013.

104.   Peterson D, Wickeham D. New challenge for academic psychiatry: the electronic health record. *Acad Psychiatry.* 2011;35(2):76-80.

105.   US Department of Justice Civil Rights Division. Statement of the Department of Justice on enforcement of the integration mandate of Title II of the Americans with Disabilities Act and *Olmstead v. L.C.* Washington, D.C.: Department of Justice;2011. http://www.ada.gov/olmstead/q&a_olmstead.pdf. Accessed December 23, 2013.

106. Price CC, Eibner C. For states that opt out of Medicaid expansion: 3.6 million fewer insured and $8.4 billion less in federal payments. *Health Aff (Millwood)*. 2013;32(6):1030-1036. Kaiser Family Foundation. State health facts: status of state action on the Medicaid expansion decision, 2014. http://kff.org/health-reform/state-indicator/state-activity-around-expanding-medicaid-under-the-affordable-care-act/. Accessed June 10, 2014.

107. Redhead, CS, Heisler EJ. Public health, workforce, quality, and related provisions in ACA: summary and timeline; May 2013. http://www.law.umaryland.edu/marshall/crsreports/crsdocuments/R41278_05172013.pdf. Accessed December 23, 2013.

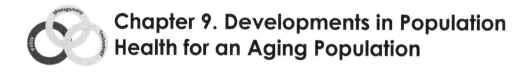

Chapter 9. Developments in Population Health for an Aging Population

William M. Altman, JD, MA

Marc D. Rothman, MD

John P. Reinhart, CPA, MBA, CNA

Kathleen Smith, MBA, MPH

"Look to your future because that is where you will spend the rest of your life."

George Burns
1896–1996
Comedian, actor, and writer

Chapter 9 Learning Objectives

- Understand how population health initiatives must take into account the physical, psychosocial, and mental status of older persons in order to be effective;

- Be able to distinguish between population health interventions that are effective with an older population from those that are ineffective;

- Become conversant with the latest government-sponsored population health initiatives through the Affordable Care Act and Medicare Advantage programs;

- Understand the range of private sector innovations in population health for an older population; and

- Understand the barriers and opportunities for effective population health for older persons in both the public and private sectors.

Part I. Introduction, Overview, and Demographics of the Elderly Population

Introduction and Overview

This chapter reviews the latest developments in population health initiatives for an older population, with special emphasis on the large and growing Medicare population. The chapter is divided into three sections: Part I gives a high-level overview of the demographics of an aging population to frame the issue of population health interventions in the context of the unique characteristics and needs of this population. Part II provides a review of key trends in population health management initiatives organized according to the distinct subsets of the aging population, from healthy community-dwelling people to those with multiple chronic co-morbidities who are high users of the healthcare system. In this section, several government-sponsored programs and "innovations from the field" are highlighted to demonstrate the high level of public and private sector activity in this area. Part III raises the issues of barriers, policy implications, and opportunities for population health management for older persons.

Discussions about population health often proceed from the widely accepted World Health Organization definition of health as "the state of complete physical, mental, and social well-being and not merely the absence of disease or infirmity."[1] As this definition relates to older persons, population health initiatives must segment the population to identify approaches that effectively address the conditions, health status, functional status, and needs of individuals to achieve the goals of population health. For discussion purposes, the older—or geriatric—population may be viewed from the perspective of both its health as well as functional status, the latter representing an important marker for defining effective population health approaches.

The importance of segmenting the geriatric population for purposes of population health is highlighted by older persons with chronic conditions. Though difficult to prevent altogether, certain chronic conditions can be delayed in an older population with appropriate interventions. Most older people will experience chronic conditions at some point in their lives, however, and population health approaches for this cohort must recognize this reality and adjust approaches and goals accordingly. Whereas in most population health approaches a high premium is placed on *preventing* diseases altogether, in older persons an important goal may be to *delay the onset* of chronic disease, while recognizing that the aging process makes the presence of chronic disease inevitable for many. Accordingly, in addition to prevention and delaying the onset of chronic disease, an important goal of population health for an older population is to manage and treat chronic diseases as an end in itself.

Characteristics of Older Populations and Implications for Population Health

It is axiomatic that the geriatric population in America is large and growing as the Baby Boomer generation enters retirement and medical advances continue to extend the life span. In 2010, Americans aged 65 and over represented 13 percent of the population, while in 2030 this percentage is estimated to be nearly 20 percent of the total U.S. population, growing from 35 million people in 2010 to 72 million people in 2030.[2]

Among the aged 65 and over cohort, the "oldest-old" (those 85 and over) is expected to grow even more significantly, from just over 100,000 in 1900 to 5.5 million in 2010. This population is projected to grow to over 19 million by 2050, or even higher if medical advances continue to lower death rates for older persons.[2] The oldest-old are high consumers of health care services and are more likely to experience multiple health problems and functional limitations; targeted population health approaches for this group are therefore needed. For example, death rates for heart disease and stroke have declined by more than 50 percent since 1981, while the mortality rate for chronic lower respiratory disease has increased by 57 percent in the same period. This finding suggests that while technology and medical advances increase life expectancy by preventing one or more diseases, a larger number of older persons will experience multiple chronic diseases and eventually die of a different cause.[3,4]

As the population ages, individuals need increasing assistance performing normal functions. Over 40 percent of people age 65 and over have a functional limitation; 25 percent have difficulty with at least one activity of daily living (ADL; e.g., bathing, dressing, eating, etc.);[5] and 12 percent have difficulty performing one or more instrumental activities of daily living (e.g., using the telephone, meal preparation, shopping, and others).[6] These functional limitations become more pronounced by residential setting. For example, over two-thirds of individuals living in long-term care facilities have limitations in three or more ADLs. As functional limitations increase, the percentage of time engaged in leisure activity declines with age, with those between the ages of 55 and 64 spending about 11 percent of leisure time socializing or communicating, while those aged 75 and over spend only 8 percent of their time engaged in these activities. This difference has significant implications for population health management initiatives, as social engagement and physical functioning can be important parts of the long-term support services needed to identify health problems early to avoid costly medical care.[7]

Population health approaches for an older population must also consider the gender, ethnic, and racial composition of the population, as interventions must be tailored to account for cultural nuances as they relate to health care services, family support, and social system dynamics. Older women outnumber older men in every age group. In 2010, older women accounted for 57 percent of those aged 65 and over, and 67 percent of those over 85 years of age.[8] Older women are much more likely to live alone than older men, emphasizing the reality that older women live longer and are often in the role of caregiver for their aging husbands, which itself can be a significant factor in population health initiatives. In 2010, 72 percent of older men lived with their spouse, while less than half (42 percent) of older women did. In contrast, older women were twice as likely as older men to live alone (37 percent versus 19 percent).[9]

In 2010, non-Hispanic whites constituted approximately 80 percent of the older population in the United States, while African Americans made up 9 percent, Asians made up 3 percent, and Hispanics accounted for 7 percent of the population. By 2050 this ethnic and racial composition is projected to be significantly altered: non-Hispanic whites will constitute 58 percent, African Americans 12 percent, Asians 9 percent, and Hispanics 20 percent of the older population.[10]

In order to improve cost effectiveness, leaders of population health management programs need to understand the sources of health care spending to better target efforts. Costs vary substantially by health status and residential setting. In 2008, individuals with no chronic conditions incurred $5,520 in annual health care costs on average. Those with five or more conditions incurred $24,658 in costs annually. Average costs among residents of long-term care facilities were $61,318, compared with only $13,150 among community residents[11], though these cost differences need to be interpreted carefully because they do not control for differences in patient condition, acuity of illness, or intensity of required services. Costs also vary by setting of care. Acute care consumes the greatest portion of health care spending for elderly people, with inpatient hospitals comprising 24 percent and physician/outpatient hospitals consuming 36 percent of health care costs. Post-acute care providers make up a much smaller portion of health care spending, with nursing homes and long-term care comprising 12 percent and home health care 3 percent of annual costs for older persons. Spending on prescription drugs is also significant, at 16 percent of health care spending.[12]

Health care costs have increased significantly for older Americans, from $9,850 in 1992 to $15,709 in 2008, although there was no increase between 2006 and 2008. Older Americans in poverty spend a proportionately higher percentage of their income on health care than do wealthier older Americans. From 1977 to 2009, out-of-pocket spending for health care services increased among those in the poor/near-poor income category from 12 percent to 22 percent of household income.[13] Between 1974 and 2010, however, there was a decrease in the proportion of older people with income below the poverty level from 15 percent to 9 percent, and with low income from 35 percent to 26 percent. There was an increase in the proportion of older people with high income, from 18 percent to 31 percent.[14]

End-of-life care is also important to consider in the context of population health for an older population. In the last decade there has been an increase in the number of older persons using hospice services at or near the end of life; a decrease in the number of people who die in hospitals; and a commensurate increase in the number of people who die at home. In the two decades from 1989 to 2009, in-hospital deaths declined from 49 percent to 32 percent, and the percent of older adults dying at home increased from 15 percent to 24 percent.[15] The percent of Medicare dollars spent on end-of-life care has decreased slightly, but still accounts for a quarter of Medicare payments for the older population.[16]

Some of the leading causes of death in the older population include, in decreasing order: heart disease, cancer, chronic lower respiratory disease, stroke, Alzheimer's disease, diabetes, influenza, and pneumonia. Although these diseases have consistently remained the most significant causes of mortality, the rate of death from these diseases has changed significantly over time, and sometimes in opposite directions. While the mortality rates for heart disease and stroke have decreased almost 55 percent and 58 percent respectively from 1981 to 2009, the mortality rate for chronic lower respiratory disease has increased 57 percent over the same time period.[17] Clearly there is still much work to be done to improve care, enhance quality of life, and reduce spending among older Americans.

Part II. Population Health Approaches for an Elderly Population

Population Health Approaches for an Aging Population in the Medicare Program

While the American healthcare system has generated tremendous advances over the past 50 years, costs have risen steadily. The United States now ranks as one of the highest in per-capita spending but lags behind other industrialized nations in several standard population health measures, including infant mortality and life expectancy.[18]

In its watershed report *Crossing the Quality Chasm: A New Health System for the 21st Century*, the Institute of Medicine (IOM) recommended a fundamental redesign of the American health care system.[19] Its central tenet—upon which much of health care innovation today is based—is the notion that payment for medical services will eventually be tied to the quality of those services and the benefit that can be shown for both individual patients and the population at large.[20] Compared with the past 40 years of American medicine, this emphasis on quality is a radical idea. Changing the focus from the volume of services to the specific and overall value of those services means that all health care agents are now called upon to link their programs, efforts, and products to measurable outcomes.

Population health programs for older persons hold great promise for being part of this transformation, but will likewise be expected to show demonstrable outcomes in all aspects. Population health programs will be scrutinized for measurable outcomes that may include: better health, increased quality of life, reduced morbidity or mortality, and reductions in overall cost. Aligning population health goals with the goals of other government programs will be important for funding, data analysis, and credibility in an outcomes-driven world.

The 2010 Affordable Care Act (ACA) includes many important demonstration projects and funding streams for testing population health initiatives and models designed to improve care, promote independence, and reduce costs for the Medicare population. Many of these initiatives draw upon a common set of elements from population health models tested in other contexts. These elements include: identifying subpopulations according to risk; promoting wellness and self-care; tailoring interventions to identified subpopulations based on risk assessments; integrating medical and nonmedical community resources to manage patient care; and monitoring health and social status as well as financial outcomes on an ongoing basis.[21] This section reviews the major population health initiatives for Medicare beneficiaries. These include population health approaches used by accountable care organizations, Medicare Advantage managed care organizations, and traditional Medicare fee-for-service beneficiaries.

Accountable Care Organizations (ACOs)

The concept of an accountable care organization (ACO) is attributed to Elliot Fisher, a physician and researcher at the Dartmouth Institute for Health Policy and Clinical Practice.[22] In general, ACOs are groups of hospitals, physicians, and other health care providers that work together to provide high-quality coordinated care to Medicare beneficiaries through a series of financial incentives designed to promote both efficiency and quality.

ACOs were developed as a method of encouraging physician and hospital care coordination by promoting accountability and shared risk among providers. The Centers for Medicare and Medicaid Services (CMS) stated that its intent in developing the ACO program was to promote accountability; improve care coordination; encourage investment in infrastructure; redesign care processes to promote high quality and efficient care delivery; and incentivize value-driven care.[23] ACO participants must define their care coordination processes across physicians and hospitals; develop methods to manage care across an episode of care; describe individualized care programs and how these programs will improve outcomes for high-risk patients and patients with multiple chronic conditions; and describe additional target populations that would benefit from individualized care plans. In many respects, ACOs will have to deploy population health approaches to care management in order to achieve these lofty goals.

There are several ACO models that have been designed and tested, as described in Table 9-1.

Table 9-1. Models for Development of Accountable Care Organizations[24,25]

Model	Characteristics	Current Examples
Integrated Delivery Networks (IDNs)	• Can include hospitals, physician practices, and insurance plans. • Incorporate financial incentives, electronic health records (EHRs), and multidisciplinary care teams.	• Geisinger Health System • Intermountain Healthcare • Kaiser Permanente • Henry Ford Health System
Independent Practice Associations (IPAs)	• Primary care practices that can incorporate medical home principles and structure. • Can have a focus on continuous quality improvement and allow for flexibility in contracting.	• Hill Physicians Medical Group • St. Francis HealthCare Partners • Continucare • Central Oregon Independent Practice Association
Multispecialty Physician Groups (MSPGs)	• May own or be affiliated with hospitals and have arrangements with health plans. • Are led by physicians and coordinate care.	• Cleveland Clinic • Mayo Clinic • Ochsner Clinic
Virtual Physician Organizations	• Small and often independent physician practices in rural areas. • Medicaid-population-focused. • Provide infrastructure for participating practices	• Community Care of North Carolina
Physician-Hospital Organizations (PHOs)	• Operate similar to MSPGs and focus on cost effectiveness. • Create partnerships with physician practices to "serve as a collective risk bearing organization."	• Advocate Health • Scripps Health • Sutter Health

The Medicare Physician Group Practice Demonstration is one of the initial federal efforts that served as a precursor to the ACO demonstrations. This five-year demonstration, which began in 2005, included ten group practices, most of them hospital-affiliated, that received bonus payments if they met certain quality standards and reduced costs by improving care coordination. Under this demonstration, CMS paid providers fee-for-service (FFS) rates, and providers were able to share in any of the Medicare savings achieved on an annual basis. The initial results from this demonstration are mixed; all participants showed improved quality but only some succeeded in reducing costs. At most, only four to five demonstration participants shared in the savings in any one year of the demonstration.[26]

In 2007, the Engelberg Center for Health Care Reform at the Brookings Institute and the Dartmouth Institute for Health Policy and Clinical Practice established an ACO collaborative to begin testing and refining the ACO model. In 2009, the Brookings-Dartmouth ACO Collaborative selected five participants for the program. Each participant agreed to take responsibility for overall quality and cost of care for their patients; partner with a private payer; and have a sufficient patient population to support comprehensive care coordination and performance measurement.* A study was conducted on four of the sites to identify factors that facilitated ACO formation and performance.† The study found that transforming from a fee-for-service environment to a coordinated care model with shared risk took time and required continued adaptation of contract and organizational structures. Another key factor was successful collaborations between providers and payers.[27]

In response to early efforts to form ACOs, section 3022 of the ACA created a permanent voluntary Medicare Shared Savings Program (MSSP), which provides financial incentives for ACOs that reduce health care costs while meeting quality performance standards.[28] CMS released a final regulation detailing the MSSP in November 2011.[29]

The regulation specifies the provider network, eligible beneficiary population, quality standards, and payment incentive structure for the MSSP. For example, the regulation defines ACOs as a group of providers and suppliers of services (e.g., hospitals, physicians, and others involved in patient care) that work together to coordinate care for Medicare fee-for-service (FFS) beneficiaries. These providers and suppliers can include group practice arrangements; networks of individual practices; or partnerships or joint ventures between hospitals and professionals. An ACO must include at least 5,000 Medicare FFS beneficiaries to participate. At the beginning of the demonstration year, CMS provides demonstration participants with a potential list of Medicare FFS beneficiaries assigned to the ACO based on where the beneficiaries receive primary care services. At the end of the demonstration year, each ACO receives a final list of Medicare FFS beneficiaries assigned to the ACO and for which the ACO is responsible for their cost of care.[30] Individual providers and suppliers participating in the MSSP continue to receive Medicare FFS payments. CMS created two risk-sharing tracks to allow providers to earn annual bonus payments from reduced Medicare spending or possibly reimburse

---

* Participants include Norton Healthcare in Louisville, Kentucky; Carilion Clinic in Roanoke, Virginia; Tucson Medical Center and affiliated physician groups in Tucson, Arizona; Monarch HealthCare, based in Irvine, California; and HealthCare Partners, based in Torrance, California.

† Carilion was not included in the study because it did not have a formal relationship with a private payer at the time of the evaluation.

CMS for any losses incurred due to increased Medicare spending compared to their spending targets.

CMS also considers a participant's performance on a set of quality metrics when determining bonus payments.[31] The participants are required to report on a set of 33 quality metrics, including patient/caregiver experience measures (7 measures); care coordination/patient safety measures (6 measures); preventive care measures (8 measures); and measures targeting populations with such chronic diseases as diabetes and heart disease (12 measures).[32]

These quality measures reflect the types of outcomes that population health approaches aspire to achieve. Though the ACO model is still at an early point in the implementation phase, CMS recently released data on ACO performance for five of these quality measures, including: (1) controlling blood sugar levels in patients with diabetes; (2) controlling blood pressure in patients with diabetes; (3) prescribing aspirin to patients with diabetes and heart disease; (4) patients with diabetes who do not use tobacco; and (5) prescribing medicine to improve the pumping action of the heart in patients who have both heart disease and certain other conditions.[33] On average, 67 percent of ACO patients with diabetes maintained a blood pressure below the target, compared with 48 percent and 47 percent percent of Medicare Advantage and Medicare FFS diabetes patients respectively. Sixty-five percent of ACO patients with diabetes maintained a blood sugar level below the target, compared with 64 percent of Medicare Advantage and 63 percent of Medicare FFS diabetes patients.[34] About 75 percent of ACO patients with diabetes avoided tobacco and took aspirin daily, and 70 percent of ACO patients with heart disease were prescribed medicine to relax blood vessels and lower blood pressure. The results varied significantly by individual provider.[35]

To date, CMS has selected over 250 organizations to participate in the ACO program (with 35 participating in the Advance Payment Model).[36] Of the initial 114 ACOs with 12-month data available, nearly half had lower expenditures than expected, and about a quarter of the organizations had lowered spending enough that they were able to share in $126 million in savings.[37]

CMS also created two additional programs which build on the MSSP: the Advance Payment ACO Model and the Pioneer ACO Model. The Advance Payment ACO Model is a subset of the MSSP that receives advance payments that are repaid from future savings earned. This model targets smaller practices and rural providers with less access to capital. From April 2012 through January 2013, CMS selected 35 organizations to participate in the Advance Payment ACO program.[38]

The Pioneer ACO Model targets organizations with significant experience in offering coordinated patient-centered care, and operating in ACO-like arrangements. In the first two years of the demonstration, the Pioneer ACO Model tests a shared savings and losses arrangement with higher levels of risk and reward than the MSSP. In Year Three of the demonstration, Pioneer ACOs can adopt a population-based model, which replaces some or all of their Medicare FFS payments with a per-beneficiary per-month payment. CMS selected 32 organizations to participate in the Pioneer ACO model.[39] Initial results from the Pioneer ACO project showed that participants demonstrated success in improving quality but results varied in reducing costs. Of the 32 Pioneer ACOs, 13 participants shared in savings and two participants shared in losses in the first year of the demonstration. As a result, nine Pioneer ACOs have already withdrawn from the program.[40]

More recently, bipartisan legislation was introduced that builds on the ACO model but has a specific focus on chronically ill beneficiaries. On January 15, 2014, Senators Ron Wyden (D-OR) and Johnny Isakson (R-GA) and Representatives Erik Paulsen (R-MN) and Peter Welch (D-VT) introduced the Better Care, Lower Cost Act of 2014. Similar to ACOs, the goal of this legislation is to encourage specialized team-based care and provide financial incentives to reduce health care costs while improving patient outcomes. Akin to the population-based approach under the Pioneer ACO Model, providers participating in the Better Care Program are paid a set amount for each enrolled beneficiary instead of the current FFS payments.[41]

Population Health Approaches Used by ACOs

ACOs have adopted a number of population health management techniques to improve quality and better coordinate care for specific subpopulations that are at high risk of readmission; have complex chronic conditions; and are generally high-cost and high-utilization beneficiaries.[42] A recent evaluation found that ACOs are using a range of population health and care management strategies, including: 1) utilizing information systems to identify high-risk patients and alert physicians; 2) engaging patients in their care; and 3) transforming care in physicians' offices.

Many ACOs have found that adoption of an electronic health record is a key component of creating an information system to classify high-risk patients and alert physicians. The EHR is essential for data sharing among providers, and facilitates data collection necessary to identify and track high-risk patients. Once

ACOs are able to identify these patients, they can then refer them to disease management programs, education, or counseling. The EHRs can also be used to keep primary care providers informed of their patients' care. For example, the NewHealth ACO Collaborative in Akron, Ohio, uses EHRs to track patients with chronic diseases and create electronic alerts to inform primary care physicians when these patients have been admitted to the hospital and provide status updates.[42]

Patient engagement in care is a second population health management technique frequently used by ACOs. Patient engagement can occur in a number of ways, such as financial incentives, personal health records, post-discharge follow-up, or call centers. For example, Arizona's Connected Care ACO has a transitional care nurse who sees the patient both in the hospital and at home after discharge to improve care coordination by reviewing medications, identifying any additional services needed, and interfacing with the primary care physician if necessary. In addition, Arizona's Connected Care ACO has a patient engagement committee and community educators to continue to engage with patients once they have returned home. The University Hospitals ACO uses financial incentives to engage patients by allowing them to earn money by identifying a primary care physician and participating in health screenings.[42]

Last, many ACOs are using population health management to transform care in physicians' offices. The physicians' offices are transforming their care models through the use of medical homes, care management, and EHRs. For example, the Cheyenne ACO in Wyoming is working toward a "patient-centered medical home neighborhood" by creating a platform to support coordinated care in the community. University Hospitals ACO in Cleveland, Ohio, helps physicians meet their goals for diabetes management and cancer screenings.[42]

Innovations From the Field: Care Management Technology
Phytel Case Study

Phytel, based in Dallas, Texas, develops technology solutions to empower physician-led population health by enabling physicians to deliver timely, coordinated care to their patients. Phytel's registry encompasses more than 30 million patients nationwide and uses evidence-based chronic and preventive care protocols to identify and notify patients due for service, while tracking compliance and measuring quality and financial results.

According to U.S. Census data and the Centers for Disease Control and Prevention, the average primary care physician's panel of 2,500 patients

Innovations From the Field: Care Management Technology

Phytel Case Study

includes 207 patients with diabetes and 162 with heart disease. Unfortunately, primary care staff members have traditionally been unable to focus on these persons with multiple chronic diseases, including maintaining personal contact; coordinating care between multiple specialists; and monitoring of signs, symptoms, or test results on a routine basis.

Healthcare organizations increasingly are turning to technology and automation to produce the best outcomes at an affordable cost. The following is an example of how physician groups are leveraging care management automation technology from Phytel to scale their care management staff and achieve significant improvements in population health.

The largest multispecialty practice in northeastern suburban Atlanta, Northeast Georgia Physicians Group (NGPG), is using Phytel's enterprise care management platform to build a patient-centered medical home and prepare for participation in accountable care organizations (ACOs). The Phytel solution aggregates and normalizes data supplied by the group's electronic health record so that care coordinators can focus on patient care rather than spend time gathering data from patient charts.

NGPG's care managers can launch a variety of automated interventions for different segments of the population, such as offering a glycemic education program to diabetic patients; scheduling patients for missed services; monitoring treatment plans; and using e-mail to communicate and coordinate with these patients. In 2013 NGPG conducted a six-month trial involving 10 clinics, with care managers using the Phytel system on a daily basis to target 860 patients with uncontrolled diabetes. At the end of the trial period, NGPG had helped 412 patients lower their A1c scores below nine points—a decrease in the uncontrolled population of nearly 50 percent. "We are extremely excited by these results," said Antonio Rios, MD, chief physician executive of NGPG. "It's a very strong example of how having the right information can really make a huge difference in improving the health of a population." Phytel has helped other health care systems accomplish similar clinical results. One practice achieved an 87 percent follow-up rate for physician visits; at another practice over 25 percent more patients are seeing their primary care physician; and at a third there was a 14 percent increase in the number of people going for colonoscopies.

Population Health in Medicare Advantage Managed Care Programs

The ACO shared savings demonstration project represents an important testing ground for population health initiatives for the elderly Medicare population. While demonstration projects represent an opportunity for innovation, it is also important to evaluate population health models that are in operation today in other parts of the Medicare program, including the Medicare Part C Medicare Advantage Program.

There has been a recent increase in the proportion of Medicare beneficiaries opting for Medicare private health plan (i.e., Medicare Advantage) coverage. The Medicare Advantage population has almost tripled from 5.3 million beneficiaries in 2003 to 14.4 million beneficiaries in 2013, or from 13 percent of Medicare beneficiaries to 28 percent.[43] Since the beginning of the Medicare Advantage program for Medicare beneficiaries, managed care organizations have been responsible for the medical care of a defined population of beneficiaries. Managed care organizations (MCOs) contract with the Centers for Medicare and Medicaid Services (CMS) to provide a defined package of benefits to members who enroll in managed care plans. MCOs get paid a set amount per member per month to arrange for the provision of care and services covered under the Medicare benefit. If the cost of care for the defined population is greater than the aggregate cost of care per member per month, the MCO loses money. But if the cost of care is less, then the MCO can achieve a profit. Accordingly, MCOs have an incentive to keep costs as low as possible but also must meet certain quality standards to avoid stinting of care.

The Centers for Medicare and Medicaid Services now publishes a rating system to assist beneficiaries in differentiating between the various managed care plans. This "star rating" system assigns one to five stars to managed care plans based on their performance on a set of quality metrics. Plans with five stars are the top performers whereas plans with one star are poor performers. The average star rating is between three and four stars, with only one plan achieving less than two stars. The metrics used to ascertain the star ratings include outcome, patient experience, access, and process measures. Some of the measures target specific populations with chronic diseases, including diabetes and heart disease.[44] Because the star ratings affect Medicare Advantage Plan payments, plans have a strong incentive to meet quality standards.

A 2010 survey showed that many MCOs are deploying population health strategies to improve care and reduce costs.[21] These population health approaches fall into five categories:

1. *Wellness promotion*, including physical activities, smoking cessation and education about healthy living. Wellness promotion also includes identifying subpopulations at risk (such as those with chronic diseases); providing targeted education to reduce risk factors; and intensive personalized care management;

2. *Focus on patients with multiple chronic conditions*, including disease-specific case management; family and caregiver education and support; telephonic monitoring; care coordination between providers; and coordination with social services;

3. *Extra attention for frail older persons*, including remote home monitoring; in-home social worker visits; medication management interventions; alteration of home environments for safety and falls prevention; and access to community social services;

4. *Reduce hospital readmissions*, including medication reconciliation on hospital discharge; home health services; and targeted home monitoring or house calls for the highest-risk patients; and

5. *Provider support and incentives*, including provider education, coordination, and incentive payments for achieving certain quality outcomes such as avoiding high hospitalization rates.

The outcomes of these interventions have not been rigorously studied, though MCO respondents to the survey report reduced initial hospitalizations, emergency room visits, and readmissions.[21]

Other Population Health Approaches in Medicare and Federal Programs

An important trend in population health for older persons in the twenty-first century will be the ongoing shift from institution-based to home-based care. This transition is in agreement with older persons' preferences,[45] and also with numerous studies showing that care in the home can be done effectively for complex and often subacute diseases, medical problems, and episodes.[45] As more care is provided in or around the home, the use of acute and postacute care services will become even more episodic than it is today. Lengths of stay in these institutional settings will continue to decline, and admissions will more likely come only after the full complement of home-based services has been either exhausted or unsuccessful.[46]

Several innovations and federal demonstration projects at the heart of health care reform and population health for older persons have at their core the concept of a medical home. The medical home model is favored by policy makers and leaders in primary care for older persons who propose an interdisciplinary team approach with a highly trained individual (a physician in the case of health care) serving as the "quarterback" or manager of the team. Implicit in this model is the notion that the skill sets of many health care workers overlap, and that highly trained individuals should no longer be doing many of the more routine or manual tasks of care. They should focus instead on highly complex issues and areas for quality improvement and decision making. Population health models for older persons will have to incorporate aspects of the medical home model and assume that vulnerable elders will have teams of health care and social service professionals caring for them in the future. In one recent evaluation of the Southeastern Pennsylvania Chronic Care Initiative—one of the earliest and largest multipayer pilot medical homes—the findings suggest that medical home interventions may need further refinement. These findings indicate that interventions did not result in a statistically significant difference in utilization or cost of care, and achieved greater performance in only one of 11 quality metrics. The researchers do caution that these findings may not generalize to other medical home interventions.[47] Several federally funded innovation projects in Medicare have been designed to further test and promote this medical home concept.

The Federally Qualified Health Center (FQHC) Advanced Primary Care Practice Demonstration tests ways in which the patient-centered medical home model can improve quality of care, promote better health, and lower costs. Specifically, the goal of the demonstration is for its participants to achieve National Committee for Quality Assurance (NCQA) Level 3 recognition as patient-centered medical homes (PCMHs). This goal entails a practice transformation process that strengthens both infrastructure, including information technology systems, and the quality of care. In evaluating this model, the Innovation Center will consider the impact of cost and quality of care for Medicare beneficiaries. Currently, there are 491 FQHCs participating in this demonstration, which includes a semiannual assessment to indicate progress toward achieving NCQA recognition.[48]

The Medicare Medical Home Demonstration allows states to provide targeted, accessible, continuous, and coordinated care to Medicare beneficiaries with chronic or prolonged illnesses requiring regular medical monitoring, advising, or treatment.[49]

The Independence at Home Demonstration is modeled after a medical home program first tested in the Veterans Health Administration (VA). Since the early

1970s, the VA provided home-based primary care (HBPC) services to veterans with complex health care needs for whom routine clinic-based care is not effective. By the mid-1990s, the VA developed standards to make the programs more uniform nationwide. These standards include the composition and responsibilities of the team providing primary care and the target population.[50]

Currently, the VA HBPC program offers participants the following services: primary care visits at home by a physician, nurse practitioner, or physician's assistant; care management through a nurse practitioner, physician's assistant, or nurse; coordination of services by a social worker; therapy visits from a physical, occupational, or speech therapist; mental health services; nutrition counseling; and medication management.[51] The average VA HBPC patient has eight chronic conditions, takes over 12 medications, and is limited in two or more ADLs. This program has expanded from about 7,000 patients in 2000 to about 25,000 patients today. The program has successfully reduced hospital days by 59 percent, nursing home days by 89 percent, and 30-day hospital readmission rates by 21 percent.[50]

Due in part to the success of the VA HBPC program and the growing interest in HBPC services, section 3024 of the ACA created the Independence at Home Demonstration. This is a three-year demonstration designed to use home-based primary care teams to improve health outcomes and reduce expenditures for Medicare beneficiaries with multiple chronic conditions by preventing emergency department visits and inpatient hospitalizations.

Demonstration participants receive Medicare FFS rates and have the potential to earn yearly bonus payments based on the participants' ability to meet quality performance targets and simultaneously reduce overall Medicare expenditures. The demonstration requires participants to meet such staffing and service standards as primary care teams including physician assistants, pharmacists, social workers, and other staff directed by physicians and nurse practitioners. In addition, the participants must have experienced home-based primary care teams able to make in-home visits; be available 24 hours per day, 7 days a week; and provide care to at least 200 eligible beneficiaries using electronic health information systems. Eligibility requirements for beneficiaries include: two or more chronic conditions; Medicare FFS coverage; two or more ADL restrictions; nonelective hospital admission within the last 12 months; and an acute or rehab service in the last 12 months.[52]

The Centers for Medicare and Medicaid Innovation released a call for applicants in December 2011, and selected a total of 18 individual practices and consortia to participate in the demonstration in April 2012 and August 2012 respectively. The individual practices include several visiting physician associations and house call programs; the consortia include the Innovative Primary Senior Care LLC, the Mid-Atlantic Consortium, and the Treasure Coast Healthcare LLC.[52]

The initial results from this demonstration are promising. HouseCall Providers in Portland, Oregon, saw hospital admissions drop from a practice average of 17 percent to 3 percent in the first 15 months of the program. One Independence at Home demonstration participant, the North Shore-LIJ Health System in the greater New York City area, was able to reduce hospital admission rates from about 13 percent to 5 percent. This demonstration participant also succeeded in almost doubling the proportion of patients who receive post-admission contact within 48 hours from 45 percent to 85 percent; and increased the proportion of patients receiving medical reconciliation within 48 hours after discharge from 63 percent to 94 percent.[53]

Innovations from the Field:
Health and Aging Care Accelerators Case Study

The aging global population offers an unparalleled opportunity for academic researchers, entrepreneurs, suppliers, and providers to collaborate. In the recent past the primary focus of both venture capital and research funding has been invested in pharmaceuticals and medical devices. Today a shift in consumer demographics is disrupting every category of health care services and driving the need for innovation. This quest for diffusion of innovation has ignited a multitude of 12-week "boot camp" acceleration programs for emerging companies since 2010. Many of these programs offer a structured process, utilizing the Lean LaunchPad methodology and the Business Model Canvas tool to facilitate the development of new ventures.

In Louisville, Kentucky, InnovateLTC partners with Nucleus to offer the LaunchIt program. The key deliverables include access to a network of mentors; initial customer exploration; developing a business plan with an elevator pitch; and a graduation event pitch for investment funding. Presently there are at least five national accelerator programs on both coasts with a growing percentage of graduates developing solutions that target the age 50+ market sectors.

Based in Louisville, Kentucky, InnovateLTC is a commercialization company that immerses graduates of accelerators and viable later-stage innovative solutions into the 50+ market sectors through a research, validate, and deliver

> ### Innovations from the Field:
> ### Health and Aging Care Accelerators Case Study
>
> methodology. Formed in 2010 through a collaboration of the State of Kentucky, the City of Louisville, the University of Louisville's Nucleus Innovation Center, and Signature HealthCARE, InnovateLTC's vision is to "Enhance both the quality of care and the quality of life for the global aging population through accelerating innovation." Together with several other entities such as the AARP, InnovateLTC has been a leader in organizing and judging at national innovation search competitions specifically aimed at innovative products, service models, and technologies for the longevity economy. Validation testing services for innovative solutions is offered by InnovateLTC through a network of test-track partners, including providers, insurers, universities (e.g., the University of Louisville and the Georgia Tech Research Institute) and consumers living in communities (e.g., the Institute for the Ages in Sarasota, Florida). The Thrive Lab is a 5,200-square-feet center in downtown Louisville slated to go live in late summer 2014. The Thrive Lab will offer simulated living environments, a research platform, programming, and a showcase for corporations, industry providers, and consumers to interact experientially with innovations in aging.
>
> Louisville, Kentucky, has the largest clustering of corporate headquarters in the United States of organizations known as the Lifelong Wellness and Aging Care sector. These organizations generate over $48 billion in annual revenue. Several of the innovations from the field case studies included in this chapter were derived from InnovateLTC's activities.

Population Health for Persons with Multiple Chronic Diseases

Population health approaches for older cohorts must account for the fact that many older people experience chronic conditions, often multiple chronic conditions, as they age.[54] Chronic diseases are long-term illnesses that are rarely cured. Such chronic diseases as heart disease, stroke, cancer, and diabetes are among the most common and costly health conditions.[55] Chronic health conditions can negatively affect an older person's quality of life; may contribute to functional decline; and can ultimately lead to institutionalization if remaining in the community becomes too difficult.[56]

It is estimated that nearly 88 percent of those 65 and over have at least one chronic condition;[57] and by 2020 nearly 157 million Americans (about 50 percent of the population) will experience at least one chronic disease.[58]

Researchers have also repeatedly documented that an increasing number of older persons will experience multiple chronic conditions. In 1999, 48 percent of Medicare beneficiaries had at least three concurrent chronic conditions and 21 percent had five or more chronic conditions.[59] These estimates may actually understate the prevalence of chronic diseases among the elderly because the administrative claims data may fail to capture the full extent of the problem.[60] People with multiple comorbidities experience poor quality of life; have higher degrees of physical and mental disability; use multiple medications; and are heavy users of the medical care system, resulting in high costs.[61] It has been estimated that approximately 10 million older American residents have four or more chronic conditions and live in noninstitutional settings. Within the Medicare program, nearly two-thirds of beneficiaries have at least two chronic conditions, accounting for 95 percent of total Medicare expenditures, while one-fourth of Medicare beneficiaries have four or more chronic conditions and account for almost two-thirds of total Medicare spending.[62]

Population health initiatives designed to improve health and reduce costs for this population must be prioritized and tailored. Researchers emphasize that effective population health approaches must identify patients with multiple chronic diseases and apply interventions designed to address the unique needs of this population. Unfortunately, efforts to develop clinical practice guidelines and other population health approaches for managing the care of this population were not developed until recently, or modified to address the needs of patients with multiple chronic illnesses or co-morbidities.[63] Instead, the more typical approach used by primary care physicians and others has been a "single-disease" approach, in which a patient's predominant medical condition, often a chronic illness, is identified and used to develop clinical practice guidelines to address that one condition. Comorbid complications are addressed only as an ancillary consideration to this traditional approach.[62]

Researchers have highlighted four fundamental shortcomings in this single diagnosis approach to primary care and population health considerations for a multi-comorbid older population:

(1) Most primary care physicians and many other health professionals have not been trained to work in teams to provide complex chronic care;

(2) Such sophisticated health information technologies as interoperative electronic health records, telemonitoring devices, and patient portals that could facilitate the essential processes of chronic care are not widely installed;

(3) Most current public and private health insurers' payment policies, which are based on fee-for-service payments, do not support the supplemental

services provided by the newer models for providing complex chronic care; and

(4) Payment for and provision of medical and social services are separate and not integrated.[63]

Boult and Wieland recently reviewed the effectiveness of population health models for chronically ill older persons, specifically their effectiveness in maintaining and improving health and well-being; reducing hospitalizations; and lowering health care spending. Three models were reviewed[63] and found to have the following common elements:

1. Comprehensive assessment of each patient to identify conditions, needs, and patient preferences;
2. Development of a comprehensive care plan based on validated clinical practice guidelines and protocols to guide practitioners in the delivery and evaluation of care;
3. Consistent implementation of the care plan over time, with appropriate modifications made to account for improved or deteriorating conditions or changed circumstances;
4. Ongoing monitoring of care plan implementation and patient adherence to the care plan for areas that require the patient's active participation in care;
5. Close coordination of care among all health providers involved in the patients' care, including inpatient, outpatient, primary, and specialty care as well as all the provider institutions involved in the patients' care; and
6. Careful management of transitions of care between health care settings, social service agencies, private support networks, and home environments.

These three models varied in their effectiveness; however, further review of them is instructive as we look to design and implement population models for the future.

The Geriatric Resources for Assessment and Care of Elders (GRACE) model was designed to provide primary health care and support services for an older low-income population to improve quality of care and reduce costs.[64] In the GRACE model, primary care physicians combined with interdisciplinary teams to conduct periodic assessments of patients, provide comprehensive primary care, and supplement this care with a variety of long-term support services not typically covered under the Medicare benefit. The GRACE program was evaluated in a randomized clinical trial and produced the following process outcomes: higher rates of flu vaccination; increased primary care visits after hospitalization; receipt of medication management lists; and higher rates of adoption of advance directives. In terms of outcomes after two years, there were no differences in functional outcome improvement measures, days spent in bed, or satisfaction with care, but there was substantial improvement in certain measures of mental functioning. The total cost of care was no different between the control and intervention groups, though Year 3 costs were lower, and costs related to hospitalizations were lower, especially for a subgroup of participants identified as at high risk of such costs. In addition, the costs for preventive and chronic care were higher for those in the intervention group.

Another population health approach for older persons with chronic diseases is called guided care. Like the GRACE program, guided care primary care physicians partner with registered nurses to provide intensive high-touch primary care to patients identified as being at high risk of using health care services in the coming year. In addition to providing primary care, the nurses are active in educating patients about healthy living and encouraging them to

> . . . engage in productive health-related behaviors by helping them to create personal action plans, referring them to 6-session chronic disease self-management courses, and using motivational interviewing during their monthly contacts.[63]

In addition to intensive patient interaction, the nurses also assess and interact with family members and other caregivers and agencies to ensure coordinated interdisciplinary care. An evaluation of guided care pursuant to a randomized clinical trial found that both patients and caregivers rated quality of care as higher compared to a control group, though caregiver depression did not differ between the two groups. Physician satisfaction and knowledge of patient condition was also higher for guided care patients, though physician ratings of other aspects of care did not differ between the groups. In terms of cost, Leff et al. found a trend towards lower health care utilization and lower costs, but the differences were not statistically significant.[65] Another study found that guided care covered not only its own costs but also reduced insurance expenditures by $1,600 per patient per year.[66]

A third population health approach is called the program of all-inclusive care for the elderly, or PACE. PACE uses many of the same approaches as GRACE and guided care, but differs in terms of the population served; the scope and frequency of services provided; and how the program is financed. PACE serves dual-eligible patients if they have been deemed appropriate for nursing home care but are able to live in the community with the supports and services provided by the PACE program. As such, PACE participants are medically complex, functionally impaired, and low-income, and typically have disabilities that are permanent and irreversible. From a population health perspective, therefore, an important goal of the PACE program is to prevent decline into chronic disease with complications as opposed to preventing the onset of chronic disease. PACE sites provide a more comprehensive array of medical and support programs than other population health approaches, including:

> . . . primary, specialty, emergency, hospital, home, palliative, and institutional long term care, case management, prescription drugs, dentistry, laboratory tests, radiology, adult day care, transportation, prosthetics, durable medical equipment, meals; and for family caregivers, respite, education and support.[63]

This comprehensive set of services is made possible because of the way PACE is financed. Each PACE site functions as a managed care plan, with funding coming from combined Medicare and Medicaid payments per PACE participant at levels that would otherwise have been spent on these beneficiaries if the PACE program did not exist.[63]

Though no randomized clinical trials have been conducted to evaluate the PACE program, several cohort and cross-sectional studies have reported preliminary findings. One study reported significantly lower hospital admissions overall, reduced preventable hospital admissions, and reduced preventable emergency room visits among PACE participants as compared with matched community-dwelling elders.[67] A 12-month cohort study compared PACE participants with patients in a Medicaid managed care plan and found that the PACE participants had fewer hospitalizations and shorter lengths of stay,[68] while a five-year cohort study found longer survival among PACE participants with a high risk of mortality as compared with a matched community group receiving nurse support services.[69]

Innovations From the Field: Effectively Managing Care Transitions across Sites of Care in an Integrated Health System
Kindred Healthcare Case Study

Kindred Healthcare is the largest provider of postacute services in the United States and is actively involved in population health initiatives for older adults. Postacute care refers to health care, rehabilitation, and social services provided to Medicare, Medicare Advantage, and other elderly patients *after* they are discharged from a community hospital and need continuing care and services in such settings as skilled nursing facilities, inpatient rehabilitation hospitals, long-term acute care hospitals, home health, and hospice. Though there are few

Innovations From the Field: Effectively Managing Care Transitions across Sites of Care in an Integrated Health System
Kindred Healthcare Case Study

incentives under today's payment systems for providers of different postacute services to coordinate care across settings, Kindred is in a unique position to test different models of coordinated care for patients through their integrated care markets.

Today Kindred is the largest provider of diversified care across the full postacute continuum, serving over 500,000 postacute care patients each year, with:

- 2,109 postacute service settings in 46 states nationwide
- 116 long-term care hospitals (LTCHs)
- 109 hospital-based and freestanding inpatient rehabilitation facilities (IRFs)
- 106 skilled nursing and rehabilitation facilities (SNFs)
- 2,051 rehabilitation sites providing inpatient and outpatient rehabilitative care
- 105 home health and hospice agencies

To prepare for the time when payment is linked to quality of services and the effective coordination of those services, Kindred has developed a three-step approach to incorporating population health approaches into its care at the local level, as illustrated in Figure 9-1.

Step One: Develop the full continuum of postacute services in local integrated care markets;

Step Two: Provide care management services to support a population health management approach for patients throughout an episode of care from hospital to home; and

Step Three: Test and implement "pay for value" and risk-based payment models.

Kindred has developed a patient-centered care management model, as illustrated in Figure 9-2. It includes key enablers of effective care coordination and improved outcomes: physician coverage across sites of care; care managers to ensure safe transitions; a health information exchange (HIE) to promote information sharing and connectivity; mechanisms that aid in appropriate patient placement and determine the appropriate length of stay; and condition-specific clinical programs, pathways, and quality measures.

The ability to have information for clinical teams *within* Kindred care settings—and to transmit information across sites of care with other providers in the continuum—is a critical element of effective care management over an episode of care. Kindred has invested in a multiyear plan to install and link electronic

Innovations From the Field: Effectively Managing Care Transitions across Sites of Care in an Integrated Health System
Kindred Healthcare Case Study

health records across all care settings. Concurrently, Kindred is developing a health information exchange [HIE], as illustrated in Figure 9-3 to facilitate the sharing of electronic patient data between Kindred sites of care and with external healthcare partners.

Figure 9-1. Steps to Advance Care and Payment Integration

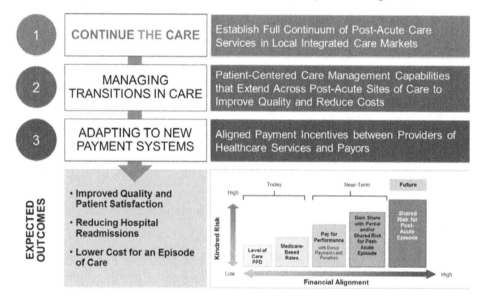

Figure 9-2. Kindred Patient-centered Population Health and Medical Home Model

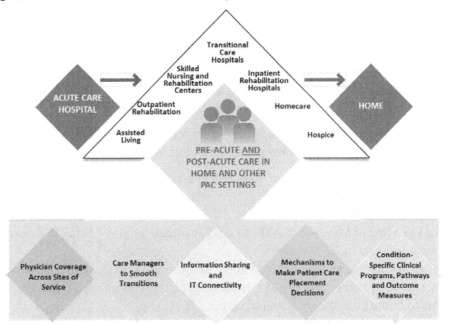

Figure 9-3. Kindred's Health Information Exchange

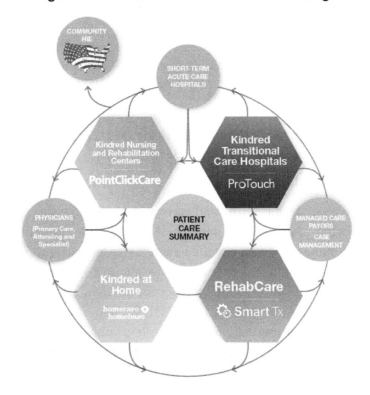

Innovations From the Field: Effectively Managing Care Transitions across Sites of Care in an Integrated Health System

Kindred Healthcare Case Study

Unfortunately, postacute care (PAC) providers were not eligible to receive federal stimulus funding for electronic health record (EHR) adoption, which has resulted in lower EHR adoption rates among PAC providers.

To date the Kindred integrated care management model has improved patient outcomes and lowered costs in key areas, including:

Reduced Rehospitalizations: From 2008 to 2012, rehospitalizations from Kindred LTCHs were reduced by more than 8 percent, and by nearly 12 percent from Kindred SNFs.

Reduced Lengths of Stay: From 2008 to 2012, average lengths of stay in Kindred SNFs were reduced by 27 percent.

Increased Discharges to Home: Since 2008, Kindred SNFs discharged 32 percent more patients to home; and in 2012, our LTCHs discharged nearly 70 percent of patients to home or to a lower level of care.

Functional Improvement Gains: In 2012, Kindred therapists were able to help patients achieve more than 78 percent improved function and independence from what they were able to do prior to admission.

As part of an effort to deliver coordinated postacute care in local communities, Kindred has been actively involved with ACOs, including Pioneer and Initial Shared Savings Plan programs, as well as managed care organizations to implement these population health strategies.[70]

Population Health for Medicare and Medicaid Dual Eligible Populations and Institutionalized Populations

Dual Eligible Populations

Older persons eligible for both Medicare and Medicaid—the so-called dual eligible population—bear a heavy burden of functional limitations and chronic diseases. More than half of dual eligible beneficiaries have at least one activity of daily living (ADL) limitation, compared with about a quarter of the nondual eligible Medicare population. A large proportion of dual eligibles have multiple limitations: nearly 40 percent of patients in this group have three or more ADL limitations. Dual eligible populations suffer higher rates of cognitive impairment (20–25 percent), diabetes (34 percent), hypertension (66 percent), heart failure (24 percent), and ischemic heart disease (35 percent) than Medicare-only beneficiaries. Because of these challenges, this population is over four times more likely to reside in an institution than the Medicare-only population.[71]

Policy makers and health advocates alike have long been concerned that care for dual eligible beneficiaries was poorly coordinated and inefficient due to the conflicting financial incentives between the Medicare and Medicaid programs. Early efforts at reforming care coordination in this population have demonstrated that improved quality could be achieved by better managing care, but results varied on reducing spending. For example, participants in PACE received a capitated payment in exchange for covering the cost of Medicare and long-term services and supports for dually eligible beneficiaries enrolled in the program.* Evaluations of the PACE program demonstrated decreased hospitalizations, comparable Medicare spending, and increased Medicaid spending. The LifeMasters program, a CMS disease management/care coordination demonstration that targeted dual eligible beneficiaries with chronic diseases, showed no effects on hospitalization or gross Medicare costs. The dual eligible Special Needs Plans (D-SNPs; Medicare Advantage plans that target dual eligible enrollees) in California have demonstrated improved costs and reduced readmissions for certain areas in California.[72]

There are about 9.2 million dual eligible beneficiaries with health care spending of about $272 billion. Dual eligible beneficiaries make up about 19 percent of Medicare beneficiaries, but account for 34 percent of Medicare spending. Likewise only 14 percent of Medicaid beneficiaries are dual eligible, but this group accounts for 34 percent of Medicaid spending overall. The dual eligible beneficiaries over age 65 comprise about 60 percent of dual eligible beneficiaries and spend about $169 billion. The remainder of the dual eligible population is primarily lower-income disabled individuals under age 65 who are able to qualify for both Medicare and Medicaid. More than half the spending comes from Medicare: $101 billion is Medicare spending and $67 billion is Medicaid spending.[70]

This disproportionate level of spending can be explained when Medicare spending levels for dual eligible and non-dual eligible Medicare beneficiaries are compared. For example, about 28 percent of the dual eligible population utilizes inpatient hospital services whereas only 18 percent of the Medicare-only population does. In addition, the average per-user spending for inpatient

---

* Eligible individuals were dual eligible beneficiaries living in the community or in nursing homes with significant activities of daily living (ADL) limitations.

hospital services is over $18,000 for dual eligible beneficiaries and over $15,000 for non-dual eligible Medicare beneficiaries. Almost 60 percent of dual eligible spending is on inpatient hospital and other outpatient care (e.g., physician, DME, hospital outpatient).[70]

Section 2602 of the ACA established the Medicare-Medicaid Coordination Office. The purpose of this office is to integrate Medicare and Medicaid benefits more effectively and improve coordination between the federal government and the states for dual eligible beneficiaries.

On July 8, 2011, CMS's Medicare-Medicaid Coordination Office released a State Medicaid Directors' letter to elicit interest in a new dual eligible initiative. The goal of the Financial Alignment Initiative is to test new payment and service delivery models that reduce Medicare and Medicaid spending while sustaining or improving quality of care. The Financial Alignment Initiative expects to achieve these goals by simplifying administrative processes, eliminating regulatory conflicts, and discouraging cost shifting between the Medicare and Medicaid programs.

The Dual Eligible Demonstration required interested states to submit a letter of intent to participate in this initiative. Of the states that submitted letters of intent, 26 submitted proposals.[73] To date, eight states have finalized memoranda of understanding (MOUs) to participate in the capitated model (California, Illinois, Massachusetts, New York, Ohio, South Carolina, Virginia, and Washington); one for the managed fee-for-service model (Washington); and one (Minnesota) for an alternative model.[74,*]

At root, states choosing to participate in the Financial Alignment Initiative will have to deploy population health strategies to effectively manage the care for this chronically ill and expensive population. It is too early to identify precisely which population health approaches states and their managed care partners will deploy, but private sector innovations from the field are already supporting these initiatives.

---

[*] The alternative model integrates Medicare skilled nursing facility programs with state Medicaid programs for dual eligibles without guaranteeing a certain level of savings.

Innovations From the Field: Dual Eligible Care Transitions
Integritas Dual Eligible Case Study

The Integritas is a transitional medical services provider group focused on serving dual eligible elderly residents who primarily reside in skilled nursing facilities (SNFs). The company has practitioners in seven states; partners with six different long-term care organizations; and makes approximately 5,500 patient encounters per month. A typical Integritas practitioner will make 10–18 visits per day. In 2013 the company filed for and successfully met the criteria to receive first-year payment in the Medicare and Medicaid Electronic Health Record (EHR) Incentive Program utilizing the Medicaid EHR Program route. Integritas invested in a certified EHR system with mobile connectivity and provided tablets to all their practitioners. The mobile EHR platform increases the accuracy of their documentation; enables timely connectivity to integrate external diagnostic test results; offers remote access to support call coverage; and integrates data for outcome-based reporting. Where Integritas has a full-time practitioner providing medical services to residents, they have observed a steady decline in unnecessary returns of recently discharged patients to acute care. The EHR also allows Integritas to pinpoint educational needs for patients, families, and their own staff.

Forming trusting relationships with patients is also an Integritas goal, and the mobile EHR system has allowed them to expand their program into patient homes and assisted living facilities, and to manage transitions from acute care over a 90-day interval. This transition management is increasingly important, as acute care hospitals are now penalized for patients who are rehospitalized.

Given ongoing legislative actions by various states to expand the roles of nurse practitioners and physician assistants, and a large unmet need for access to primary care services, especially for the elderly population, the Integritas model is well positioned to provide needed services in a mobile, effective, and integrated way.

Institutionalized Populations

There are over 15,000 nursing facilities nationwide, and at any time up to 2.2 million Americans are receiving their daily care in such facilities.[71] This population requires assistance in multiple activities of daily living (ADLs) on a daily basis, and is at high risk of such adverse health outcomes as falls, malnutrition, pressure ulcers, and multiple hospitalizations at or near the end of life. As this group represents high utilizers of in-hospital services and are frequently readmitted to acute care hospitals after discharge, efforts to reduce adverse outcomes and reduce potentially avoidable hospitalizations have been under way for several years.

Innovations From the Field: Reducing Unnecessary Hospitalizations
INTERACT 2 Case Study

The Interventions to Reduce Acute Care Transfers (INTERACT™) is a quality improvement program that has been adopted by hundreds of nursing facilities throughout the United States.[75] INTERACT[76] is designed to decrease unnecessary hospitalizations among nursing home residents using five key strategies:

(1) Principles of quality improvement, including measurement, tracking, and benchmarking of clearly defined outcomes with feedback to all staff; and root-cause analyses of hospitalizations.

(2) Early identification and evaluation of changes in a patient's condition before they become severe enough to require hospital transfer.

(3) Management of common changes in condition when such management is safe and feasible without hospital transfer.

(4) Improved advance care planning and use of palliative or hospice care when appropriate and the choice of the resident (or their health care proxy) as an alternative to hospitalization.

(5) Improved communication and documentation within the nursing home; between the nursing home staff and families; and between the nursing home and the hospital.

INTERACT was initially tested in a collaborative quality improvement project involving 30 nursing homes in three states (Florida, New York, and Massachusetts).[77] Among the 25 homes that completed the project and for which baseline and intervention hospitalization rate data were available, there was a 17 percent reduction in all-cause hospitalizations; among the 17 homes rated by the project team (masked to hospitalization rates) as "engaged," the reduction was 24 percent.

Following its initial success, INTERACT was revised by a group of national experts in nursing home care; INTERACT Version 3.0 tools are now available free for clinical use at http://interact.fau.edu. The newer version of the program is currently undergoing rigorous evaluation in a randomized, controlled quality improvement implementation project involving approximately 250 nursing homes. The project is supported by the National Institute of Nursing Research of the National Institutes of Health.

Innovations From the Field: Reducing Risk of Pressure Sores
Signature HealthCARE Case Study

Despite decades of effort on the part of nursing home clinicians, pressure ulcers remain a scourge of long-term care, causing suffering and pain for residents, and contributing to complicated medicolegal issues for providers. It is estimated that over 21 percent of individuals in long-term care facilities for a minimum of two years will experience at least one pressure ulcer over the course of their stay. Eleven percent of patients with stage 1 pressure ulcers progress to a more advanced stage.

Routine and regular repositioning has been shown to decrease the incidence of pressure ulcers. The BAM™ Labs TLC Smart Bed Technology is a noninvasive device used to track position changes. The BAM™TM Labs TLC Smart Bed comprises a commercially available mat that has been fitted with a highly sensitive transducer which collects any movement while the resident is in bed. As the resident breathes or moves, motions detected by the sensor are transmitted wirelessly to a cloud-based program in which they are filtered, analyzed, and returned to the caregiver on a mobile device. Caregivers are able to review a resident's heart rate, breathing rate trends, and the intensity and duration of movement.

The BAM™ position change application enables caregivers to set an individual resident's turn schedule; then record the directional position changes, (right, left, up); determine the time elapsed since the last position change; and receive automated reminders for the next position change. Whether the turn was actually done, missed, late, or falsely recorded can also be captured. The data generated help to improve turn compliance by providing real-time feedback to certified nurse assistants and senior staff.

Initial studies have been promising. Over a 12-week period, use of BAM™ systems resulted in better compliance from staff for turning patients, from 13.0 percent to over 48 percent. BAM™ Labs is partnering with InnovateLTC to bring the BAM Labs TLC Smart Bed technology to a wider market.

Signature HealthCARE, based in Louisville, Kentucky, is a leading provider of services operating approximately 100 communities in nine states, primarily in the Southeast. In addition to skilled nursing facilities, Signature has diversified operations that include home health, community-based services, medical services, and a critical access hospital. Their organizational culture is based on three pillars: learning, spirituality, and intra-preneurship.

Goodmark Medical, LLC,™ based in Orlando, Florida, was established to identify and commercialize new, unique, and innovative products and services for the healthcare markets. Goodmark's mission is to build and sustain medical market

Part III. Policy Implications and Conclusion

Policy Implications of Population Health for the Elderly

Population health initiatives for older persons hold great promise for improving quality of care, promoting lifelong wellness, enhancing quality of life, and reducing the cost of health care. The projected demographic wave of older persons—the "silver tsunami"— in the United States compels a concerted effort to identify those population health strategies tailored to the unique needs of an older population that are effective, so that limited public resources can be appropriately targeted. We have documented the extensive public sector support for population health through the ACA and other federal mechanisms. We have also described exciting innovations from the field that are led by the private sector. These activities must be accompanied by a robust research agenda regarding population health programs for older persons to analyze rigorously what works and what does not. Specifically, as discussed in this chapter, research should systematically test and evaluate different population health approaches based on the unique characteristics, needs, resources, and capabilities of subsets of this population—from independent community-dwellers, to those with multiple chronic conditions, to people living in institutions.

For their part, policy makers should focus on aspects of our current payment and care delivery system that inhibit the implementation of effective population health approaches by adopting a HiAP approach. For example, the current Medicare fee-for-service payment system contains disincentives for providers to coordinate care across settings, resulting in lower quality, a higher number of hospital readmissions, and higher costs. Policy makers should incrementally adopt policies that promote care coordination and reward providers for the value rather than the volume of services provided. In addition, there is a disparate set of quality metrics used across the Medicare program that makes it difficult to compare outcomes. MedPAC has been discussing the feasibility of using a small set of population-based quality measures to compare quality across fee-for-service Medicare, Medicare Advantage plans, and Medicare ACOs.[78] By making outcomes more comparable, evaluators will be able to compare the effectiveness of population health programs across Medicare. Likewise, policy makers should continue to fund such innovations as the use of EHRs in population health, and extend funding to all providers, including postacute providers, so that adoption of EHRs is more widespread.

While technology and innovation are key enablers of effective population health initiatives, ultimately success will also depend critically on an adequate, well-trained, and well-paid workforce. It is well documented that there is a current and projected shortage of primary care physicians to lead such population health strategies as patient-centered medical homes.[79] Initiatives to support the training of more primary care physicians (including geriatricians) are necessary but not sufficient to advance population health efforts. Expanding the scope of practice for such other providers as advanced nurse practitioners, physician assistants, registered nurses, pharmacists, and others will also be necessary to meet the growing demand for services for the older population. Likewise, such other personnel as mental health professionals, care managers, and aides play a critical role; they must also be trained and supported as part of a comprehensive effort to construct an adequate workforce to advance population health for the elderly.

Conclusion

It is vitally important to empower older people themselves, their families, and social support systems for population health to realize its potential to improve care, improve quality of life, and reduce costs. For older persons with intact cognitive abilities, education about healthy living, prevention, adherence to care guidelines, and medication compliance has proven to be effective, such as in the guided care model reviewed in this chapter.[66] Even for cognitively impaired older persons, targeted interventions can facilitate participation in care and informed health care decision making.[80] Including family caregivers and other sources of social support is likewise important for population health for older persons, with a particular focus on caregiver burnout, as caregivers are often older and sometimes frail themselves. Therefore, policymakers should ensure that both health and social support services are included in population health approaches for all older persons.

CHAPTER 9 DISCUSSION QUESTIONS

Discussion questions are provided for team building or class exercises. Answers for all questions are provided in Appendix C.

Question Number	Question
1	Describe why it is important to take into account the unique physical, mental, and psychosocial characteristics of older persons when designing population health approaches.
2	Describe the goals of population health interventions for older persons in general, including goals for those with chronic diseases.
3	Describe at least two innovations from the private sector that you think are key enablers of effective care management, and why.
4	What are some limitations identified by researchers in population health approaches for an older population?
5	Discuss some of the policy implications of population health for an elderly population.

CHAPTER 9 SUMMARY

- It is axiomatic that the geriatric population in America is large and growing as the Baby Boomer generation enters retirement and medical advances continue to extend life span. Population health approaches for an older population must consider this population's needs for assistance in performing normal functions; the gender, ethnic, and racial composition of this population; and sources of health care spending, as interventions must be tailored to meet the needs of the elderly population.

- Population health programs for older persons hold great promise for being part of the transformation of Medicare from a volume-driven to a value-driven system; but will likewise be expected to show demonstrable outcomes. The ACA includes many important demonstration projects and funding streams for testing population health initiatives and models designed to improve care, promote independence, and reduce costs for the Medicare population.

- An important trend of population health for older persons in the twenty-first century will be the ongoing shift from institution-based to home-based care. Several innovations and federal demonstration projects related to health care reform and population health for older persons have, at their core, the concept of a medical home, which facilitates home-based care.

- Population health approaches for older cohorts must account for the fact that many older people experience chronic conditions, often multiple chronic conditions, as they age. Researchers emphasize that effective population health approaches must identify patients with multiple chronic diseases and apply interventions designed to address the unique needs of this population.

- Older persons eligible for both Medicare and Medicaid—the dual eligible population—bear a heavy burden of functional limitations and chronic diseases. Policy makers and health advocates alike have long been concerned that care for dual eligible beneficiaries was poorly coordinated and inefficient due to the conflicting financial incentives between the Medicare and Medicaid programs. Early efforts to reform care coordination for this population have demonstrated that improved quality could be achieved by better managing care, but results varied on reducing spending.

- This chapter has documented the extensive public and private sector support for population health initiatives. These population health activities must be accompanied by a robust research agenda to rigorously analyze what works and what does not. Policy makers should attempt to address aspects of our current payment and care delivery system that inhibit the implementation of effective population health approaches.

CHAPTER 9 REFERENCES

1. World Health Organization. Preamble to the Constitution of the World Health Organization. Geneva, Switzerland: World Health Organization;2002:61-66.

2. Federal Interagency Forum on Aging-Related Statistics. *Older Americans 2012: key indicators of well-being (Older Americans 2012).* Hyattsville, Md.: Federal Interagency Forum on Aging-Related Statistics;2012. p. 2 and Indicator 1.

3. Federal Interagency Forum on Aging-Related Statistics. *Older Americans 2012: key indicators of well-being (Older Americans 2012).* Hyattsville, Md.: Federal Interagency Forum on Aging-Related Statistics;2012. p. 26 and Indicator 15.

4. James BD, Leurgans SE, Hebert LE, Scherrr PA, Yaffe, K.,, Bennett DA. Contribution of Alzheimer disease to mortality in the United States. *Neurology.* 2014;10:1212.

5. Katz S. Assessing self-maintenance: activities of daily living, mobility and instrumental activities of daily living. *J Am Geriatr Soc.* 1983;31(12):721-726.

6. Federal Interagency Forum on Aging-Related Statistics. *Older Americans 2012: key indicators of well-being (Older Americans 2012).* Hyattsville, Md.: Federal Interagency Forum on Aging-Related Statistics;2012. p. 32 and Indicator 20.

7. Federal Interagency Forum on Aging-Related Statistics. *Older Americans 2012: key indicators of well-being (Older Americans 2012).* Hyattsville, Md.: Federal Interagency Forum on Aging-Related Statistics;2012. pp. 46-47 and Indicator 28.

8. Federal Interagency Forum on Aging-Related Statistics. *Older Americans 2012: key indicators of well-being (Older Americans 2012).* Hyattsville, Md.: Federal Interagency Forum on Aging-Related Statistics;2012. p. 3 and Indicator 1.

9. Federal Interagency Forum on Aging-Related Statistics. *Older Americans 2012: Key indicators of well-being (Older Americans 2012).* Hyattsville, Md.: Federal Interagency Forum on Aging-Related Statistics;2012. p. 8 and Indicator 5.

10. Federal Interagency Forum on Aging-Related Statistics. *Older Americans 2012: key indicators of well-being (Older Americans 2012).* Hyattsville, Md.: Federal Interagency Forum on Aging-Related Statistics;2012. p. 4 and Indicator 2.

11. Federal Interagency Forum on Aging-Related Statistics. *Older Americans 2012: key indicators of well-being (Older Americans 2012).* Hyattsville, Md.: Federal Interagency Forum on Aging-Related Statistics;2012. pp. 52-53 and Indicator 30.

12. Federal Interagency Forum on Aging-Related Statistics. *Older Americans 2012: key indicators of well-being (Older Americans 2012).* Hyattsville, Md.: Federal Interagency Forum on Aging-Related Statistics;2012. p. 53 and Indicator 30.

13. Federal Interagency Forum on Aging-Related Statistics. *Older Americans 2012: key indicators of well-being (Older Americans 2012).* Hyattsville, Md.: Federal Interagency Forum on Aging-Related Statistics;2012. p. 57 and Indicator 33.

14. Federal Interagency Forum on Aging-Related Statistics. *Older Americans 2012: key indicators of well-being (Older Americans 2012).* Hyattsville, Md.: Federal Interagency Forum on Aging-Related Statistics;2012. p. 13 and Indicator 8.

15. Federal Interagency Forum on Aging-Related Statistics. *Older Americans 2012: key indicators of well-being (Older Americans 2012).* Hyattsville, Md.: Federal Interagency Forum on Aging-Related Statistics;2012. p. 66.

16. Riley GF, Lubitz JD. Long-term trends in medicare payments in the last year of life. *Health Serv Res.* 2010;45(2):565-576.

17. Federal Interagency Forum on Aging-Related Statistics. *Older Americans 2012: key indicators of well-being (Older Americans 2012).* Hyattsville, Md.: Federal Interagency Forum on Aging-Related Statistics;2012. p. 115 and Indicator 15.

18. WHO Department of Health Statistics and Informatics. *World health statistics 2013.* Geneva, Switzerland: World Health Organization;2013:132-141.

19. Insitute of Medicine.. *Crossing the quality chasm: a new health system for the 21st century.* Washington, D.C.: National Academies Press;2001.

20. Berwick DM. Launching accountable care organizations—the proposed rule for the Medicare Shared Savings Program. *N Engl J Med.* 2011;364(16).

21. Tompkins C, Higgins A, Perloff J, Veselovskiy, G. Population health management in Medicare Advantage. *Health Aff Blog.* http://healthaffairs.org/blog/2013/04/02/population-health-management-in-medicare-advantage/. Accessed May 16, 2014.

22. Berenson RA, Robert Wood Johnson Foundation. Next steps for ACOs: will this new approach to health care delivery live up to the dual promises of reducing costs and improving quality of care? 2012; http://healthaffairs.org/healthpolicybriefs/brief_pdfs/healthpolicybrief_61.pdf.

23. Centers for Medicare and Medicaid Services. Shared Savings Program. 2014; http://www.cms.gov/Medicare/Medicare-Fee-for-Service-Payment/sharedsavingsprogram/index.html?redirect=/sharedsavingsprogram. Accessed March 27, 2014.

24. Shortell SM, Casalino LP, Fisher ES. How the Center for Medicare and Medicaid Innovation should test accountable care organizations. *Health Aff (Millwood).* 2010;29(7):1293-1298.

25. Flareau BF, Yale K, Bohn JM, Konschak C. Chapter 3. The lens of leadership. *Clinical integration: a roadmap to accountable care.* Virginia Beach, Va.: Convurgent Publishing;2011:59-72.

26. Centers for Medicare and Medicaid Services. Medicare Physician Group Practice Demonstration: Physician groups continue to improve quality and generate savings under Medicare Physician Pay-for-Performance Demonstration. Washington, D.C.: Centers for Medicare and Medicaid Services; July 2011.

27. Larson BK, Van Citters AD, Kreindler SA, et al. Insights from transformations under way at four Brookings-Dartmouth accountable care organization pilot sites. *Health Aff (Millwood).* 2012;31(11).

28. Office of the Legislative Counsel for the U.S. House of Representatives. Patient Protection and Affordable Care Act: Health-related portions of the Health Care and Education Reconciliation Act of 2010. Washington, DC: U.S. House of Representatives;2010.

29. Centers for Medicare and Medicaid Services. Medicare Program; Medicare Shared Savings Program: Accountable Care Organizations; Final Rule. http://www.gpo.gov/fdsys/pkg/FR-2011-11-02/html/2011-27461.htm. Accessed June 10, 2014.

30. Robert Wood Johnson Foundation. *Health policy snapshot: what are accountable care organizations and how could they improve health care quality?* Princeton, N.J.: Robert Wood Johnson Foundation;2011.

31. Centers for Medicare and Medicaid Services. Summary of final rule provision for accountable care organizations under the Medicare Shared Savings Program. 2012; http://www.cms.gov/Medicare/Medicare-Fee-for-Service-Payment/sharedsavingsprogram/Downloads/ACO_Summary_Factsheet_ICN90 7404.pdf. Accessed March 27, 2014.

32. Centers for Medicare and Medicaid Services. Accountable Care Organization 2013 Program Analysis: quality performance standards narrative measure specifications. Baltimore, Md.: Centers for Medicare and Medicaid Services;2012.

33. Centers for Medicare and Medicaid Services. Quality data added to Physician Compare website [press release]. Baltimore, Md.: Centers for Medicare and Medicaid Services;2014.

34. National Committee for Quality Assurance. Improving quality and patient experience: the state of health care quality 2013. [press release]. Washington, D.C.: National Committee for Quality Assurance;2013.

35. Rau, J.. Medicare data show wide differences in ACOs' patient care [press release]. *Kaiser Health News*, February 21, 2014. http://www.kaiserhealthnews.org/stories/2014/february/21/medicare-data-shows-wide-differences-in-acos-patient-care.aspx?referrer=. Accessed March 27, 2014.

36. Centers for Medicare and Medicaid Services. Fast facts:All Medicare Shared Savings Program ACOs;2013. http://www.cms.gov/Medicare/Medicare-Fee-for-Service-Payment/sharedsavingsprogram/Downloads/All-Starts-MSSP-ACO.pdf. Accessed March 27, 2014.

37. Department of Health and Human Services. Medicare's delivery system reform initiatives achieve significant savings and quality improvements—off to a strong start. 2014; http://www.hhs.gov/news/press/2014pres/01/20140130a.html. Accessed March 27, 2014.

38. Centers for Medicare and Medicaid Services. Advance Payment Accountable Care Organization (ACO) Model. 2013; http://innovation.cms.gov/Files/fact-sheet/Advanced-Payment-ACO-Model-Fact-Sheet.pdf. Accessed March 27, 2014, 2014.

39. Centers for Medicare and Medicaid Services. Pioneer Accountable Care Organization Model. 2012; http://innovation.cms.gov/Files/fact-sheet/Pioneer-ACO-General-Fact-Sheet.pdf. Accessed March 27, 2014.

40. Centers for Medicare and Medicaid Services. Pioneer accountable care organizations succeed in improving care, lowering costs [press release]. Baltimore, Md.: Centers for Medicare and Medicaid Services;2013.

41. Wyden R. Summary: The Wyden-Isakson-Paulsen-Welch Better Care, Lower Cost Act. Washington, D.C.: U.S. Senate;2014. http://www.wyden.senate.gov/download/?id=7f456cdf-edae-4dcb-ba64-c33f0fcc21ce&download=1. Accessed March 27, 2014.

42. Silow-Carroll S, Edwards JN. Early adopters of the accountable care model: a field report on improvements in health care delivery. New York, N.Y.: The Commonwealth Fund; 2013. http://www.commonwealthfund.org/Publications/Fund-Reports/2013/Mar/Early-Adopters-Accountable-Care-Model.aspx. Accessed March 27, 2014.

43. Gold M, Jacobson G, Damico A, Neuman T. Medicare Advantage 2013 spotlight: enrollment market update. 2013; http://kaiserfamilyfoundation.files.wordpress.com/2013/06/8448.pdf. Accessed March 27, 2014.

44. AISHealth. Fact sheet 2014 Star Ratings. 2014; http://aishealth.com/sites/all/files/2014_star_ratings_factsheet_092713.pdf. Accessed March 27, 2014.

45. Fried TR, van Doorn C, O'Leary JR, Tinetti ME, Drickamer MA. Older person's preferences for home vs hospital care in the treatment of acute illness. *Arch Intern Med.* 2000;160(10):1501-1506.

46. Gill TM, Baker DI, Gottschalk M, Peduzzi PN, Allore HBA. A program to prevent functional decline in physically frail, elderly persons who live at home. *N Engl J Med.* 2002;347(14).

47. Friedberg MW. Association between participation in a multipayer medical home Iintervention and changes in quality, utilization, and costs of care. *JAMA.* 2014;311(8):815.

48. Centers for Medicare and Medicaid Services. FQHC Advanced Primary Care Practice Demonstration. http://innovation.cms.gov/initiatives/fqhcs. Accessed March 29, 2014.

49. Centers for Medicare and Medicaid Services. Details for title: Medicare Medical Home Demonstration. 2007; http://www.cms.gov/Medicare/Demonstration-Projects/DemoProjectsEvalRpts/Medicare-Demonstrations-Items/CMS1199247.html. Accessed March 27, 2014.

50. National Health Policy Forum. Medicare care for the elderly living at home: home-based primary care (HBPC) and hospital-at-home programs. 2011; http://www.nhpf.org/library/forum-sessions/FS_07-22-11_HomeCareElderly.pdf. Accessed March 27, 2014.

51.   U.S. Department of Veterans Affairs. Home-based primary care.
       http://www.va.gov/geriatrics/guide/longtermcare/home_based_primary_care.
       asp#. Accessed March 29, 2014.

52.   Centers for Medicare and Medicaid Services. Independence at home fact theet.
       2013; http://innovation.cms.gov/Files/fact-sheet/IAH-Fact-Sheet.pdf. Accessed
       March 27, 2014.

53.   Commonwealth Fund. *Quality Matters* newsletter. In focus: making house calls
       to improve care of patients with advanced illnesses. Washington, D.C.: The
       Commonwealth Fund; February/March 2014.
       http://www.commonwealthfund.org/publications/newsletters/quality-
       matters/2014/february-march/in-focus. Accessed March 27, 2014.

54.   Boyd CM, Fortin M. Future of multimorbidity research: how should
       understanding of multimorbidity inform health system design? *Public Health
       Rev.* 2010;32(2):451-474.

55.   Federal Interagency Forum on Aging-Related Statistics. *Older Americans 2012:
       key indicators of well-being (Older Americans 2012).* Hyattsville, Md.: Federal
       Interagency Forum on Aging-Related Statistics;2012.

56.   National Center for Chronic Disease Prevention and Health Promotion. *The
       power of prevention: chronic disease . . . the public health challenge of the 21st
       century.* Atlanta, Ga.: Centers for Disease Control and Prevention;2009.

57.   Hoffman C, Rice D, Sung HY. Persons with chronic conditions: their prevalence
       and costs. *JAMA.* 1996;276(18):1473-1479.

58.   Wu S, Green A. *Projection of chronic illness prevalence and cost inflation.*
       Washington, D.C.: RAND Health;2000.

59.   Anderson G, Horvath J. *Chronic conditions: making the case for ongoing care.*
       Princeton, NJ: Robert Wood Johnson Foundation Partnership for
       Solutions;2002.

60.   Foley SM, Daley J, Hughes J, Fisher ES, Heeren T. Comorbidities, complications,
       and coding bias: does the number of diagnosis codes matter in predicting in-
       hospital mortality? *JAMA.* 1992;267(16):2197-2203.

61.   Boyd CM, Darer J, Boult C, Fried LP, Boult L, Wu AW. Clinical practice guidelines
       and quality of care for older patients with multiple comorbid diseases:
       implications for pay for performance. *JAMA.* 2005;294(6):716-724.

62.   Wolff Jl, Starfield B, Anderson G. Prevalence, expenditures, and complications of
       multiple chronic conditions in the elderly. *Arch Intern Med.* 2002;162(20):2269-
       2276.

63.   Boult C, Wieland GD. Comprehensive primary care for older patients with
       multiple chronic conditions: "Nobody rushes you through." *JAMA.*
       2010;304(17).

64.   Counsell S.R., Callahan CM, Clark D.O., et al. Geriatric care management for low-
       income seniors: a randomized controlled trial. *JAMA.* 2007;298(22):2623-2633.

65.   Leff B, Reider L, Frick KD, et al. Guided care and the cost of complex healthcare:
       a preliminary report. *Am J Manag Care.* 2009;15(8):555-559.

66. Boult C, Reider L, Frey K, et al. Early effects of "Guided Care" on the quality of health care for multimorbid older persons: a cluster-randomized controlled trial. *J Gerontol A Biol Sci Med Sci.* Mar 2008;63(3):321-7.

67. Kane RL, Homyak P, Bershadsky B, Flood S. Variations on a theme called PACE. *J Gerontol A Biol Sci Med Sci.* 2006;61(7):689-693.

68. Nadash P. Two models of managed long-term care: comparing PACE with a Medicaid-only plan. *Gerontologist.* 2004;44(5):644-654.

69. Wieland D, Boland R, Baskins J, Kinosian B. Five-year survival in a Program of All-inclusive Care for Elderly compared with alternative institutional and home- and community-based care. *J Gerontol A Biol Sci Med Sci.* 2010;65(7):721-726.

70. Medicare Payment Advisory Commission, Medicaid CHIP Payment Access Commission. Data Book: Beneficiaries Dually Eligible for Medicare and Medicaid. MedPAC; December 2013.

71. U.S. Department of Health and Human Services, National Center for Health Statistics. *Health, United States, 2012, with special feature on emergency care.* Atlanta, Ga,: National Center for Health Statistics;May 2013.

72. Kaiser Family Foundation. Best bets for reducing Medicare costs for dual eligible beneficiaries: Assessing the Evidence. October 2012; http://kaiserfamilyfoundation.files.wordpress.com/2013/01/8353.pdf. Accessed March 29, 2014.

73. Centers for Medicare and Medicaid Services. The financial alignment initiative. http://www.cms.gov/Medicare-Medicaid-Coordination/Medicare-and-Medicaid-Coordination/Medicare-Medicaid-Coordination-Office/FinancialAlignmentInitiative/FinancialModelstoSupportStatesEffortsinCareCoordination.html. Accessed March 29, 2014.

74. Centers for Medicare and Medicaid Services. Approved Demonstrations— Signed MOUs.   http://www.cms.gov/Medicare-Medicaid-Coordination/Medicare-and-Medicaid-Coordination/Medicare-Medicaid-Coordination-Office/FinancialAlignmentInitiative/ApprovedDemonstrationsSignedMOUs.html. Accessed March 29, 2014.

75. Ouslander JG, Bonner A, Herndon L, Shutes J. The Interventions to Reduce Acute Care Transfers (INTERACT) quality improvement program: an overview for medical directors and primary care clinicians in long term care. *J Am Med Dir Assoc.* 2014;15(3):162-170.

76. INTERACT. Interventions to Reduce Acute Care Transfers. http://interact2.net/. Accessed March 29, 2014.

77. Ouslander JG, Perloe M, Givens JH, Kluge L, Rutland T, Lamb G. Reducing potentially avoidable hospitalizations of nursing home residents: Results of a pilot quality improvement project. *J Am Med Dir Assoc.* 2009;10(9):644-652.

78. Medicare Payment Advisory Commission. Measuring quality across Medicare's delivery systems. Washington, D.C.: MedPAC;2013.

79.   Schwartz MD. Health care reform and the primary care workforce bottleneck. *J Gen Intern Med.* 2012;27(4):469-472.

80.   Altman WM, Parmelee PA, Smyer MA. Autonomy, competence, and informed consent in long term care: legal and psychological perspectives. *Vill L Rev.* 1992;37:1671.

SECTION III. Health Technologies: Enablers of Change

Executive Editor,

James H. Taylor, DMan, MBA, MHA

Section III Overview

Health Technologies: Enablers of Change
(Technological Innovation)

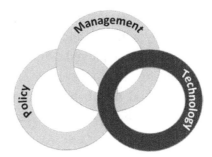

The four chapters that make up Section III present important information and raise significant issues related to the role of technology in discussions of population health. Chapter 11 considers the language used to talk about terminology and the vital role terminology plays in communication that is fundamental in making technology accessible to clinicians, researchers, and individual health seekers. Chapter 12 addresses the use of personal health data; examines the highly charged issue of privacy and control of personal health data; and reviews alternative approaches to making personal health data available to individuals and to those with a population health perspective. Chapter 13 offers a primer on Big Data through a review of Big Data terminology; a brief history of data mining and data warehousing; and examination of the mechanics of Big Data and of the issues raised by its use in population health research. Chapter 10 presents a case study of an attempt to establish a state-run health information exchange (HIE), which reminds the reader that issues of technology are often less technical than political and relational; and that failure to understand that reality can quickly derail highly promising technology-based opportunities.

Advances in health technology present heretofore unavailable opportunities to improve both individual and population health. Individuals will have new and compelling ability to take charge of and positively affect their personal health status from EMR/EHR-enabled data. These individual patient-generated data, when made available in aggregated states and properly protected, offer the potential to transform public health practitioners' ability to identify, understand, and address both isolated nonrecurrent events and systemic and evolving endemic conditions.

Today's health technology can be an enabler of true change, offering unprecedented capabilities to understand individual and population-based problems, needs, and opportunities. Policy makers, managers, and technology experts must, however, remain always aware that technology is a tool used by people who must deal successfully with one another's needs, issues, and politics before the technology will ever be deployed. Inability or unwillingness to recognize that without attention to these basic relational fundamentals, technology will enable nothing; and health policy and management of health resources will be far less robust and unable to realize the promises that technology presents.

James H. Taylor, DMan, MBA, MHA
Special Advisor to the Executive VP for Health Affairs
University of Louisville
and
CEO of University Medical Center

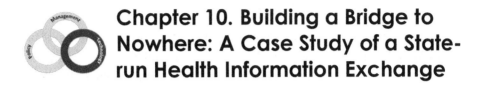

Chapter 10. Building a Bridge to Nowhere: A Case Study of a State-run Health Information Exchange

John Tobin, DMan, MPH

James H. Taylor, DMan, MBA, MHA

"National eHealth programs rarely unfold as predicted, especially when carefully planned out in advance. Of course, that is because they are complex and unpredictable. But policymakers often persist in thinking things will go better next time."[1]

Greenhalgh T, Russell J, Ashcroft RE, Parsons W.
Milbank Q. 2011;89(4)

Chapter 10 Learning Objectives

- Understanding the history of the Connecticut Health Information Exchange (HIE) up to its current status as an example of other state-run HIE initiatives.

- Understanding a case example of a state-level HIE and its role of governance and planning activities.

- Understanding the complexities of designing and establishing an HIE at a state level and the challenges associated with it.

- Gaining insights to the complex social processes that can be both inter- and intra-organizational over a multiyear period for establishing large-scale health information technology systems.

- Learning the importance and roles of leadership, technology, and policy, and their interplay in designing and implementing HIEs.

- Gaining hospital CEO-level insights on the impact of such strategic-level HIE initiatives and their potential impact on efforts to improve population health.

Introduction: A Case Study with a Twist

Analyses of failure are rare in the business literature, and admissions of failure in the public sphere are even rarer. We have no doubt that any open-minded and industrious researcher with an interest in politics and public policy will find many examples of government programs that have had consequences unintended by their authors; have failed to solve the problems they were intended to solve (or even made things worse); and yet (assuming no malfeasance, of course) seem to linger indefinitely in federal or state bureaucracies. As of this writing, it appears that the Connecticut Health Information and Technology Exchange (HITE-CT), one of many attempts to develop statewide health information exchanges funded by the Health Information Technology for Economic and Clinical Health (HITECH) Act of 2009, is headed for just such an outcome. Can we as leaders and policy makers learn from the HITE-CT's experience so that we might in fact do better next time?

Health care reform, in which information technology is considered by most policy makers as a critical enabler, remains a subject of intense political debate. But what interests us here is not political ideology—although that is an important element—but rather the patterns that emerge from our political processes before our eyes and over and over again, despite both repeated warnings from credible sources and contemporary analyses of programs gone awry.

In the case of state-run health information exchanges (HIEs), experts recognized early on that financial self-sufficiency is essential to the long-term success of these enterprises; they also identified the requirements for a business model that would provide such financial independence. The National Association of State Chief Information Officers (NASCIO) published an analysis in September 2011, which posed the following questions in Table 10-1:

Table 10-1. NASCIO Questions on State-run HIE Viability

NASCIO September 2011 HIE Analysis Questions
As state CIOs continue to consider innovative ways of providing viability to state-run HIEs, there are several questions that should be considered:
How long will grant funding last and what are key revenue streams that will augment associated costs?
How will the HIE integrate into the existing state architecture?
Will your state's privacy policies become a hindrance to participation?
Would an opt-in versus an opt-out model limit possible revenue?
As the HIE market becomes more competitive, what added services could be offered that complement the core services?
What technical requirements will need to be met and what costs will be associated with providing those services?
Will your state consider multistate collaboration as a way to cut costs and provide further value?
What staff augmentation will be needed to have the proper workforce in place to plan, implement, and sustain a state-run HIE?
What services do competing HIEs offer that the state could leverage?
Have you reached out to nonhealth entities for financial support?

For example, states may establish agreements with agencies or departments about using a master person index (MPI) for the HIE, as well as the index for all state transactions. States have been given an unprecedented opportunity to make substantial leeway in developing a sustainable model for an HIE. The federal funds granted to the states are generous, but the funds are not sufficient to sustain state-run HIEs. State CIOs and state policy makers will need to be diligent in allocating public funds for planning and implementation costs, but ultimately a well-thought-out business plan and innovative services for building revenue will promote success. While states have progressed at different rates, sustainability will be paramount for a state-run HIE to flourish.[2]

Three years later, financial sustainability for HIE remains an elusive goal, and state HIEs have answered those questions with mostly limited success. Three studies recently published in *Health Affairs* document the rapid growth—fueled by federal money—in the adoption of health information technologies and participation in HIEs; but also note that larger hospital systems and physician practices account for most of the growth, while resource-poor smaller and rural hospitals were lagging.[3,4] Only 44 percent of hospitals had what the authors defined as a "basic" electronic health record system. One study focused specifically on the sustainability issue and reported that (as of 2012) "Most health care providers, including two-thirds of hospitals and 90 percent of physician practices, are not yet participating in these (state-run HIE) efforts"——primarily because they derive no great benefit.

> Long-term financial sustainability for organizations facilitating health information exchange appears to be the most pressing challenge. The fact that three-quarters of efforts cite developing a sustainable business model as a major barrier is a warning to policy makers that the growth in health information exchange will likely falter unless these efforts become self-sustaining or there is a long-term public commitment to their financing.[5]

Methodology

In developing this chapter, the authors drew inspiration from "Why National eHealth Programs Need Dead Philosophers: Wittgensteinian Reflections on Why Policymakers Refuse to Learn." In this interesting and somewhat unusual paper, Greenhalgh et al. offer a spirited defense of the value of case studies "with an *n* of 1" in trying to understand complex social processes and draw lessons that are actually generalizable, even though each study represents a single situation. In their words[1]

> . . . to understand a complex social situation, we must understand, first and foremost, the many and varied social practices of which it is made up, and the different (and perhaps conflicting) ways in which particular words, phrases, lists, instructions, taxonomies, gestures, behaviors, and the like are actually used by different groups. These practices are necessarily particular to the case. Indeed, it is only by grasping their contextual significance that we can understand the case.

and

> While it is possible to theorize national eHealth programs with the goal of analytic generalization, this may be less practically useful at the policy level than the approach described here. That approach is to achieve through the detailed study of particular programs the ability to reflect and deliberate on the complex, interdependent social practices that make such programs unique. A scholarly analysis of the case-of-one is engaged and interpretive rather than abstracted and representational. It depends on what has been called theory's ineradicable dependence on the dynamics of the life-world within which it has its currency.

Thus with the foregoing in mind, the authors will depart somewhat from the common notion of a case study. The typical business school case focuses on a specific problem faced by leaders of an organization, together with relevant data and sufficient background material to define the context within which the problem had to be addressed. Students are then invited to "solve" the problem themselves with the information provided, and the ensuing classroom discussion develops a critique of the decisions made by the subject organization's leaders. Usually there is what amounts to a correct answer or a particular lesson the students are expected to derive from the case.

Rather than exploring a specific problem and a preferred solution, our interest is in presenting for study and discussion the complex dynamics of social processes that unfold over an extended period of time. Thus, while the leadership group we are studying had a specific task/problem to solve—the creation of a statewide HIE—we are more interested in exploring and decoupling the following issues throughout the remainder of this chapter:

- The composition of the HITE-CT leadership group;

- How the leadership group came into being;

- Complexity themes that emerged through the interactions of the players;

- The extraneous influences on the proceedings and any unintended consequences that emerged;

- The effect on population health in the region where the scenario unfolded;

- The relationship to health policy and Health in All Policies (HiAP) issues as addressed throughout this book.

Our perspective on complexity is grounded in the theory of Complex Responsive Processes developed by Professor Ralph D. Stacey and colleagues at the University of Hertfordshire in the United Kingdom (UK). The reader is invited to consider the insights that might arise in considering problem solving from this perspective, which will be explained in the following sections.

When the Connecticut Department of Public Health (DPH) became the federal government's "designated agency" to develop an HIE, Dr. Robert Galvin, the Commissioner of Public Health at that time, formed an interdisciplinary advisory board and required verbatim transcripts to be prepared on each meeting of the HITE-CT. The advisory board oversaw and advised DPH during the first year of the project. When the advisory board was replaced by the board of directors of HITE-CT, the quasi-public agency formed to manage the project, DPH remained the lead state agency for the project, and the practice of verbatim meeting transcripts continued in 2013. There are now roughly 40 such transcripts from late 2009 until the present, posted on the HITE-CT website and available to anyone interested:

http://www.ct.gov/hitect/cwp/view.asp?a=4277&q=504376.

The transcripts can be difficult to follow, not only because of the give-and-take of conversation, incomplete sentences, insider references and the like, but also because they often involve commentary on slide presentations and other documents that may no longer be available.

What the transcripts provide is a raw record of conversations over a three-and-a-half-year period. While they do not provide a coherent narrative, the transcripts give a sense of the emerging conversation, significant and recurrent themes, and impressions of the participants.

The transcripts reflect a real-life situation with which both authors (and, we suspect, many readers) are familiar. Nonprofit organizations typically have boards of directors who volunteer their services. Meetings occur at regular intervals, but usually a month or more apart, and thus produce discontinuous conversations over time. Some issues are carried over from meeting to meeting, while others may recur at meetings after an interval of months has elapsed. The level of commitment and preparation of individual members varies, as does the level of participation in meeting discussions, committee work, and attendance. Finally, as in any social process, what is not said is just as important—in some cases, more important—than what is said. All these dynamics are evident in the transcripts.

While having the opportunity to talk with a few of the participants in this process, we opted not to try to construct an oral history. These ancillary conversations and other public documents allowed us to fill in some gaps, confirm impressions, and reconstruct a timeline. Our narrative is limited to themes, impressions, and reactions derived from review of the transcripts, which posed some limitations but provided an evidence-based approach rooted in public record documentation.

In collaborating on this chapter, and in the spirit of its analytical approach, the authors engaged in several conversations via e-mail, telephone, and video conference, including two video conferences for which written transcripts were developed. These conversational reflections are provided in the second half of the chapter titled, "Thinking Aloud: A Conversation," and offer insights (from the perspective of two recently retired hospital CEOs) on how healthcare organizations may assess and address the complexities associated with health information technology and HIE issues on the journey toward improving the population health in our communities.

The Connecticut Health Information Technology Exchange

The concept of a health information exchange (HIE), a system for the electronic storage and transfer of health information among patient care providers, regulatory and public health agencies, government and private insurers, and so forth, is not new. Providers and insurers have been making significant investments in increasingly sophisticated information technology systems for decades, and the Office of the National Coordinator for Health Information Technology (ONC) was formed by executive order in 2004 under the Bush Administration, to encourage the development of a national HIE infrastructure, develop intraoperability standards, and so forth. During the latter half of the first decade of the twenty-first century, several Connecticut provider groups were exploring possibilities for regional HIEs.

The real impetus for HIE formation, however, came with the enactment of the HITECH Act as part of the American Recovery and Reinvestment Act (ARRA) of 2009, commonly referred to as the 2009 stimulus program. The HITECH Act legislatively mandated the ONC, and provided substantial funding under several grant programs for HIE infrastructure development. One of the objectives of HITECH was the creation of statewide HIEs that would ultimately connect with the national information exchange system. Only states could apply for funding; in Connecticut, the state Department of Public Health (DPH) became the state's designated agency for HIE development.

The DPH, under Commissioner Robert Galvin, MD, sponsored legislation that created a multi-stakeholder advisory board to assist the department in seeking grant funding and in deploying any monies received toward development of an HIE. In a process that is not unusual in Connecticut, the legislation not only spelled out the composition of the advisory board but also the appointing authority for each member not ex officio by virtue of being a state official. So, for example, the representative of Connecticut's hospitals was chosen by the speaker of the Connecticut House of Representatives, while the representative of the Federally Qualified Health Centers was chosen by the President pro tempore of the Senate. Although this process is intended to ensure broad representation, it invariably introduces a significant political element; and by including a disproportionate representation of state officials, essentially guarantees domination, if not control, by the state.

The advisory board began its activities in fall of 2009, and the verbatim transcripts of each meeting were entered into the public record beginning in December of that year.

The department applied for and eventually received an ONC grant of approximately $7.28 million under the State HIE Cooperative Agreement Program, one of the several programs established under the HITECH Act. It is important to note that the state had to meet certain milestones in order to receive funding; the total amount was not disbursed by the federal government as a lump sum. It appears that approximately $2,000,000 of the grant funds were earmarked to support DPH staff committed to this project, and the balance was used as described below.

The first order of business was creation of a strategic plan. The state issued a request for proposal, and the department, with the involvement of the advisory board, selected the Gartner Group, an information technology research and advisory firm located in Stamford, Connecticut, in the spring of 2010. The strategic plan was completed in December 2010.

The state opted for a hybrid model that would include a clinical data repository, a variety of such services as a patient record locator, and a master record index; and would provide the infrastructure whereby electronic health records (EHRs) could be transferred among providers, could capture and transmit laboratory results, and could handle electronic drug prescription processing. Figure 10-1 illustrates the conceptual HIE model that HITE-CT adopted.

Figure 10-1. HITE-CT Hybrid HIT Model (push/pull)

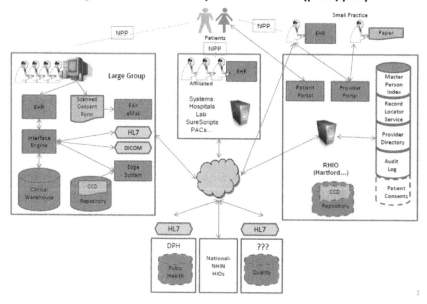

HIE could achieve Meaningful Use status for their individual electronic record systems, thus qualifying for federal incentives under the HITECH act. The goals for CT-HIE were identified as:

CT-HIE Goals
The State of Connecticut plans to transform its health care system by HITE-CT to improve the quality, efficiency, and accountability of health care in Connecticut.
HITE-CT will establish and manage a statewide health information exchange to attain substantial and measurable improvements in several key areas, including but not limited to:
• Patients' access to health care and their medical records • Continuity and coordination of care • Quality of care, medical outcomes, and patient experience • Effectiveness and efficiency of health care delivery • Public health outcomes

One of the significant issues with an HIE of any sort involves the confidentiality of sensitive records, which is a complex issue being addressed at state and national levels due to its importance. Those responsible for the Connecticut project—DPH and later HITE-CT—selected a so-called "opt-out" model in which patient records would be sent to and housed in the HIE data repository unless the patients took active steps to prevent the inclusion of their records. Consumer representatives on the HITE-CT board advocated for an "opt–in" model, in which consumers would have to agree to have their records included in the HIE. Limitations in technology made obtaining of patient consents complicated and difficult for either model.

DPH and its advisory board recognized that the HIE would not be supported by grant funds alone. A roughly estimated "sustainability" plan was incorporated into the operating plan. It was assumed that providers, in order to achieve Meaningful Use to qualify for federal incentives and avoid federal penalties after 2016, would be willing to pay for HIE services on a subscription basis. The operating plan assumed such revenues would begin to flow in in the fall of 2011.

DPH and the advisory board determined that the best vehicle for managing the state-HIE would be a quasi-public agency similar to a public utility, and sponsored legislation to put such an agency in place. The governor signed the law creating HITE-CT in November 2011. As with the advisory board, the legislation spelled out both the composition of the board of directors and the appointing authority for each nongovernment stakeholder representative. Several nongovernment members of the advisory board were carried over to the HITE-CT board, but there were additions, notably two designated "consumer" representatives. The new board began its work on January 1, 2011. Figure 10-2 provides an overview of the spectrum of stakeholders involved in the HITE-CT.

Figure 10-2. HITE-CT Stakeholders

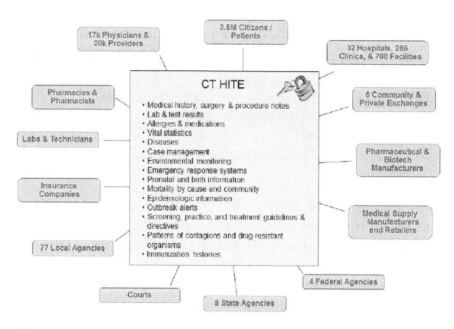

All of this occurred toward the end of Dr. Galvin's tenure. A new commissioner, Jewel Mullen, MD, MPH, MPA, became chair of the HITE-CT board of directors; other state officials and staff support also changed with the election of a new governor in 2011. Some members were carried over. The new HITE-CT board carried on its work with no change in direction, still following the Gartner Group's strategic and operating plan. In November 2011, the board also engaged David Gilbertson as executive director.

The new HITE-CT Board, working with various subcommittees, developed a request for proposal (RFP) to build the HIE. Axway, a global software and services company, was selected to build the HIE; it entered into a contract in December 2011 and commenced work on infrastructure at that time. HITE-CT opted for a remote hosting approach with hardware and software located at the Axway facilities in Phoenix, Arizona, rather than in Connecticut.

Although it was understood that hospital participation in the project would be essential to the HIE's success, there was pushback from the hospital industry almost from the beginning. An adversarial relationship existed between the Connecticut Hospital Association (CHA) and the Department of Public Health, and hospitals were skeptical of the state's ability to manage the HIE. Evidenced by the transcripts, outreach to hospital stakeholders was minimal until sustainability issues started to emerge in early 2012.

This situation continued to deteriorate through 2012, and Axway's work on the project ceased in lieu of the sustainability challenges. The HITE-CT board looked into possible grant funding through the Medicaid program, but this option turned out to be a blind alley. There was also increased discussion of Project Direct (Direct), a secure messaging system championed by ONC, possibly in recognition of the several failed attempts to create sustainable state HIEs around the country.[6] In light of the sustainability challenges, board members reluctantly accepted the reality that Direct was the only option they actually had sufficient resources to attempt.

During this time frame, there was considerable discussion of what had gone wrong. Possible causes cited in the meeting transcripts included:

- Lack of support from the state;

- Inadequate resources;

- Lack of public and political recognition of the HITE-CT effort; and

- Acknowledgment that for three years HITE-CT had stuck to a "grand plan" without having had the resources or expertise to execute it.

In addition to financial problems and lack of provider support, HITE-CT had never been able to resolve the confidentiality and the opt-in versus opt-out controversies.

Gilbertson announced his resignation in July 2012; his responsibilities were assumed by the chief technology officer, John DeStefano, and Chris Kraus, the operations officer. After Gilbertson's departure, the process for establishing the HIE was "losing energy." Meetings became shorter and more frequently canceled. It became the practice of the HITE-CT Board to go into executive session—and thus off the record—as soon as each meeting was convened, presumably to discuss the sustainability challenges and the Axway relationship.

DeStefano was asked to develop a revised strategic plan. At the January, 2013, meeting, he gave a succinct assessment of what the key failure of HITE-CT had been,[7]

> Part of the issue, premise of HITE/CT is, you know, its name. It says Health Information Technology Exchange of Connecticut. And I really firmly believe that this problem is less about technology. I think it's, you know, in some ways the name. It doesn't really reflect what we should be doing. This is a business problem. Unless we can go out to our business customers and give them what helps them, some return on investment for what we have, some improvements to their work flow, some future that they can see in all of this, that's what we have to give them. Giving them technology, this is commodity technology now. It's been commodity technology for a while. After about 2005, Health Exchanges existed all over the place and they were dissolved all over the place too. It was never about the technology and it still isn't.

As of mid-year 2013, DeStefano had recommended a revised strategic plan focused on Direct, the secure messaging system discussed above. At this point, efforts were made to engage the hospitals, but to no avail. It was also apparent that providers, including nonhospital ones, had little interest in Direct. Participants in some secure messaging pilot projects were being paid, so even if Direct were eventually to be adopted by the providers, it was obvious that it had little promise as a revenue source. Although the HITE-CT board recognized that the HIE project as originally envisioned was a failure, the organization, under DeStefano's direction, continued to look into other ways in which HITE-CT could continue to have some function and relevance.

HITE-CT Timeline

A timeline of the activities as discussed in the prior section is provided as a chronology of events in Table 10-2.

Table 10-2. HITE-CT Timeline

Date	Activity
2007–2009	• DPH designated to develop a state HIE plan with standards and protocols. • DPH creates an advisory board to assist with the effort. • Public Act creates a legislatively appointed advisory board.
February 2009	• HITECH bill enacted as part of the American Recovery and Reinvestment Act (Stimulus Bill) of 2009. DPH directed to apply for funds under the Act.
March 2010	• Patient Protection and Affordable Care Act (ACA) enacted.
March 2010	• Gartner project to develop a strategic plan begins. This project ultimately includes an operations plan, also developed by the Gartner Group.
April 2010	• DPH receives $7.29 million grant to plan and create a statewide HIE that can interface with a national HIE.
June 2010	• Bill creating Health Information and Technology Exchange of Connecticut (HITE-CT) signed into law. HITE-CT becomes the state's designated HIE agency.
September 2010	• Version 1 of the HIE strategic and operating plan submitted to ONC.
December 2010	• Version 2 submitted 12/2; ONC comments received 12/20—sustainability issue an ONC concern. Plan for that developed, among other corrections.
January 1, 2011	• HITE-CT begins operations. New state administration takes office; new commissioner of DPH as well as some DPH staff changes.
February 2011	• Version 3 submitted, eventually approved by ONC.
April 2011	• Request for proposal (RFP) issued for HISP; goal is to deploy to "willing providers" by September 1, 2011. RFP issued by state Department of Information Technology on behalf of HITE-CT.
November 2011	• David Gilbertson hired as executive director.
December 2011	• Axway selected as HIE vendor.
January 2012	• First mention of financial challenges: running up Axway bills; no revenue; and grant cash flow problems.
July 2012	• Gilbertson resigns.

Date	Activity
May 2012	• Decision to shift direction from a full HIE to secure messaging only (Direct Project).
November 2012	• Indebtedness to Axway reaches $2.5 million.
November 2012	• First mention of Axway's "claim" (according to the transcripts, this claim is never explicitly identified as a lawsuit).
Present	• As of late 2013, the lawsuit with Axway remained unresolved; the status of the HIE infrastructure remains uncertain (because HITE-CT has not paid Axway for its services); there are few if any active participants in the secure messaging program; and Connecticut hospitals and health systems continue to develop their own HIEs.

Board Composition and Influence on Process and Outcomes

As discussed above, there was an original advisory board established for 2009–10, and a revised board membership adopted in 2011. Tables 10-3 and 10-4 provide a list of the positions and stakeholders that were engaged on the board along with identifying the appointing authority.

Table 10-3. 2009–10 DPH Advisory Board Composition

Position	Appointing Authority
Lieutentant Governor	Governor
Representative of medical research organization (University of Connecticut School of Medicine)	Governor
Insurer or health plan representative	Governor
Attorney with privacy, data security, or patient rights experience	Governor
Private health information exchange or health information technology entity experience	President pro tempore of the Senate
Public health experience	President pro tempore of the Senate
Hospitals, an integrated delivery network, or hospital association representative	Speaker of the House
Expertise with Federally Qualified Health Centers	Speaker of the House

Position	Appointing Authority
Private-practice physician using an EHR system	Majority Leader of the Senate
Expertise with Federally Qualified Health Centers	Speaker of the House
Consumer or consumer advocate	Majority Leader of the House
Pharmacist or other provider using an electronic information exchange	Minority Leader of the Senate
Large employer or representative of a business group	Minority Leader of the House
Ex officio (or their designees) without vote:	
Commissioner of Public Health	Per statute
Commissioner of Social Services (Medicaid agency in Connecticut)	Per statute
Commissioner of Consumer Protection	Per statute
Commissioner of the Office of Health Care Access (Certificate of Need agency in Connecticut)	Per statute
Chief Information Officer of the Department of Information Technology	Per statute
Secretary of the Office of Policy and Management (executive branch budget director)	Per statute

Table 10-4. 2010–11 to Present, HITE-CT Board Composition

Position	Appointing Authority
Lieutentant Governor	Governor
Representative of medical research organization (University of Connecticut School of Medicine)	Governor
Insurer or health plan representative	Governor
Attorney with privacy, data security, or patient rights experience	Governor
Private health information exchange or health information technology entity experience	President pro tempore of the Senate
Public health experience	President pro tempore of the Senate
Hospitals, an integrated delivery	Speaker of the House

Position	Appointing Authority
network, or hospital association representative	
Expertise with Federally Qualified Health Centers	Speaker of the House
Private-practice physician using an EHR system	Majority Leader of the Senate
Expertise with Federally Qualified Health Centers	Speaker of the House
Consumer or consumer advocate	Speaker of the House
Pharmacist or other provider using an electronic information exchange	Minority Leader of the Senate
Large employer or representative of a business group	Minority Leader of the House
Licensed physician who works in a practice of not more than 10 physicians, and who is not employed by a hospital, health network, health plan, health system, academic institution or university	President pro tempore of the Senate
Commissioner of Public Health (Chair)	Per statute
Commissioner of Social Services	Per statute
Commissioner of Consumer Protection	Per statute
Chief Information Officer of the Department of Information Technology	Per statute
Ex officio (or their designees) without vote:	
Secretary of the Office of Policy and Management	Per statute
State Healthcare Advocate	Per statute

Thinking Aloud—A CEO Conversation: Insights on Complexities

With that overview of the HITE-CT project details and timeline behind us, let us direct our attention to the social processes that unfolded. The remaining sections provide a brief overview of complexity theory that informs our thinking followed by our reflections in a conversational format. In addition to our complexity perspective, we also bring to the conversation our experience with health care information technology and the public policy processes governing HIEs as hospital stakeholders.

A Complexity Primer

Complexity science offers a different way of viewing experience of the physical world from that of the dominant perspective informed by a Newtonian cause-and-effect linear approach to understanding how the world works. This dominant perspective is so much a part of Western thinking that it is seldom questioned; we take it for granted that there is a cause for every effect and if we can find that cause, explanation, predictability, and replicability are the rewards for our efforts. Decades ago, physical and computer scientists began to consider phenomena that were not predictable and for which no identifiable cause could be found for particular outcomes. Previously, such phenomena were considered outliers and of no scientific significance. Scientists began to study the activities of autonomous, often interdependent, and diverse agents. They observed unpredictable emergent, self-organizing activity for which a scientific explanation failed to explain what was occurring.

From this work, the complexity sciences and the concept of complex adaptive systems (CAS) evolved. A CAS approach started being applied to physics and biology as well as human organizations in the twentieth century. CASs are characterized by the emergent, self-organizing activities of autonomous agents, be they inanimate matter, living organisms, or human organizations. Further, the results of interaction are influenced by the degree of diversity of agents; are stable and unstable at the same time; and are largely unpredictable.

Many organizational scholars have argued that human organizations are CASs, and that using CAS theory helps better explain organizational behaviors and outcomes. They posit that an organization is a discrete system, albeit made up of subsystems and interacting with other organizational and societal systems. These scholars have extended systems theory with imported concepts from the complexity sciences. They have contributed to presenting an alternative way of thinking about organizations from the dominant, largely mechanistic perspective.

Using the complexity sciences as a source domain, Ralph Stacey and his colleagues at the University of Hertfordshire in the United Kingdom have introduced a theory, Complex Responsive Processes, which seeks to explain human interaction, especially organizational, in a way that makes sense of everyday experience. They have drawn on concepts from psychology, sociology, anthropology, and philosophy to bring theoretical understanding to the complex dynamics of humans in interaction with others and themselves.

Complex Responsive Processes theory is concerned with the local, largely conversational interaction of people; power relations; ideology as the basis of choice; and the social background of people's interactions. People, the diverse agents from a complexity perspective, interact locally in the present in ways that are unpredictable and with unknowable outcomes, which may be both stable and unstable at the same time. In seeking to understand what is really happening in human organizations, Complex Responsive Processes theory pays close attention to the dynamics of people in interaction; to the ubiquitous power gradients that exist between people and the way that power is used; to the ideologies people bring to their interactions with one another and how those ideologies influence choices that are made; and to how social background (called culture and habitus) influences human interaction.

In the framework and terminology of Stacey's theory, leaders can and do make gestures into a group of intended followers—goals, policies, directives, explanation, rhetorical persuasions, and so forth—but the leader has no control over how those gestures will be understood, interpreted, and acted upon by those would-be followers. Some will enthusiastically support; some will "play the game"; some will actively resist; some will resort to subversion; and some will represent every nuance in between. Moreover, those responses will develop and evolve through countless interactions—person-to-person conversations, various forms of correspondence, physical actions, and, in the case of public policy, news media and blogosphere accounts and analyses, and so on.

Carrying this line of thinking into the realm of politics and public policy, our reality is that powerful individuals, often with the best of intentions, devise plans and strategies, establish programs and processes, and write and enact laws and regulations. But these inevitably get caught up in ideological struggles, power politics, the election cycle, the ups and downs of the economy, and a host of other factors; and are subject to the interpretation and actions (or lack thereof) of countless individuals both within and outside of government. And these complex dynamics, whereby these strategies and programs "morph" into unintended consequences, have, perhaps, a greater impact on us than the laws and regulations themselves.

It is not our intention in this brief chapter to make anyone an expert in complexity or the theory of Complex Responsive Processes. We emphasize, as does Stacey, that this perspective "is a way of thinking about what we already do. It is not about prescribing what people ought to be doing, or about labeling what they are doing as futile or foolish." What we are trying to do—through a somewhat different approach to the analysis of a failing health information exchange project—is to strengthen awareness of the complex phenomena that are all around us in the hope that that awareness will have a positive impact on each reader's thinking and actions in the future.

We hope that the reader also will conclude as we have, that

The complexity of contemporary health care, combined with the multiple stakeholders in large technology initiatives, means that national e-Health programs require considerably more thinking through than has sometimes occurred. We need fewer grand plans and more learning communities.[1]

Conversational Discovery

An online conversation led to the central idea behind this chapter: how two recently retired hospital CEOs who share decades of experience in health care management and an intense interest in the application of concepts from the complexity sciences to leadership and organizational change might be thinking about the massive changes sweeping our field. We decided to focus on one specific element of that change: the rise of health care information technologies and Big Data; and in keeping with the themes of this book, their implications for leaders and policy makers.

In articulating his theory of Complex Responsive Processes (described in some detail in the Complexity Primer above), Stacey draws heavily on the thought of the pragmatist philosopher and social psychologist George Herbert Mead (the mechanism of human communicative interaction on a small scale) and the process sociologist Norbert Elias (human interaction on a population-wide scale) to explain the emergence of the global patterning of social processes solely through the interaction of simultaneously collaborative and competitive intentions of individual persons at a local level. The theory provides a unique way of understanding a variety of social issues that include:

- the emergence of the self;
- personality and social controls;
- culture;
- ethics;
- knowledge formation;

- power relations; and others.

As Stacey and his colleagues have continued to develop this social science-oriented approach to complexity in organizations, they have taken up other important scholars' contributions to this way of thinking: the philosopher John Dewey (ethics); the physician/biologist Ludwik Fleck (thought collectives and the social construction of scientific knowledge); the philosopher/historian Michel Foucault (power and knowledge); the anthropologist Clifford Geertz (culture); the sociologist Pierre Bourdieu (the concept of habitus); the philosopher Hans Joas (norms and values); and the social theorist John Shotter (the "politics" of everyday conversation), to name some of the more important ones.

Collaboration on this project was made possible by many conversations via electronic media—e-mail, telephone, and videoconference—and two such conferences were recorded and transcribed. We have attempted to capture the essence of these conversations in the section that follows as a way of illustrating our perspective on complexity and some relevant effects on population health initiatives in the twenty-first century.

The authors cannot hope to do justice to this rich body of work in the space of a chapter.[8,9] We are not theorists by training or experience—our interest lies in bringing this way of thinking to everyday practice: understanding how organizations function; and understanding what leaders do and how they do it. In the conversational vignettes that follow, transcribed conversations are organized around certain complexity themes of relevance to the HITE-CT case. Many of the vignettes are structured, starting with a "CEO Insight" that is meant to provide a complexity background/context point of view shaped by the theories and writings of Stacey and colleagues, followed by our conversation on each topic.

Methodology

CEO Insights

One of the most basic ideas in the theory of Complex Responsive Processes is that leadership/managerial work is a conversational activity—we do what we do by talking to other people, and meaning emerges in the interactions. Even written communication is a form of conversation between writer and reader, and has no meaning outside of that interaction (except for the mental "conversation" the writer has with him- or herself). But the ideal form of conversation—especially in a world of e-mails and tweets—is among human

> **CEO Insights**
>
> bodies in the same physical space in which all have full access to facial expressions, body language, subtle changes in tone of voice, and so forth.
>
> A second important Stacey theme touched upon here is the paradoxical nature of human interaction. Anyone experienced in organizational life knows that co-workers exhibit a variety of paradoxical "faces" simultaneously: competitive and collaborative, altruistic and self-serving, helpful and obstructive, to name a few. Paradoxical behavior is a reality that leaders must accept, not try to resolve.

Jim: Our chapter is organized around a case study that John has produced, based on his review of the transcripts of the activities of groups of people in Connecticut trying to put together a statewide health information exchange. We are going to discuss those efforts from a perspective that we both bring to this conversation. It is a complexity-informed perspective. Our approach is influenced by our studies with Ralph Stacey and his colleagues at the University of Hertfordshire. So maybe, John, we should start with the general declaration that for us a complexity approach brings a particular interest in the process by which people in interaction go about their work.

John: Right. One thing we want to avoid in our discussion is a critique of individual participants. Instead we want to focus on the process and how the process itself shapes its own development. Ralph Stacey writes about "enabling constraints," the paradoxical way in which a social process simultaneously enables and constrains its participants. The fact is that all of us are enmeshed in very complex social processes all the time, and what we can do and what we can't do is affected by our interaction with other people who have agendas and needs of their own. We're lucky we have these transcripts providing a verbatim record of three years' worth of meetings—what people said (and didn't say). It's a good opportunity to study a conversational process in a way that one can't do from summary records of conversations, such as meeting minutes.

Jim: We should also recognize up front that there are limitations to examining a process through transcripts. Not being present for the actual interactions that went on, we can't see facial expressions, we can't see gestures and body language, and we can't see how people respond bodily to certain words. John, you did have the opportunity, however, to interview a few people who were either involved directly in the process or who observed it from the outside.

John: Right; and again, I tried to use that opportunity as a way to fill in some of the blanks, but we decided to focus almost exclusively on the transcripts and what is in them. They were done specifically to establish a public record of what transpired, and so one would expect the transcripts to have accounts of committee reports and other formal meetings, and also give some sense of what went on behind the scenes. From our complexity perspective, we know that work in organizations gets done through many, many casual conversations in the workplace and elsewhere, and you can't capture that in monthly meetings.

More on Methodology

Jim: As I'm listening to our conversation so far, I think it's interesting that we we are talking about the process by which this activity emerged over several years. We're not necessarily talking about the substance of what they were designing, nor the specifics of the strategic plan. We're paying attention to the way in which they went about their work; which, given our complexity perspective, is what seems to us most important if you're going to learn anything from this "case of one."

John: If we can capture the process in a way that makes sense, the value should be some insights that might be helpful in choosing what might be a more fruitful approach in a similar scenario in the future. Another important aspect of our perspective is that each of these situations is unique, and each process has its own dynamics. You can't necessarily say "they did these things wrong, or if they went about their work in a certain other way, things would have come out better." But you certainly can look at the process in terms of the group dynamics such as composition, accountability, leadership, resources, and political context, and think about how those might have affected the outcome.

Jim: Our contention is that by looking at this one example, understanding its limitations, the reader reflecting about this situation and the process that went on can learn from this case of one. It is our hope that as the reader participates in their own organizational processes, he/she will have some expanded ways of thinking about what's going on and have a positive influence in their own processes.

John: We know from the literature that this this kind of outcome has happened in other states, and from readings that that the National Health Service (NHS) in the UK, which is a well-developed national system already, failed in a hugely expensive project to create a national EHR system. That certainly raises a general question as to the effectiveness of a government process as a vehicle for a very complex technical project that required, as it turns out, a lot of nontechnological skills. The NHS relied on a consultant to develop a strategic plan and then hired a service provider to actually build the system, and simply assumed that hospitals and other essential stakeholders (i.e., Figure 10-2) would buy in and use the system. The outreach and "diplomacy" required to engage major constituents could have been better—and stands as a lesson learned for future large-scale health information technology projects. Likewise, the HITE-CT board seemingly never fully understood either the technology-related issues or the relational issues associated with gaining constituent support.

A Composition of a Group and the Context within Which It Works

CEO Insights

The emergent quality of complex social processes arises from the interactions of the participants. Participants' individual actions and contributions to the process shape and are shaped by those interactions. The diversity of the group and the ever-present possibility of unnoticed or barely noticed differences in understanding or interpretation of the actions of others create the possibility for conflict, surprise, and novelty. Thus our interest in the composition of the DPH advisory board and later, the HITE-CT board that were both engaged in a complex social process. No one person or small group can control the outcome of evolution and emergence—as the HITE-CT experience amply demonstrates—but more powerful people have relatively more impact on the process than the less powerful. Consequently, the interactional dynamics of the people in this process, such as how leadership is or is not experienced, power relations, and shared or conflicting ideologies matter a great deal.

Mainstream organizational theory conceives of organizations as systems. Although this orientation has been responsible for significant advances in organizational theory, Stacey points out that system thinking has some negative consequences. One is the tendency to think of group processes as self-contained entities working in isolation.

Continuity

Jim: As we look at the Connecticut experience, it seemed a lack of continuity of the process greatly influenced what happened and what didn't happen. The HITE-CT process went on over a long period of time—years, with many different people being involved, and with different people being in charge, sometimes from meeting to meeting. This lack of continuity of process has had an influence on leadership, policy, and even technology.

John: I agree. Both of us have extensive experience working with not-for-profit boards or other groups that were not constituted by politial appointment as this board was, but they were, nevertheless, groups of volunteers assembled to oversee an organization or project. All of the organizations in our experience have had a management individual or team to provide continuity for the governing body populated by volunteers.

At the beginning, an advisory board and the State Department of Public Health were supposed to run the project. They were mostly focused on getting federal funding. Project implementation was to be, and eventually was, handed over to a quasi-public entity. There was some carryover of board members but not all; and so there was a significant change in board membership. There was also an election in the middle of this multiyear initiative that resulted in a new governor and a change in all of the commissioners in the state administration. There was really no focal point for any kind of ongoing continuity. At least in the organizations with which we're familiar, a professional management team provides that continuity. Here, because of a lack of funds, they did not hire an executive director until, I think, the middle of 2010, when the process had been under way for more than a year. And then the new executive director left after several months. One could argue that the lack of professional management was one of the flaws in this process.

Lack of Diversity and the Domination of Certain Ideologies

Lack of Accountability (as it would be experienced in the private sector)

Jim: It seems to me that there are other related factors contributing to the process not being successful. If you look at the composition of both the advisory board and then the HITE-CT governing board, even though there was a legislative mandate that it be open, transparent, and inclusive, it is predominantly composed of governmental employees from various agencies, resulting, perhaps, in a lack of diversity of perspectives. Some government employees may have similar perspectives and come from a common experience, in contrast to private-sector organization employees. So there was a lack of diversity and, perhaps, a lack of either robust input or the ability to question the purpose of the activity or the process as it went along. Where was the accountability for expenditure of taxpayer funds and ensuring progress on the HIE initiative?

John: Another consequence of the board appointment process is that everybody on each of the boards was chosen by a different political officeholder. So where should we expect their loyalty to lie, the process or the appointing official? That's why I think it's important for us to resist the temptation to do what typically happens in organizations: say "somebody screwed up here," when in reality there was no one, no one person, accountable. The best evidence of that is they had a federal grant and they spent it, even though they knew that when money ran out, that was it. Their sustainability depended on developing services that they could sell to providers, but even when it became clear that wasn't going to happen, no corrective action was taken.

Something for policy makers to consider, then, is there really is a difference between the way government officials think and act (versus private sector analogs) and that accountability also differs from what one would experience in the private sector. Was the way the state chose to organize this project appropriate for the kind of project they ultimately had to accomplish?

Context-bound, "stuck"

Jim: Everybody, from the beginning as you have said, recognized that government wasn't going to fund this effort long term, and there needed to be enough value to users for them to be willing to pay for the services after the government HIE start up funding ended. Yet sustainability wasn't a focus until very late in the process. How did this process allow what amounted to denial to prevail?

John: Although it would be speculation on my part—reading between the lines—I believe there was always an underlying assumption, even though they talked about sustainability over and over again and actually developed a fee-for-service model, that eventually more government money would be made available. The State never stepped up to provide financial support; the insurance industry in Connecticut never stepped up; and my interpretation of the record is that the federal government actually made it fairly clear that the $7.8 million was all there was going to be from that source.

Jim: Or, if not government grants, there would be government mandates to provider or user communities that would deal with the issue.

John: It's worth noting the overall context within which this apparent denial occurred. The Obama administration came in with significant money in the 2009 stimulus package earmarked for health care IT. Then came the enactment of the ACA. A lot of us in health care believed that with health care reform, mandates for health information exchanges was [sic] going to happen. But, as time went on, and it became increasingly clear that the implementation of the ACA was not going to follow a clear or certain path, that the federal government wasn't going to fund HIEs beyond startup funding, and that states were not going to fund it or mandate the providers to do so. From a complexity standpoint and from a policy standpoint as well, it's important to appreciate that processes like this one don't happen as isolated events. This is not just some little group doing something in a room someplace. What's going on in the broader economy, what's going on elsewhere in government, really affects how this kind of project plays out.

Power Dynamics

CEO Insights

Power differences are integral to all social relationships, and complex social processes are patterned by power dynamics—how power is exercised by some and responded to by others. According to Elias, power differences between individuals are rooted in interdependence. If you have, and can withhold, something I need or desire, you have power over me. Interdependence and, therefore, power imbalances, has increased as role specialization has increased in modern society. In organizations, power can be based on formal position within a hierarchy; knowledge or expertise others need; personal charisma; political connections; and many other factors. Power, because it is based in interdependence, is fluid—relative power is context-dependent. Power exercised to excess—domination—tends to provoke acts of resistance that may be overt, covert—or both.[10]

Resistance

John: One of the more interesting process issues in this case is that the most outspoken members of the group on the opt-in/opt-out problem were the so-called consumer advocates, and they never gave up on their position. The HIE board ended up revisiting this issue over and over again. One of the consumer advocates actually made a PowerPoint presentation outlining the reasons for her opposition to an opt-out versus an opt-in model. After review by a special committee recommended the opt-out approach, the board voted to stay with the original opt-out plan. We know the two consumer representatives continued to oppose the opt-out approach and worked to undermine the board's position by talking to legislators and other influential parties.

The board spent a lot of time talking about the mechanism by which one could opt in or opt out—how the paperwork would be handled because there were technical limitations. This is a very emotional and personal issue for a lot of people, not just a technology one. The privacy of personal information has become a significant issue in our society in general. And they just never were able to deal with that.

Jim: Think about how the power dynamics played out. The committee and then the board, both made up overwhelmingly of governmental employees, said to the consumer members, "We've heard you but we don't want to do it that way." And in response, we know from your conversations with various people close to the process, the consumer advocates lobbied legislators and talked to the media, all behind the scenes, in an attempt to either at best change the approach the committee and then the board were pursuing, or at worst, to undermine credibility and chances for a successful implementation. So, consumers weren't on board and providers had essentially been excluded. Those who would most benefit from the broad availability of health information and those who would fund the effort to make it happen were alienated. At this point, what chance did this process have of success?

John: That's true. From our experience in other settings, boards like this one, because they are made up of volunteers who have no personal skin in the game, have a very hard time dealing with tough issues, having "let it all hang out" debates—and you can see that in the transcripts. People would make statements, give opinions, and, just as you say, the response from the chair or other members is more or less "we hear you," but then ignore it, and leave things just hanging in the air.

Disciplinary Power and Accountability

CEO Insights

The philosopher/historian Michel Foucault wrote extensively about power, a particular form of which—disciplinary power—had its origins in eighteenth-century social reformers' ideas about "humane" prisons and mental hospitals, but which is now a taken-for-granted characteristic of modern institutions, government, and large business corporations. Disciplinary power is exercised by controlling human behavior through the organization of work spaces; clothing (uniforms—including business suits); time (schedules, deadlines); work standards evaluated through examination (including goals, incentive programs, etc.); and surveillance by "hidden" eyes (surveillance cameras seem to be everywhere). One of the authors had an unsettling experience while reading Foucault's Discipline and Punish—*realization of the similarity in design between the hospital he worked in and the ideal prison! Stacey agrees with Foucault that disciplinary power is necessary for the functioning of a complex society, but notes it is also easily abused. The transformation of discipline into domination and coercion is the well-known slippery slope.*

Jim: I've thought about the proposition here that a group of people could come together and a policy that was the best for the stakeholders involved would emerge for the benefit of improving the health of the regional population. That hasn't happened. How does one make sense of what happened or, really what didn't happen? Toward my own sense-making, I would like to take up the idea of accountability. One of the reasons we think this process didn't work very well was the lack of accountability. Accountability has to do with being held responsible. Considering Foucault's concept of disciplinary power seems useful to understanding why there seemed to be no accountability in the HITE-CT process. Foucault sees organizations as being able to get things done through the use of disciplinary power. For disciplinary power to be effective, there must be structure within which people go about their business. He notes the key elements of disciplinary power are surveillance, normalized judgment, and examination. My translation is that expectations are set, organization members are monitored, and periodical review is conducted to compare results to the expectations previously established. Accountability is the setting of expectations and the monitoring of performance where there are consequences to meeting or not meeting expectations. With the HITE-CT process, I don't see a structure designed to support the elements of disciplinary power. So as I look at how this process was organized, accountability simply doesn't seem to be a realistic expectation. Without accountability, it is highly unlikely anything difficult or important can be achieved.

John: It comes back to policy and the fact that we live in a federal democracy. That's the broader issue here. How, in a country like ours, where the federal government has certain powers and responsibilities and the states have certain powers and responsibilities, how do you implement a national program where policy is crafted in such a way that the federal government really can't hold a state agency directly accountable for results? As you say, in the private setting, accountability is clear. If you don't produce, you actually put your livelihood at risk. That kind of accountability is rarely exercised in government bureaucracies.

Jim: If I were put into this situation, I'd participate in the process in a way to try to early on have the group identify differences in ideology; seek to have the process embrace a value proposition that would resonate with all constituents; seek to establish accountability (or perhaps accountabilities) for the governing body; and personally try to facilitate some collective sense-making of those involved in the process.

John: From a complexity perspective all anyone in a leadership role can do is participate as effectively as you can in the process, by just dealing with the process as it emerges.

Ideology

Jim: Remembering that we have been asked to keep the themes of leadership, policy, and technology as a focus of our discussion, I have been considering how to think about policy in this process, and what policy making in this situation might have to do with the lack of attention to the value proposition in that consumers and providers were not engaged. The advisory committee and then the board were faced with making decisions about what to do and how to do it as they sought to bring a health information exchange into being. Policy is about decisions, and decisions are about choices. When thinking about choice, the concept of ideology as the driver of choice comes to mind. Joas wrote about ideology being driven by norms and values, where norms are societally directed what is right and values are individually felt what is good, understanding that the societal and the individual are both the result of processes of interaction of human persons. With the HITE-CT process, I would suggest that an ideologic norm existed with members of the advisory committee and the board that negated any sense of need for attention to consumer or provider buy-in. The largely governmental members did not question the rightness of a centralized, opt-out-based HIE. Plus, the federal government's funding of a state-run HIE reinforced the ideologic rightness of what they were doing. Here policy was driven by the ideology of what was right, mainly a centralized, opt-out state-run HIE.

John: As we've talked about ideologies from time to time, one thing we saw in this group is that it was dominated by people from state agencies—state officials—and you and I believe that there is a kind of bureaucratic mindset. This isn't meant in any way as a criticism, it's just the way work gets done in a state bureaucracy. As this group approached its task, it did so from that perspective. Just as you said, "It's going to be this way and it's going to be a centralized health information exchange, it's going to be controlled by the state, everybody's in it unless they do something specific to opt out." They never really took into account the other interests, hospitals for example, that perhaps should have been involved more fully in the process. So the dominance of a certain kind of ideology clearly shaped how this process played out.

Technology and Cult Values

Jim: We haven't talked very much about technology, and it seems the reason is because leadership and policy are the real issues in this case study. The technology either wasn't a real issue or the group never got to it, because the process didn't get to a place where the technology and the implementation of it became important. There was never agreement on the need for the technology.

John: A couple of things you said prompted some "complexity" thoughts on my part. One could make the case that in our society, this whole idea of health information exchanges, Big Data, has become idealized, which is really what cult values ultimately are about. An ideal that everybody agrees is a good thing without really thinking much about it, but then when you try to implement the ideal in a real-life situation, it doesn't always turn out to be that way.

Jim: What we see here is what happens when the idealized (what Mead called a cult value) concept of a centralized, state-run HIE that is seen to be essential to population health management is addressed by different people with different ideologies, experiences, and needs. It is messy, and what seemed a given-for-granted good is lived out as a conflict between what different people value and need.

John: Exactly. If you believe that what people do, rather than what they say, is what they really believe—it is evident that the providers with the wherewithal believe in this technology. Hospitals and big medical practices and some other providers are making huge investments in health information technology and are also investing in local information exchanges. So the issue wasn't whether the players believed in the technology or in the concept of the health information exchanges. It was *this* approach to a health information exchange that they had a problem with: who owns and who runs the state information exchange? And what's in it for the providers if they are expected to pay for that system? I think that's where this got off track. It really had to do with power, control, and trust as do so many things in organizations, rather than the technology itself.

Conclusion

For the authors, the process of writing this chapter—research, extensive reading, multiple conversations, writing, and editing—was an essential part of our own journey toward becoming truly reflexive practitioners. Our knowledge of, assumptions about, and biases toward health information exchanges and the Connecticut experience evolved as the project evolved, and we ended up in a very different place from where we began.

It is easy to be objective—or judgmental—concerning the behaviors and performance of individuals when one stands outside a social process than it is when one is directly engaged. The authors understand, from decades of experience, what it is like to be in a leadership role where the leader is as much caught up in, and both enabled and constrained by, the web of power relations, conflicting ideologies, conflicting norms and values—in short, the everyday politics of organizational life.

For retired executives, it is also easy to be more accepting of the implications of complexity than it is when one is actively working in a leadership role in an organization. An interesting post by Richard Straub in the *Harvard Business Review* Blog Network on May 6, 2013, "Why Managers Haven't Embraced Complexity," attracted a significant number of responses. An equally thoughtful one, "Why We Shouldn't Be Surprised That Managers Don't Embrace Complexity," by Greg Satell, appeared on the *Forbes Magazine* website on May 18, 2013. Both Straub and Satell reach essentially the same conclusion because the entire management enterprise, who we are and what we do, not to mention the authority we wield, is rooted in the presumption that we, as executives, have the ability to accurately anticipate the future and to control events as they unfold. As Satell puts it,

> . . . I don't believe managers will ever embrace complexity to a great extent. Complexity is messy and uncomfortable. It's fine and well to enjoy thinking about complexity as an intellectual exercise, but when you are accountable for results, it's a nuisance.[12,13]

He goes on to sum up and agree with Straub's reasons why this is so, namely, that managers like to be in control; the tools we've had haven't handled complexity well; and the new technologies of nonhuman decision making are unnerving.

So what conclusions can we fairly draw from our "case of one"? The themes of this book are technology, policy, and leadership, and their nexus, as shown by Esterhay and Bohn's model 1-4 in Chapter 1. We shall comment briefly on each.

Technology: We do believe it is unnecessary to say more about the information technology itself—the hardware and software. The technology works. It is possible today to cost-effectively accumulate, store, transmit, organize, and analyze vast amounts of information.

In our conversations, however, we talked about technology as a *cult value*-- a society-wide ideal that has meaning only when actualized by flesh-and-blood human beings working in real organizations in the present moment.[14] We argue that health information exchanges have become cult values in their own right, at least for some in leadership roles in government and health care, and at least as far as the technology's altruistic goals are concerned. We saw in the transcripts that the groups we were studying considered health information exchanges a good thing—with the expectation that others would see the matter the same way—without any real understanding beyond the purely technical of what would be required to make a functional health information exchange a reality in Connecticut. Turning the idealized concept into a working reality turned out to be a business problem that required the ability to collaborate with consumers and the leaders of provider organizations; the ability to work through such difficult areas of conflict as the opt-in and opt-out problem; and other skills that neither group exhibited to any great degree.

Policy: The policy implications of this case have been woven through our narrative both explicitly and implicitly. Our main point is that there can be a disconnect between policy makers' intentions and how those intentions are actualized at the local level because neither "end" controls the process—no matter how much they believe they do.

In our conversations, we discussed at some length aspects of this process that were in our opinion problematic: the lack of accountability; the composition of the group with its illusory inclusiveness and transparency; and the government mindset that seemed to be exhibited by many of the players in a group that was effectively dominated by state officials.

We found the the manner in which the boards were created by statute particularly troubling. Simply putting a group of people on a board or committee and labeling it "inclusive" or "transparent" doesn't make it so. The characteristics of any group, and the social processes in which it is engaged, will emerge from the interaction of the interests and intentions of each individual member. Those intentions in turn will be shaped by the goals, aspirations, values, and ideologies each individual participant brings to the process and the role(s) each chooses to play within the group.

As we worked our way through this process, and because we know that state-run HIE projects in several states have had similar outcomes, there was a powerful temptation to conclude that a government bureaucracy is not the right vehicle for such a complex project. By virtue of their functions, government bureaucracies are hierarchical, compartmentalized, rule-governed, and risk-averse. But in reality, most established organizations, especially bigger ones, become at least to some degree, hierarchical, compartmentalized, rule-governed, and risk-averse—and the people who work in private-sector organizations are just as committed to their ideologies, norms, values, power, control, and trust differences—albeit different ones, perhaps—as are people in government. There have been high-profile failures in both public and private sectors—the catastrophic global upheaval in financial services in 2007 and 2008; the *Deepwater Horizon* oil spill in the Gulf of Mexico in 2010; and the recent bankruptcy of the city of Detroit, to name just a few. At the same time, the number of profitable, innovative private companies is legion, and the many government programs and services that work well are simply taken for granted.

The space program is ample evidence that government agencies can successfully develop and manage large-scale, incredibly complex technological projects. We do not believe that organizational form, in and of itself, is a determining factor— but in this particular case, it was an important one that should give policy makers something to ponder, especially in light of the importance of striving toward improving the health of the population of each community and our nation as a whole.

Leadership: All of this brings us back to the theme that is of most interest to us— leadership. We begin by recommending to the reader Stacey's recently published 2012 book, *Tools and Techniques of Leadership and Management* (especially Chapter 9), a brief and accessible account of Stacey's thinking on leadership. For Stacey, the essence of leadership is "practical judgment" (*phronesis*), the expertise that a leader develops over time through the experience of leading. The development of practical judgment requires actually doing the work of leading, and practitioners will benefit greatly from the tutelage of mentors or role models who are more expert. Although Stacey sees practical judgment as the only "tool" of any real use to leaders in a world of complex social processes replete with "mess" and contingency, he warns against idealizing practical judgment. Even the best leaders make mistakes and must deal with the consequences of those mistakes as they arise. Ideally, practical judgment requires that personal integrity and an ethical sense are present. History tells us, however, of powerful and successful leaders whose practical judgment was not characterized by societal norms of morality. Phronesis doesn't necessarily result in "good" leadership. "Good" leaders require personal integrity and a well-developed ethical sense as interdependent individuals continually negotiate what each can accept as fair and just. Finally, the exercise of practical judgment in complex social processes requires highly developed conversational and rhetorical skills.

> The techniques of practical judgment encompass a well-developed sensitivity to group dynamics; an ability to judge when to hold ongoing conversation open and when it is necessary to reach temporary closure; an ability to improvise; and an ability to engage in the organizational game of politics in persuasive and effective ways.[15]

Mintzberg[16] has criticized business schools for emphasizing analytical rather than so-called "soft" skills in their curricula. He argues, and we agree, that many business schools are producing technocrats better trained for consultancy than for leadership roles in our organizations. However, while we would like to see a greater emphasis on the kinds of skills Stacey and Mintzberg are talking about, we tend to agree with Stacey that for leaders, experience is in fact the best teacher.

Network Leadership: In the opening chapter, Esterhay and Bohn mentioned the importance of network leadership in the highly interconnected and interdependent world that is emerging all around us and in which all of us are destined to participate. In spite of its potential importance, the concept of network leadership has not been well developed, and there is little to go on in the current literature. From our perspective, we must not treat leadership, networked or otherwise, in isolation. Leaders and led are enmeshed in the same process and one has no meaning without the other. Thinking of organizations as systems leads us to think of organizations as freestanding when they are actually linked in a variety of ways now—in common economic and political circumstances, multiple business interdependencies, communications networks, and the broader society/culture in which they are embedded. Information technology and social networks are only accelerating the evolution of organizations.

In the further development of the notion of network leadership, Stacey's ideas on leading complex social processes are the best starting point we know of. We are on the threshold of radically rethinking what organizations are, how they function, and how they are to be led in this era of emerging networks.

Our final comment on this topic is to stress that we must resist the temptation to posit some ideal organization or some network leadership ideal. Complexity science tells us we cannot manage emergence. Complexity science also tells us that the interplay of conflicting intentions—the "mess" of complexity—is what gives rise to novelty and creativity along with stabilizing and destructive forces. Whatever form organizations may take and however leadership roles and functions may develop, all any of us can—or should—do as individuals is engage, as skillfully as we can, in the work we do—and keep an open and reflexive mind.

Trust: While we did not deal explicitly with trust in this chapter, we offer a brief commentary because it was an important theme in the HITE-CT process. Furthermore, the complex responsive processes theory perspective on trust— what the term means and what role it plays in organizations—is quite different from that found in mainstream management discourse. Trust is a very value-laden term in our culture. Our trust in others implies a belief in their integrity, reliability, competence, commitment to common goals, and so forth, and our own trustworthiness implies those same characteristics in ourselves.

Mainstream management theorists tend to view trust in this way, where trust is good and mistrust is bad. Furthermore, discussions of leadership often cite trustworthiness as an essential attribute of leaders, and assign leaders responsibility for creating trust in organizations.

By contrast, we believe trust emerges in interaction with others; and through practical experience, we have come to understand trust to be mainly about predictability and consistency of response and action in others with whom we interact. We also see trust as emerging from a process of interaction between interdependent people in which leaders actively participate but cannot control. No one person "creates" trust in organizations. Stacey points out that in everyday lived experience, trust is not an absolute. In our relationships, we trust (however one chooses to define the term) others along a constantly emerging continuum from not at all to completely, based on our previous and current interactions. Stacey argues that trust, as understood in our broader culture, can become a cult value in that it is generalized and idealized. Overemphasis on trust in this idealized form, blind trust, discourages reflectivity—really thinking about what we are doing and why—and leads to passive acceptance and inaction in situations where active engagement is called for.[16,17]

A Case of One: Finally, we want to come back to our own thoughts about our case "with an *n* of one":

Jim: We started the chapter with the idea of a case of one. The reader must be wondering about the usefulness of a case-of-one approach and the HITE-CT case we've been discussing. To me, the usefulness of this methodology to the reader comes from thinking about what happened in this case and then taking it to their own experiences in different settings; looking at the way the process happened; in looking at the process of how leadership and policy and technology were addressed; and reflecting on how the underlying currents of power, control, trust, and ideology influenced the process, knowing that they will be important whatever your case of one is.

John: Right. All we can do is raise questions. What if? What if the federal government had provided all the money, what would have happened? What if there had been a different kind of leadership? What if the state had taken a stronger role? What if there had been a more compelling reason for the major providers to participate in funding?

We don't know. I mean, that to me is the essence of complex social dynamics. You really don't know how those things will play out, but at least you can step back, analyze our case of one, learn what we can from similar projects in others states, and gain whatever insights that effort may offer. We have examined the Connecticut HIE case and understand that something similar to this has happened in other states. Undoubtedly some factors are the same. Funding levels and an unarticulated or poorly articulated policy on the part of the federal government played an important role. Then you have all the local characters, their histories and relationships with one another, and where the (various) providers are in their own technological journeys. You can look at only one case at a time. Extract what you can out of it and the next one, and the next process is going to be another case of one.

We began this chapter with a quote on the importance of thoughtful reflection as a prelude to action, and we have attempted to introduce the reader to ideas from one group of scholars who are wrestling with these difficult issues. We conclude with a closing quote from Professor Stacey:

> All anyone can do, no matter how powerful, is engage intentionally and as skillfully as possible in local interaction, dealing with the consequences in an ongoing manner as they emerge.[13]

CHAPTER 10 DISCUSSION QUESTIONS

Discussion questions are provided for team building or class exercises. Answers for all questions are provided in Appendix C.

Question Number	Question
1	The methodology used in this chapter is "a case study with with an *n* of one." What do you see as the strengths and shortcomings of this approach?
2	State-sponsored health information exchanges were described as having been given "cult value" status in practice. Explain this concept. Do you agree with the authors that HIEs are an idealized "taken-as-good" by the governmental and research elements of the healthcare sector?
3	Accountability is a theme considered by the authors. Discuss what accountability means to you and what is necessary to have someone feel accountable.
4	From your own experience, choose a situation in which the result of an interactive process of people was not what was planned or intended. Reflecting on the process, how do you make sense of what happened?

CHAPTER 10 SUMMARY

- The HITE-CT case example provides an example of detailed lessons learned that offer insight into other state-run HIEs in development.

- The outcome of a process of interactive, interdependent humans cannot be predicted but is influenced by how the interdependent humans interact in the process. Leaders cannot control such complex social processes, but leaders can influence the trajectory of an evolving process. The skills needed for leaders of complex processes are qualitative and experience-based rather than quantitative and analytical.

- Ralph D. Stacey is a thought leader in a perspective on complexity theory that is rooted in philosophy and the social sciences—sociology, group psychology, and anthropology among others—as well as the natural sciences. Stacey's ideas are especially relevant and accessible to management practitioners. Exploring the richness of complexity thinking, particularly Stacey's work, should be a priority for healthcare leaders to support their awareness of evolving relationships and actions.

- There is a spectrum of stakeholders impacted in all HIE initiatives. The population health-level impact should be studied and understood from a policy- and community health-level perspective.

CHAPTER 10 REFERENCES

1. Greenhalgh T, Russell J, Ashcroft RE, Parsons W. Why national eHealth programs need dead philosophers: Wittgensteinian reflections on policymakers' reluctance to learn from history. *Milbank Q.* 2011;89(4):533-563.

2. National Association of State CIOs. *Sustainable success: state CIOs and health information exchange.* Lexington, Ky.: NASCIO; 2011.

3. Hsiao CJ, Jha AK, King J, Patel V, Furukawa MF, Mostashari F. Office-based physicians are responding to incentives and assistance by adopting and using electronic health records. *Health Aff (Millwood).* 2013;32(8):1470-7.

4. Desroches CM, Charles D, Furukawa MF, et al. Adoption of electronic health records grows rapidly, but fewer than half of US hospitals had at least a basic system in 2012. *Health Aff (Millwood).* 2013;32(8):1478-85.

5. Adler-Milstein J, Bates DW, Jha AK. Operational health information exchanges show substantial growth, but long-term funding remains a concern. *Health Aff (Millwood).* 2013;32(8):1486-92.

6. Office of the National Coordinator for Health Information Technology. The Direct Project. www.directproject.org. Accessed August 25, 2013.

7. Connecticut Department of Public Health. Verbatim Proceedings. Department of Public Health. Connecticut Health Information Technology and Exchange. East Hartford, Conn.: Connecticut Department of Public Health; January 7, 2013.

8. Various authors. Various complexity topics. *Complexity and Management Centre*;2013. http://complexityandmanagement.wordpress.com/. Accessed June 10, 2014.

9. Reflexive practice. Reflexivepractice weblog;2013. http://reflexivepractice.wordpress.com/. Accessed June 10, 2014.

10. Scott JC. *Domination and the arts of resistance : hidden transcripts.* 1st ed. New Haven, Conn.: Yale University Press; 1992.

11. Mead GH. Scientific method and the moral sciences. *Int J Ethics.* 1923;23:229-247.

12. Satell G. Why we shouldn't be surprised that managers don't embrace complexity. *Forbes Blog.* http://www.forbes.com/sites/gregsatell/2013/05/18/why-we-shouldnt-be-surprised-that-managers-dont-embrace-complexity/. Published May 18, 2013. Accessed December 25, 2013.

13. Stacey R. *Strategic management and organisational dynamics: the challenge of complexity to ways of thinking about organizations.* 6th ed. Upper Saddle River, N.J.: Prentice Hall; 2011.

14. Stacey R. *Strategic management and organisational dynamics: the challenge of complexity to ways of thinking about organizations.* 6th ed. Upper Saddle River, N.J.: Prentice Hall; 2011.

15. Stacey R. *Tools and techniques of leadership and management: meeting the challenge of complexity.* New York, N.Y.: Routledge; 2012.

16. Mintzberg H. *Managers, not MBAs: A hard look at the soft practice of managing and management development.* San Francisco, Calif.: Berrett-Koehler Publishers; 2005.

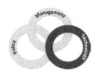

Chapter 11. Using Terminology Standards to Count the Healthy and Sick

Mark Samuel Tuttle, AB, BE, FACMI

Stephanie Suzanne Lipow, MLIS

". . . it is no easy matter to make a computer behave as a clerk."[1,2]

C.W. Churchman
The Design of Inquiring Systems: Basic Concepts of Systems and
Organization, *1971*

"[The Unified Medical Language System is] designed to help improve the retrieval of machine-readable information across systems, and in particular, to overcome the variety of ways that the same concepts are expressed in machine-readable and human language in different systems."[3]

R. Kleinsorge, J. Willis, and S. Emrick.
UMLS Overview—AMIA Tutorial 2007

Chapter 11 Learning Objectives

- Learn why 1) terminology is about communication, and the goal of standard terminology is to name important things in a comparable, scalable, and reusable way; 2) evolution didn't prepare us to do the latter; and 3) computers can help.

- Learn the language used to talk about terminology and terminology standards.

- Learn why we don't yet have interoperation-by-meaning in healthcare.

- Appreciate a population health objective requiring the use of standard terminology.

- Gain an understanding of the important healthcare terminology standards: ICD-

9-CM, ICD-10-CM, SNOMED CT, RxNorm, LOINC, and CPT.

- Prepare to meet certain realities concerning the use of terminology instances in electronic health records.

- Get started with terminology-based predictive analytics.

Introduction

The premise of this chapter is that the health of a population is exactly the sum of the health of the individuals in it, and we get this sum by counting. This premise is not intrinsically true; we can imagine other ways of assessing the health of a population, but for practical reasons it is true enough currently. This fact then poses the questions, "What, exactly, do we count? And when and how? And what do we do with the results?" In contrast to earlier eras, an explicit subtext here is that we want all this counting to scale to the nation and to the world. Fortunately, health terminology and supporting processes have evolved and are evolving to answer these questions. That evolution is accelerating rapidy because of the increasing availability of technology, especially but not limited to electronic health records. Recently, technology has begun to drive the standardization of health terminology, particularly the terminology used in electronic health records. Not coincidentally, the same globalization that is supported by advancing technology also supports the rapid evolution of such diseases as influenza, putting yet more stress on the means we use to name them.

This chapter takes on the longstanding challenge of naming the things we want to count when assessing a population, and the emergent challenge of counting in a way that can exploit the opportunities enabled by technology. As implied, the observations that lead to names—the labels generated by observations of individuals—need to scale in a useful manner with the size of the population, and this scaling must be graceful and productive. Naming diseases has always been difficult; and as will be illustrated, it is still difficult. Naming the increasingly numerous and volatile repertoires of laboratory tests, medications, and procedures poses additional challenges. A major part of the challenge is that the observations that make up the counts must be comparable across human observers—think diagnoses; and machines—think lab tests. In most cases these humans and machines don't "know" one another. They will generally be separate and connected only at the moment the counts are aggregated. Increasingly, we want these counts to be aggregated as close to the time the relevant observations were made as is practical—the better to try to intervene, if that is called for.

At this writing the proportion of each electronic health record or any record of health status that is "standard" is small, but increasing rapidly. Thus, this chapter will attempt to prepare the reader to make use of the full gamut of forms of information about health: from narrative to genomics, from the International Classification of Diseases (ICD) to the Systematized Nomenclature of Medicine (SNOMED), from the informal (local templates) to the formal (Logical Observation Identifiers Names and Codes [LOINC] and RxNorm), and from paper to Big Data enabled by Meaningful Use. Leveraging all this will require continuous learning. As we learn from Zen, all change is opportunity. These changes will enable public health students and practitioners—those who read this book—to see more and do more than has ever been possible.

To make all this as real as possible, this chapter begins with a scenario. The way to get the most out of this chapter is to put yourself inside it.

Why You Need This Chapter...!

You are called to the office of the chief medical officer (CMO) of your institution. You are not surprised to find that the CMO is an elderly male veteran of many decades of healthcare and institutional crises. He dispenses with pleasantries and says. . .

> "You have been recommended as an interdisciplinary problem solver and communicator. I want our institution to develop a Distant Early Warning system[*] for metabolic syndrome.[†,‡]
>
> I cannot get my doctors to agree on whether or not there is such a thing, but it doesn't matter. It is clear we are going to be responsible for a population in

---

[*] The United States built a DEW Line (distant early warning system) in Alaska, Canada, and other "distant" locales during the Cold War. While a triumph of technology, the DEW Line is also remembered for generating false positives.

[†] A sample definition of metabolic syndrome can be found at: Wikipedia contributors. Metabolic syndrome. Wikipedia, The Free Encyclopedia. November 14, 2013, 13:09 UTC. Available at: http://en.wikipedia.org/w/index.php?title=Metabolic_syndrome&oldid=581623575. Accessed November 16, 2013.

[‡] This challenge is adapted from conversations with Brennan O'Banion on March 28, 2013. O'Banion is an experienced practitioner of public health who presently works with the Kentucky Health Information Exchange (KHIE). He focuses on utilizing the KHIE to improve statewide public health surveillance and reporting.

which—we don't really know this with any accuracy—we have emerging epidemics of hypertension, type 2 diabetes, hyperlipidemia, obesity, and related chronic conditions.

We have a large current database of patient electronic medical records collected over the years. I have a computer science class ready to work on the problem, but they don't know where to start. They have determined the first problem is formulating a computable definition of the syndrome. My geneticists face the same challenge: how to define the phenotype? Both groups think they are going to put the hospital's data in the cloud and have automated applications generate answers. If they get an answer I won't know whether I will believe it.

I know there are problems with the data, but these conditions don't develop overnight. There must be clues that predict them, and some of the clues should be in the observations we have recorded. If you can help us predict which patients to focus on, we can start experimenting with interventions. We know about the demographic and socioeconomic predictors. We want you to focus on the opportunities we anticipate to emerge associated with our participation in the Centers for Medicare and Medicaid Services (CMS) Meaningful Use of Electronic Health Records (EHRs) incentive program[4]—specifically, the support for interoperation that includes encoding of diagnoses, laboratory test results, medication administration, procedures, and other information using terminology standards. We should be able to access the primary care records of patients who end up here, whether or not our affiliated doctors created the records.

Tell me what I should do to start measuring and predicting, starting as soon as possible. Assume records are accumulating that contain standard terminology. And then tell me if this Unified Medical Language System (UMLS) thing can be used to look at pre-Meaningful Use records. I will have our health information management staff contact you.

If you come back with a plan in a week, I will think you are not ready. If I don't see you in a month I will worry that you are not getting anywhere.

Any questions?"

So what do terminology and standard terminology have to do with your assignment? In this context, *terminology empowers humans*, enabling them to name and talk about the many aspects of metabolic syndrome; and *standard terminology empowers computers*, enabling them to count the occurrence of certain potentially relevant patient descriptions in electronic health records (EHRs). There are feedback loops in both directions. If humans can communicate with one another clearly and productively, they are more likely to record care descriptions accurately and usefully. If computers can count and aggregate these descriptions in a fast, scalable, and reproducible way, then they make it easier for humans to understand what is going on in the population being studied. Alternatively, if the care descriptions are not comparable, then counting the population will be difficult and the result less useful. Further, if the aggregations used are not reusable throughout the population, then analyses will not be comparable. Whatever hypotheses we have about the definition and utility of the label "metabolic syndrome," it will be easier to test if we have a scalable, comparable assessment of care descriptions of potentially relevant patients.

A few hours after your meeting with the CMO you get a text message from him that says, *"I want to detect whatever is detectable in real time."*

Learning the Lingo...

We begin this chapter with a review of terms used to communicate about terminology. It is focused on understanding the way various relevant constituencies talk and think about the subject.

> *Questions of terminology go back at least as far as the Garden of Eden, according to the book of Genesis*: "So out of the ground the Lᴏʀᴅ God formed every animal of the field and every bird of the air, and brought them to the man to see what he would call them; and whatever the man called every living creature, that was its name." Old Testament, Genesis 2:19 (Hebrew Bible)

In 1988, the first author was told while on the road giving terminology presentations, "We know how to do terminology here," implying that a federal effort to connect extant terminologies wasn't relevant. Twenty-five years later, national (and international) terminology standards are a requirement for most uses of information technology in healthcare.

Because your efforts regarding metabolic syndrome will be intrinsically interdisciplinary, the words and phrases defined below are certain to arise. Your success will depend on understanding the ideas so named and your ability to communicate productively in the face of their—occasionally disruptive—use.

Most of the work that led to today's standard terminologies was undertaken using preindustrial methods. Some observers would argue that there was a kind of technological determinism at play. Computing resources were scarce and expensive. Visionaries saw the potential of information technology but lacked the infrastructure and therefore the experience to scale what they were doing. For this and other reasons, terminology development was slow to make appropriate use of the Internet, and it trailed rather than led the use of the World Wide Web (WWW).

Anticipating a later section of this chapter and in accord with the explicit population health objective of this book, the Unified Medical Language System (UMLS)[5] built by the U.S. National Library of Medicine was the first large terminology project undertaken using modern information technology. Tools now taken for granted and widely used in computer science and other fields were nearly absent in health care and population health studies for many years. These included the Internet, UNIX, relational databases, client-server architecture, workstations, bitmapped displays, laser printers, personal computers, direct manipulation software development, digital projectors, and the like, all of which proved essential to the early development of the UMLS. Each of these technologies improved communication among a geographically distributed interdisciplinary team, and therefore accelerated improvement in the quality of the content produced. Whatever else the UMLS project has done, it has raised the collective consciousness regarding the creation, deployment, use, and maintenance of terminologies.

Until recently, small groups worked on terminology development and maintenance for decades, sometimes producing high-quality artifacts, but almost always in isolation. No larger consensus on important and fundamental definitions of the terms used to describe terminologies was ever reached. Any collective sense of irony on this failure—a failure to agree on "terminology terminology"—was overcome by the larger evolutionary role of language in supporting local communication and productivity. Local language can improve productivity locally, but a side effect is that it defines group identity and the latter inhibits the discovery and exploitation of commonality across groups. This is the first of several terminology challenges posed by our sociobiology; that is, that sometimes our behavior is the result of evolution.

Nevertheless, certain critical ideas emerged over and over again even though different groups named them differently. It is helpful to understand these ideas, even if the use of their names in some contexts may evoke emotional and antagonistic reactions. Thus this section opens with a paradox: it is important to understand the things being named, but we suggest that you not use many of these names in interdisciplinary contexts. Instead, use deliberately simple, deliberately unpretentious words like *vocabulary*, *name*, *field*, *record*, and *standard*, along with—and this is important—specific examples, so that listeners can understand what you mean and not take offense. For one thing, the definitions appearing here may not appear anywhere else.

Finally, some would argue that the emergence and deployment of standard terminologies in health care will make the kind of intellectual and conceptual background described below obsolete. Alternatively, assessing health care at scale, using population health assessment across diverse settings and using diverse sources of information, will make these ideas even more important than they are now. The astute reader will observe that they are not part of a coherent structure, and that is part of your challenge (and opportunity) and a comment on the domain wherein you will need a tolerance for ambiguity. The reader is invited to impose his or her organization on these entries as a way of helping them to remember them.[*]

A helpful way to think about these words and phrases and the ideas they name is to remember that each one is the answer to a relevant question. And it's the questions that are important! You are sure to be in interdisciplinary meetings as part of your assignment. If someone uses a word X that you don't understand or that you think is confusing, one stratagem is to ask politely, "If X is the answer, what was the question?" You are asking for a definition in a way that attempts to focus on why you should care. In that spirit, this entire chapter is a response to "If terminology and standard terminology is the answer, what was the question?" Further, in each case we'll usually add our opinion on whether the ideas matter in this context. Again, the questions matter more than the answers. Finally, sometimes it's better to just ignore usage unless it proves critical. For example, if someone uses the word *ontology* in an interdisciplinary context, then asking them to define it will derail the meeting. If your project moves into bioinformatics, the same thing may happen when such words as *gene* and *allele* are used in such settings.

What do we call a unit of thought, and why do we care? A concept is a unit of thought, like *metabolic syndrome*. Some concepts have names, sometimes more than one name. Sometimes *concept* refers to a unit of representation in a

---

[*] See Question 1 at the end of this chapter.

computer. Regardless, it's very important to be able to talk about units of meaning independent of the names of those units, because the meaning of words can distract folks when the focus should be on the ideas. For example, *jaundice* and *icterus* are "just" the Latin and Greek words for *yellow*, respectively; but sometimes local convention treats their meanings differently. Similarly, *hypertensive* is sometimes a label for a patient whose blood pressure is controlled by medication, and sometimes not. The important point is that there are units of meaning, and there are words and phrases that are names for these units, and they are not the same thing. In this context, it's the meanings and names that are important and not the words in the names. This observation leads to the next question.*

How are concepts, symbols, and the things the symbols name related? The **Meaning Triangle**[6,7] explains that the connection between a symbol—here, the phrase *metabolic syndrome*—and a category of patients who have some specific things in common—is a *concept*. The concept is the apex of the triangle. The symbol and the category of patients are the two other vertices of the triangle, the point being that there is no direct connection between them; that edge of the triangle is a dotted line. This diagram is a very powerful idea, but a distraction in the context of your assignment. You should be prepared, however, if someone brings it up. Figure 11-1 illustrates the Meaning Triangle with the concept or unit of thought we call *metabolic syndrome*.

Figure 11-1. The Meaning Triangle for Metabolic Syndrome

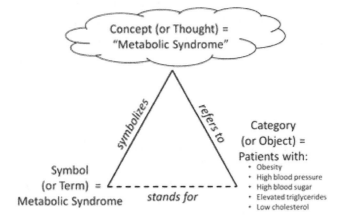

---

* There will be many links in this chapter to Wikipedia. It is an example of a powerful complexity management strategy, used by terminology developers – it represents its entries homogeneously while linking to relevant heterogeneous sources. All Wikipedia links were tested during October, November, and December of 2013.

What defines the universe of named things? An **ontology**, literally (Greek again) "the study of that which exists," has come to mean in the context of this chapter, a formal collection of category names[*] with defining relationships among them. To oversimplify, a relevant ontology would assert that metabolic syndrome is something that exists and that it is a kind of disease. Depending on what we think about it, we could assert that it's a kind of metabolic disease. The tough part of creating an ontology is that one is then obligated to distinguish metabolic syndrome from all other diseases, or all other metabolic diseases, using relationships to still other categories. Computer programmers want ontologies so that they can create programs that can reason about named things, but—as implied—ontologies are very hard to create and maintain at the scale required for health care and biomedical research. Narrowly speaking, there are no large health care ontologies of interest at this point, although, as will be described below, some terminologies are more "ontologic" than others. Note that we are beginning to focus on properties of health care descriptions, instead of on the characteristics of health care. The interplay of the structure of descriptions and the structure of the world they describe is explored in Blois (1984), referenced earlier. The subtitle of that book is *The Nature of Medical Descriptions*.

What distinguishes information that is comparable, reusable, and scalable? A unit of information that is **formal** has certain qualities. The most important is that its equivalence is testable. That is, the names *metabolic syndrome* and *syndrome X*[†,8] name *concepts*. Are those concepts the same or different? If there is a communicable way to say "yes" or "no," then we could assert that those names are formal. Some would argue that formality also requires some notion of explicit relatedness. For example, is there a way of specifying how the name *abdominal obesity–metabolic syndrome*[‡] is related to either or both of the other

---

[*] The alert reader will note that this definition includes important words – *formal, category*, and *relationship*—not yet defined as some definitions will be circular.

[†] As late as the year 2000 a book was published – Reaven G, et al. *Syndrome X – overcoming the silent killer that can give you a heart attack.* New York, N.Y.: Simon & Schuster; 2000. However, no extant terminology uses the term *syndrome X* today, as it has been replaced by more descriptive names.

[‡] This is the name of a relevant entry in OMIM (Online Mendelian Inheritance in Man). Available at:
http://www.omim.org/entry/605552?search=metabolic%20syndrome&highlight=syndromic%20syndrome%20metabolic. Accessed online December 17, 2013.

names? The problem with formality is that the quality does not predict utility; that is, whether we care. This is one reason that projects that start out with formalization as a goal can fail. Because there are many reasons for this kind of failure, one must be very careful with the tradeoffs implicit here. Not too long ago, an argument in favor of the ontologic approach to medical terminology used the "nine planets" as a model of what a healthcare ontology ought to be—failing to remember that this proposal was made after Pluto had been demoted to the status of dwarf planet, and officially, there are only eight planets—although nothing in the physical world had changed. Instead, our naming changed because we came to know more about the many Pluto-like objects, now called plutoids, in our solar system. The field of artificial intelligence struggled with this challenge for decades. In contrast, the discipline of engineering often eshews formality because it focuses first on fulfilling human needs. An example with which we are all familiar is the Google search engine, for which formalization generally tends to follow success rather than precede it.

What do we call the process by which one computer exchanges information with another autonomously? **Interoperation** is a capability possessed by two or more computers by which they can exchange information with one another. By implication the process is at least semiautomatic, allowing, for instance, information about a patient stored in one computer to be transferred and stored in another computer. Not surprisingly, there is also an implication that the receiving computer can do something useful with the information received as well as just storing it.

How do we explain what to represent or not, or what is represented or not, in some artifact? As the late statistician George Box put it, "all models are wrong, some models are useful."[9] **Models** make certain things explicit, and hide or ignore certain other things. In this context, models are abstractions of some reality. Ideally, a model allows us to focus on what matters in a specified context. Three models are of immediate use to us, and it's worth remembering the differences among them. They are named *reference model, information model,* and *terminology model.*

How do we compare two things that cannot be put side by side? How is a computer enabled to do this? A **reference model** is something that we "refer to" as a way of assessing some quality, typically for purposes of comparing what we have with something we don't have.[*,10] For example, to tell whether person A is

---

* The Wikipedia definition covers the use of the term *reference model* in software architecture. See ... Wikipedia contributors. Reference model. Wikipedia, The Free Encyclopedia. October 17, 2013,

taller than person B, we could have them stand beside eachother and assess the outcome by inspection. Alternately, we can use a tape measure—a reference model—to measure A's height, then measure B's height, then compare that result. If A and B are children, the reference model has the added benefit of generating results that are comparable across time; we can tell how much each child grew over some period of time. Thus reference models are about comparability, particularly comparability in computers. As we will see below, Systematized Nomenclature of Medicine—Clinical Terms (SNOMED CT) attempts to be a reference model for, among other things, diseases; sometimes it can tell us some ways in which different diseases are related to one another.[*]

What do we do when important relationships between concepts become more complex? An ***information model*** relates concepts that depend on one another in potentially complicated ways. For example, something that will prove important in our pursuit of metabolic syndrome is the concept *body mass index* (BMI). Sometimes a patient's record will contain a BMI value, and sometimes not. If the record contains the patient's weight and height, the BMI can be computed. An information model would make explicit the relationship between weight, height, BMI, the units for weight and height, and a time stamp for the measurements. Thus information models are distinguished from terminology models in that the latter specifically limit what can be expressed and the former can have potentially unbounded complexity. For example, a terminology model may not permit the representation of the (theoretical) constant 703.06957964 . . . used in some BMI computations; an information model pragmatics lets us decide to use 703. In summary, a typical information model is a simple extra-terminologic complexity management artifact. Its cost is the introduction of nonhomogeneous, potentially noncomparable, semantics inside the model. In summary, we do whatever we want in an information model, and then put a box around it. Usually, the box has a "standard" output, and often standard inputs, but ad hoc innards.

11:34 UTC. Available at: http://en.wikipedia.org/w/index.php?title=Reference_model&oldid=577558540. Accessed December 18, 2013. That definition focuses on the use of reference models in support of "clear communication" and "standards," which is a more general view of reference models than that used in this chapter.

[*] See Question 8.

What determines what can and cannot be represented in a given terminology? A ***terminology model*** is an abstraction that makes explicit what can and cannot be represented in a terminology that adheres to that model. For example, by definition a terminology contains terms; and by implication, those terms name concepts. (While only rarely are terminology models explicit, often they can be inferred by inspection.)[*,11] Usually, the most important thing the terminology model does is specify whether or not concept-ness—"Do two different terms name the same concept or not?"—is explicit. (Most terminologies in healthcare are now what is called "concept-oriented," meaning that concept-ness is explicit, but a few terminologies consist of terms not connected by concept-ness.) Similarly, the terminology model specifies what kinds of relationships, if any, connect the terms or concepts, and whether concepts have narrative definitions, associated (nonlinguistic) codes, and other attributes. Thus terminology models generally prohibit relationships sufficiently complex to represent such things as BMI computations. Increasingly, terminology models contain information about the status of terms and concepts in time—maintenance information, in other words. For a computer scientist, a terminology model explains a terminology to a computer. Sometimes a terminology model explains why terms in one terminology are not easily compared with terms in another. Regardless, a typical terminology model specifies the repeatable element, informally called an entry, enabling the terminology to scale (in principle) without limit. This specification is very important for computers, so that programs can rely upon each terminology entry specified by the terminology model to have a predictable structure. In summary, terminology models specify what can be exploited computationally.[12] To look ahead here, as with novels by Ernest Hemingway, the rules are easy to make up but hard to live by.

How should time be represented in a computer, or in a terminology? A ***temporal model*** would capture for a computer when events happen relative to one another. Unfortunately, representing time in a general way proves to be very difficult at present. Initially, theoretical computer science sought to deal with time as an explicit variable. These efforts failed, and were replaced by models that represented only the *order* in which symbols were seen, as opposed to when they were seen. This simplification proved profoundly productive, but—of course—much was lost. For example, databases are good at

---

[*] Some "knowledge" resources, including some terminologies, are now released in *RDF* (Resource Description Framework). See ... Wikipedia contributors. Resource description framework. Wikipedia, The Free Encyclopedia. Such (advanced) formats are themselves close to the notion of a terminology model described here.

representing what is called *transaction time*; that is, when something was first stored in the database. But such seemingly simple notions as "during" prove to be more difficult to handle in a straightforward, reproducible, and scalable way. Sometimes an information model can capture the fact that one event—a medication adverse event, say—happens during another event like the patient's being on a specified medication. But as observed, facts in one information model may not be readily aggregatable with facts in another information model. For example, the difficulty of detecting the so-called Vioxx signal—that a widely used anti-inflammatory medication was associated with cardiac events in a certain class of patients—was partly due to a lack of standard ways of interpreting and therefore aggregating temporally based data.[13] Therefore, you should represent temporally based concepts in as simple a way as is practical, and not be surprised if things get more complicated than you anticipated, and that you have to try again—a subject we shall revisit below.

What do we call the part of the field of medicine devoted to the classification of disease? **Nosology** is the practice of classifying diseases.[14] Disease classifications are probably as old as civilization; Indian, Chinese, and Greek cultures each had their own classifications. Not surprisingly, these classifications evolve with our understanding of diseases, and can be guided by quite different objectives. An early objective was predictive value: is the disease contagious, or not? Later nosology was driven by the desire to count the dead by cause of death in a scalable way. More recently, public health nosology has been focused on the organization of diseases by etiology, or what causes them. Defining metabolic syndrome poses additional challenges. Understanding the history of nosology helps one understand that terminologies are purpose-built, but over time they may support whatever else they end up being used for. In the future, nosology may be hidden as healthcare focuses on outcomes for individual patients, predicted by a combination of "-omics" and lifestyle.[*,†,‡,15] Current pressures on

---

* See remarks by John Mattison at StrataRx 2012 Conference. Panel discussion titled *Disruptors: Panel on What Healthcare Will Look Like in 2020*. San Francisco, California, October 16–17, 2012. http://www.youtube.com/watch?v=1i_xD3djctw. Accessed online December 18, 2013. Mattison argues that "the future of medicine is the single patient multi-omic profile."

† A contrary view is that some nosology is driven by pharmaceutical regulation.

‡ See the following presentations. Atul B. Transforming a trillion points of data into diagnostics, therapeutics, and new insights into disease (slide #29). Society for Clinical Trials Annual Conference, Boston, Massachusetts, May 2013. http://www.slideshare.net/atulbutte/2013-05-society-for-clinical-trials. Accessed online December 18, 2013. Nelson S. Sifting through sand for nuggets: understanding big data in the face of changing nosology (Slide #4). 2013 NIHI

nosology include advances in genomics and the need to predict responses to therapy.[*] Both these pressures are sure to affect the evolving definition of metabolic syndrome.

Which terminology models attempt to enable reproducible counting? A **classification**[†] is a terminology designed to place each classified thing in exactly one class. More formally, the classes are intended to be mutually exclusive and exhaustive. Thus at the risk of over-implifying, every patient gets at least one name (label); whether that patient gets more than one depends on the granularity and identity of the categories naming any additional maladies (comorbidities). Usually, a classification places each named category in a hierarchy. In this context, ICD-9-CM and ICD-10-CM (see later) are classifications; both name diseases and place individual diseases in a hierarchy of "similar" diseases. They also include human-readable instructions on how to decide whether a diagnosis belongs in one category or another. In practice, however, problems arise, especially in regard to what is similar to what. For example, here is the current ICD-9-CM hierarchy containing "Dysmetabolic syndrome X":[‡,§]

Symposium on Big Data in Healthcare, Auckland, New Zealand, October 2013. http://www.nihi.auckland.ac.nz/sites/nihi.auckland.ac.nz/files/pdf/informatics/bigdata/Sifting%20through%20sands%20for%20nuggets%20-%20Stuart%20Nelson.pdf. Accessed online December 18, 2013.

[*] See, the following presentations. Atul, B. Transforming a trillion points of data into diagnostics, therapeutics, and new insights into disease (slide #29). Society for Clinical Trials Annual Conference. May 2013. http://www.slideshare.net/atulbutte/2013-05-society-for-clinical-trials. Accessed online December 18, 2013. Nelson, S. Sifting through sand for nuggets: understanding big data in the face of changing nosology (Slide #4). 2013 NIHI Symposium on Big Data in Healthcare, Auckland, New Zealand, October 2013. http://www.nihi.auckland.ac.nz/sites/nihi.auckland.ac.nz/files/pdf/informatics/bigdata/Sifting%20through%20sands%20for%20nuggets%20-%20Stuart%20Nelson.pdf. Accessed online December 18, 2013.

[†] There is no Wikipedia entry for "Classification." Instead Wikipeidia has a long list of types of classification, one of which is "Medical classification." Wikipedia contributors. Medical classification. Wikipedia, The Free Encyclopedia. October 25, 2013, 06:28 UTC. Available at: http://en.wikipedia.org/w/index.php?title=Medical_classification&oldid=578655801. Accessed December 19, 2013. This article hints at longstanding and ongoing national and international disputes about the artifacts used for classification in healthcare.

[‡] A theory as to why hierarchies are harder to create and maintain as one ascends (increasing in generality) their levels is presented in Blois MS. Medicine and the nature of vertical reasoning. *N Engl J Med*. 1988; 318(13):847-51.

[§] See the following web page: http://www.icd9data.com/2013/Volume2/M/Merycism-to-Metalliferous.htm (accessed online December 18, 2013). The index to ICD-9-CM indicates that "Metabolic Syndrome" is to be coded as 277.7. In turn, the preferred name for that code is

> *2013 ICD-9-CM Diseases and Injuries Codes*
> * - Endocrine, Nutritional And Metabolic Diseases, And Immunity*
> *   Disorders (240-279.9)*
> *   - Other Metabolic And Immunity Disorders (270-279.9)*
> *   - Other and unspecified disorders of metabolism (277)*
> *   - Dysmetabolic syndrome X (277.7)*

As remarked already, hierarchies like this are not scalable: they are difficult to create and hard to maintain, especially in the face of advancing knowledge. It is easy to be critical but hard to do better.[16,*] For one thing, the many versions of ICD and its predecessors have been in use since the late nineteenth century—initially for counting causes of death in a comparable manner. Today, ICD is used for health and morbidity statistics and reimbursement, and it supports such analysis as that which your hypothetical CMO has asked you to undertake. Maintenance of the ICD-9-CM hierarchy was made more difficult because the curators ran out of space for codes; the fixed decimal structure did not allow for enough digits for "new" diseases. Thus we cannot tell whether lumping "immunity disorders" into one of the classes above was the result of science or of maintenance expediency. This lumping was changed in ICD-10-CM, which, after an adoption delay, may be in broad use in the United States some months after this book is published. Here is the analogous hierarchy for this version.

> *2013 ICD-10-CM Codes*
> * - Endocrine, nutritional and metabolic diseases (E00-E89)*
> *   - Metabolic disorders (E70-E88)*
> *   - Other and unspecified metabolic disorders (E88)*
> *   - Other specified metabolic disorders (E88.8)*
> *   - Metabolic syndrome (E88.81)*

Even after the disappearance of the "immunity disorders" appendage from the ICD-9-CM hierarchy, we are still left with uncertainty about what is and is not going to be "similar" to "metabolic syndrome," given only the names of the

---

"Dysmetabolic Syndrome X." ICD-9-CM does *not* tell us whether the two terms are synonymous, or just "similar," or just to be counted as the same thing.

[*] A theory as to why hierarchies are harder to create and maintain as one ascends (increasing in generality) their levels is presented in Blois MS. Medicine and the nature of vertical reasoning. *N Engl J Med.* 1988; 318(13):847-51.

categories. Put differently, medical coders have to understand how to use ICD-9/10-CM comparably, and this understanding requires extensive knowledge and experience. Readers with some familiarity with ICD disease names should ask themselves whether such category names as "other and unspecified metabolic disorders" are a necessary feature of a classification or not. This topic will be revisited below during the discussion of "face validity." Put differently, the many versions of ICD (International Classification of Diseases) have been about labeling the dead and the health state of those alive with one or more categories in a reproducible way, and less about the names of those categories. Looking ahead, one place we might care very much about how a category name looks is in a patient's problem list. The focus on categories over names is in contrast with the opposite objectives of nomenclatures, as will be described below. In our opinion, competing terminologies are evolving toward one another, and differences that affect your assignment may diminish in number. For instance, ICD-11, scheduled for release in 2015, has explicit connections to SNOMED CT.[17,18] For the present, these connections are a good thing. One remaining difference, however, between a classification and other kinds of terminologies is the tendency to name the "other" elements in a category. Thus in ICD-9-CM, the code 277.9 is named "unspecified disorder of metabolism." In order to understand what might be in this class, one must understand what is named by all the other more explicitly named members of the class.[*]

Are some classifications more structured than others? Often, a **taxonomy** is a classification created using some explicit set of principles.[19] While a taxonomy seems to be useful when categorizing plants, beetles, and other species, analogous principles for disease classification have proven to be elusive, and we know of none in broad use. Taxonomies usually have a dual objective: coherent naming and coherent classification; ideally this coherence produces a kind of predictability lacking in "pure" classifications. Note that this observation is as much about properties of descriptions as properties of the world so described.

How should things be named? A **nomenclature** is a collection of names and rules for creating names.[20] Again, biology leads the way.[21] As with taxonomies, we know of no system of rules for creating the names of diseases, although the terminology model for SNOMED CT (see later) has a lot to say about this. But again, the point of a nomenclature is to have coherent, predictable, and

---

[*] When encountering a large number of such codes, consult the local medical coder for guidance. Ask, for example, what NOS (not otherwise specified) and NEC (not elsewhere classified) mean in the context of metabolic syndrome.

understandable naming. A result of such naming is then intended to be a useful classification. The current SNOMED CT hierarchy for metabolic syndrome is not particularly revealing, but it does make explicit that four other disease names are considered synonyms.[*]

> *SNOMED CT Concept*
>   *- Clinical finding*
>   *- Disease*
>   *- Metabolic disease*
>   *- Metabolic syndrome X*
>   *+Dysmetabolic syndrome X*
>   *+Insulin resistance syndrome*
>   *+Metabolic syndrome*
>   *+Reaven's syndrome*

As of this writing, the current version of SNOMED CT lists 52 other metabolic diseases as hierarchical "siblings" of "metabolic syndrome X" —that is, they are in the same "class"—and many of these diseases are differentiated from metabolic syndrome through relationships to anatomic sites, morphology, and the like. These relationships are the result of the rules used to name things in SNOMED CT; it's just that these rules are hard to apply to diseases like metabolic syndrome. SNOMED CT says that "Metabolic syndrome X" IS_A "metabolic disease," but nothing else; of course this is both an observation about the difficulty of applying the rules, and about the uncertainties surrounding the disease. Simply put, *the category names in ICD "look" very different from the category names in SNOMED, and yet the same world is being described.* Further, unlike the case in ICD, the SNOMED CT class of diseases—"metabolic disease"— does not contain an "Other" element. Instead, there are the 53 explicitly named maladies. One has the option of labeling a patient with the name "metabolic disease" if none of the 53 are appropriate.

What do we call the study of terms and their use? Etymologically, we should use the word **terminology** to name the study of terms and their use.[22] But this meaning has been all but extinguished from common parlance. In this chapter we bow to convention and use *terminology* to refer, typically, to an organized collection of names of categories—an artifact, in other words—of use in some specified domain.[23] This is the same development that has happened to the term

---

[*] Here the "+" sign labels synonyms of the preferred name of the concept.

ontology—it was originally the "study of . . . " and now it's used generally to refer to an artifact. Again, in both cases, the implication is that the artifact—terminology or ontology—is associated with some domain.

What is an example of a terminology that is not a reference terminology? An **interface terminology** tries to connect user-friendly, or at least user-useful, names with names in a reference terminology or other terminology endpoint. As observed above, sometimes the functional objectives of a terminology interfere with the creation of names that are both convenient to use and readily understood in some context. The endpoint could be a term used for reimbursement, a lab order, a medication order, an input to a decision support program, or health statistics. An interface terminology provides locally recognizable names, sometimes including abbreviations (such as MetSyn) or shorthands for the desired endpoints. These names can suffice locally because the local context limits the universe of discourse. Emergency rooms, pediatric clinics, and pathology labs, all make use of vernaculars that can enhance productivity. In contrast, a major challenge facing the likes of ICD and SNOMED is that they try to support all these uses simultaneously. Current terminology best practices argue that the use of acronyms and abbreviations in electronic health records is a bad idea; the opportunity for ambiguity is too great. For example, humans would be unlikely to confuse COPD (chronic obstructive pulmonary disease) with COPD (dyphylline, guaifenesin), a drug used to treat it, but a computer might have a tough time. Fortunately, **RxNorm** and other standard terminologies are very clear on which is which. The reader is invited to compare the use of *metabolic syndrome*, "MetSyn,", and "MetS" in Medline and on the Web.

What do we call a terminology that didn't go to college? A **controlled vocabulary** seems to be a terminology without a pedigree. Most healthcare informatics cognoscenti use the terms interchangeably, however, and thus you should avoid reading too much into these labels. Be forewarned, though, that some disciplines, such as information retrieval, prefer to use *controlled vocabulary*[24] and regard *terminology* as overkill. As with most matters in this chapter, what you call it matters little; what it *is*, is almost everything.

How is the ongoing responsibility for a terminology named and formalized? In the context of this chapter, *provenance* has come to mean two things. First, in analogy with the **provenance**[25] of a work of art, the provenance of a term indicates where it came from, and by implication, why we might care about it. Sometimes a term's provenance has a formal name, and this name includes a version number or date. Second, terminology provenance can name the group responsible for the creation and maintenance of the terminology; often this group is referred to as the *authority*.

What do we call a group of things with something in common? Most, but not all, terms in terminologies name categories. To say, however, that a **category** is a group of things with something in common is not to say much unless we care about what makes them common, even if the commonality condition is made explicit. For example, medieval libraries organized books by size; and therefore, the books on a given shelf were in a common category. Most, but not all, names in health care and biomedical terminologies are category names; categories often name collections of categories. As we've seen, "metabolic disease" is the name of a category containing "metabolic syndrome" and many other categories. SNOMED CT assures us that this membership is about meaning and not about words. The words suggest the relationship but do not confirm it.

What is an example of a cognitive organizing principle in the domain of healthcare and biomedical research? As can come up on day one of medical school the notion of a **disease** can prove elusive. One definition is that a *disease is a cognitive organizing principle*. This definition proves useful in the context of health care terminology: the names of diseases become the names of categories, and most of these categories are defined by attributes. Rarely are definitional attributes required; instead, the attributes form a constellation that may prove useful. *Metabolic syndrome* is an example of a category with no required attributes as yet.

What is an example of a term that is not a category name? An **instance** can have a name. The two authors of this chapter are instances—unique individuals; Mark and Stephanie are not categories, though, of course, our occupations place us in categories. The National Library of Medicine maintains a terminology called MeSH (medical subject headings): it names what people write about in biomedicine. Along with the names of diseases, chemicals, microorganisms, and the like, there are also many names of instances. For example, geographic designations—the United States, states, cities, and regions, all might appear in a public health journal article—are all instances. There is only one city called Louisville, Kentucky. Instances can make use of necessary definitional attributes, making equivalence testing easier. Latitude and longitude values and zip codes can be definitional; it is relatively easy to explain to a computer that Lexington, Kentucky, is not another name for Louisville, Kentucky. The information in electronic health records is a mixture of category names (diagnoses) and instance names (a particular laboratory testing result). Often, instance names have equivalency tests, making them formal, or at least formalizable.

Is there a way to leverage more than one terminology at a time? The National Library of Medicine's **UMLS** "integrates and distributes key terminology, classification and coding standards, and associated resources to promote creation of more effective and interoperable biomedical information systems and services, including electronic health records."[5] It does this by providing data—"knowledge sources"—and tools—for lexical processing and browsing. Importantly, these resources are well documented, well maintained, and have a predictable release schedule.

What is a collection of terms organized by meaning? A **thesaurus** is a reference work—a reference model in our parlance—organized by meaning, with synonyms, antonyms, and related terms located in categories. Traditionally, it contrasts with a dictionary, a reference work in which entries are listed orthographically and the focus is on narrative definitions.[*]

Where do we find the authoritative terms related to metabolic syndrome? The core resource of the UMLS is the **Metathesaurus**.

> The Metathesaurus is a very large, multi-purpose, and multi-lingual vocabulary database that contains information about biomedical and health related concepts, their various names, and the relationships among them. ... [It] is built from the electronic versions of various thesauri, classifications, code sets, and lists of controlled terms used in patient care, health services billing, public health statistics, indexing and cataloging biomedical literature, and/or basic, clinical, and health services research. . . . [It] is organized by concept or meaning. In essence, it links alternative names and views of the same concept and identifies useful relationships between different concepts.[26]

For example, as preparation for your meeting with an endocrinologist you study the Metathesaurus entry named "metabolic syndrome X" and discover that some, but not all, sources treat "insulin resistance syndrome" as the same thing, and that the Metathesaurus agrees that they are synonyms. The endocrinologist disagrees, explaining how they differ, but you are now in a position to understand better what you're going to find in paper charts and electronic health records. The Metathesaurus began as an explicitly concept-based synthesis of important health care and biomedical terminologies when few terminologies were concept-based. Further, it pioneered efforts to make its

---

[*] See Question 4 at the end of this chapter.

terminology model explicit. Being concept-based and schema-explicit made potential users uncomfortable; they felt that such a representation abused whatever truth and beauty was in the constituent terminologies, especially their terminology. Particularly controversial was the fact that the Metathesaurus made both intra- and inter-terminology synonymy (or lack thereof) explicit.

How do terminologies evolve? By definition, the authorities responsible for a terminology are responsible for maintaining it. ***Terminology maintenance*** includes keeping pace with our understanding of the world and with the uses to which the terminology is put. Everyone understands that scientific reductionism generates new concepts by splitting categories previously thought to be homogeneous, but experience shows that such changes constitute the minority of terminology updates observed to date, important though they may be. Instead, most changes to large terminologies tend to be clerical in nature: formatting errors, spelling corrections, changes in punctuation, capitalization, abbreviations, and adding and eliminating so-called entry terms are examples of the kind of changes resulting from problems detected during machine processing. As the machine processing of terminologies becomes more common, these data improvement changes will decline in frequency; terminologies will be more likely to get myriad details right the first time. Another trend is the increasing influence of genotyping on the classification of, say, microorganisms; this causes a reorganization of the relevant hierarchies. Increasingly, "the market"—terminology consumers—is concerned with the operational challenge of keeping abreast of the new versions of deployed terminologies. Sometimes new knowledge causes terminologies to merge concepts previously thought to be different. An example of such a merger is the ancient—and at the time, problematic—emergence of the knowledge that the morning star and the evening star are the same thing: the planet Venus. Of a more practical note is the emergence of the relationship between land animals, e.g., pigs, and whales, once we understood, with confirmation from genotyping, that whales are descended from land animals. You should expect a reorganization of the neighborhood containing metabolic syndrome during your career, but not necessarily soon. If some of your team looks forward to being "done" with the terminology part of the project, explain that 1) "We'll never be done"; and that 2) "That's a feature." Terminology maintenance is a very difficult topic for the uninitiated to appreciate. One way you can explain it is to compare a large terminology with a glacier. At any given moment, it's hard to see any movement, but if you climb on it, you can hear it moving; and if you come back in a year, the front edge may be in a different place entirely. Further, the front edge may be receding while the back is getting bigger, or vice versa. The key is to embrace the changes, however they manifest themselves.

How does one tell if one terminology is better than another? Measuring **terminology quality** and utility is currently problematic. Most attempts at measuring terminology quality focus on the formal properties: does the terminology follow its own (or any) schema? And are the data "clean"?* But these qualities may be orthogonal to utility. Conversely, a terminology that represents a domain well may lack ease-of-use properties that enable it to be widely deployed. Worse, the more current a terminology, the harder it may be to use, as laboratory testing and medication terminologies have shown. In the extreme, available lab tests and medications may change every day. During the life of this book, genotyping of flu strains may change daily, and the genotyping of flu viruses yields instances.† A good dramatization of the latter—birds "weaponizing" the flu, and the resulting mutations of the virus—is in the movie *Contagion* cited previously. The multiple constituencies that terminologies serve further complicate this dilemma. First among these is reimbursement and regulation. Add to this various administrative, educational, and research agendas; and, as has been observed, terminologies must serve multiple masters. Ultimately, market forces will determine relative quality and utility. There is no easy way to assess, much less measure, these things prospectively at present. Regardless, emerging pressure, from Meaningful Use[27] and from competitive forces, will reinforce terminology that supports the assessment of care quality.‡

How does one manage the use of terminologies that change over time? All widely used terminologies change over time. Those who maintain them, however, have had an ambivalent attitude toward their past history. To oversimplify, "that was then, and this is now," implying that past versions are "wrong" in some sense and thus not to be discussed. This ambivalence is understandable; those who maintain terminologies always try to make each version better. And perhaps they are embarrassed by something in a previous version. This reticence, however, makes it difficult for those of us trying to study

---

* See the following webpage for an example. BioPortal. Systematized Nomenclature of Medicine-Clinical Terms. http://bioportal.bioontology.org/ontologies/SNOMEDCT?p=summary . Accessed online December 18, 2013. These metrics are constructive and informative, but they do not tell us whether SNOMED CT is useful.

† Personal conversation with James Case, DVM, PhD, on November 20, 2013.

‡ See Question 6 at end of this chapter.

terminologies and patients longitudinally. ***Time travel*** has come to mean an ability to compute what an obsolete term or code meant when it was in use, and what if anything has replaced it at present. Similarly, time travel enables a computation of how a current concept used to be named and coded. While MeSH has represented such information for librarians for several decades, only recently have terminologies made such inter-version information explicit and therefore computable. The Metathesaurus is designed to keep track of concept splits and mergers; but in general, formalizing this kind of thing across all important terminologies is still a work in progress. The reader is referred to the discussion of "codes" below.

Is there a standard way to process the narrative text in an electronic health record? Predictors of metabolic syndrome may exist in care narratives collected in a data repository. While we encourage data exploration, we advise against the reinvention of text processing software. For one thing, the results may be remarkably sensitive to the computable definition of a ***word***. For example, is "X" a word? Is "x"? The UMLS provides some text processing tools that answer this question in a consistent way. Your institution may already have projects that process clinical narrative as part of data mining, and these projects will use open-source or proprietary text processing tools that you will want to investigate. So while there is no standard (computational) definition of a "word," there is a considerable body of experience and several repertoires of open-source tools that you should access before engaging in the unilateral development of text processing software.

What is a term and how do we know when a word or words constitute a term? In our context, a ***term*** is a noun or noun phrase, one or more words, usually without an embedded verb, that names something in a specified domain. Sometimes the usage is specialized so that the meaning of a term in a terminology may deviate from the meaning of the term in natural language. We care about this definition here because terms are what we want to look for in the narrative text describing a patient.

What do we call a term whose meaning is understandable independent of context? We say that a term has ***face validity*** when we as humans can understand the meaning of the term (the concept the term names) without reference to the context of the term in the terminology. Clearly, this is a relative quality; some terms have better face validity than others. For example, the term *metabolic disease* has a degree of face validity that the term "other and unspecified metabolic disorders" does not. As observed above, the latter term depends on understanding the meaning of the neighboring terms in the hierarchy. Similarly, the term *MetSyn* can be divined if we know the context, but out of context it may prove mysterious, and out of context *MetS* is hopelessly ambiguous. Interestingly, terms with a greater degree of face validity—again for humans—prove to be more useful to computers also; for one thing, matching them to words and phrases in narrative text, or in, say, a problem list is easier and more productive. And the words in a term may suggest relationships with other terms. As implied above, problem lists place special demands on face validity.

How do I decide whether two terms name the same thing? As we saw with SNOMED CT above, some terminologies assert that different terms are synonyms—not just diseases that get classified the same way, but different names for the same disease. Similarly, the Metathesaurus can agree or disagree with what its constituent sources call a **synonym**. As observed, all this inconsistency causes considerable angst in the community at large. You should be aware of this sensitivity, but avoid entrapment and the associated productivity cost. Remember the earlier admonition about the danger of focusing on words rather than on meanings—the concepts the words name. If you are goal-oriented—predicting metabolic syndrome, and the like—you can avoid methodologic disputes. Ideally, your data can tell you when to lump or split concepts, and synonymy or relatedness will be an emergent property.

Why do colleagues attach more importance to codes than they do to terms? An overreaction to the "words-are-bad" observation is the near-reverence that some practitioners and professionals attach to codes. Simply put, a **code** is a nonlinguistic name for a concept. As shown above, ICD-9-CM codes "Dysmetabolic syndrome X" as 277.7. ICD-10-CM codes "Metabolic syndrome" as E88.81. SNOMED CT has two identifiers—codes—for the disease: (historically) DB-61052 and (going forward) 237602007. As asserted in the Wikipedia entry for "Medical classification," numerical codes are a goal. "Medical classification, or medical coding, is the process of transforming descriptions of medical diagnoses and procedures into universal medical code numbers."[28] To a degree, codes are easier to manipulate computationally, and storing them requires less computer memory; but over time and at scale, pursuit of this simplicity is counterproductive and sometimes fatal. The biggest problem with codes is well understood by medical librarians. Discovering the meaning of any sufficiently old code is a (human) research problem. Even if—and we are waiting for this to happen—every code is accompanied by an authority name and version number, there can be intra-version updates to codes that may confuse the situation.

Whatever the problems with (linguistic) names for concepts, at least they can represent what the person (or program) doing the coding might have "thought" at the time. Codes are not helpful in problem lists, obviously. Further, building hierarchical information into the code is now considered a bad practice for technical reasons. Again, it's easy to observe all this now that computing resources are so cheap—relatively. But codes are still used for reimbursement. The problem is that readers of this chapter will be faced with the cost of the use of codes in electronic health records for some time to come. Part of the aforementioned reverence attached to codes is evidenced by the fact that the Wikipedia entry referenced above fails to mention either of these shortcomings, namely that codes do not age well, and that building semantics (meaning) into the codes in a nonlinguistic way proves to be inadvisable. Nevertheless, an important use of codes are the *Concept Unique Identifiers (CUIs)* in the Metathesaurus; these are "the names that never change," which each concept acquires when it is first introduced and which are sustained across name changes—exactly what has happened to the name *metabolic syndrome* in the past.

How should one construct human-readable, narrative definitions for concepts? Sometimes even well-constructed concept names are ambiguous; or, in an effort to eliminate ambiguity, names can become too technical. Especially when naming novel concepts or renaming poorly named concepts, a human-readable **narrative definition** can make all the difference. This observation prompts the question, "What is a definition that is not a narrative definition?" Ontologies can contain defining relationships that are to a degree understandable by a computer. A straightforward discipline to apply when constructing definitions was articulated by Aristotle. In this context a narrative definition of X can say, "X is a member of the class Y, and is distinguished from the other members of the class because it has qualities A, B, and C"—the implication being that Y, A, B, and C are defined elsewhere. While your CMO may be happy with a "Magic Box" (see later) predictor of metabolic syndrome, if it works, he will be a lot happier if the predictions are built on predicates with human-readable definitions, especially Aristotelian definitions.

The hypothesis implicit in this section has been that you will be more productive in your terminology-related professional life if you understand, or at least have some appreciation of, the ideas described above. Nonetheless, one of our favorite software engineering quotes is "One line of working code is worth 500 of specification."[29] Translated into our context, understanding and leveraging the information, and any terminology in, let us say, one electronic health record is more important than being able to recite these definitions.

Interoperation by meaning, not yet. . . so what should you do?

While time is on your side, at present you will find the proportion of medical encounter records in any large context that are fully compliant with Stage 2 of Meaningful Use to be disappointing. This will be true even if the records are stored in a single-vendor system. In the records that are fully compliant, you will find standard terminology that can be exported in a standard format. Before proposing how to deal with the shortfall, it is helpful to understand why this predicament has evolved in the United States.

There are two schools of thought on this situation, and not much ground in between. The first, and traditional, explanation is that medicine is too complex for interoperation. There are too many subtleties, too many ambiguities, and "every patient is different"; or alternatively, "my patients are different." Further, physicians evolve their own ways of taking care of patients and they are unlikely to change these ways in the absence of compelling forces. One kind of compelling force, however, is almost any kind of new imaging technology. In spite of forces trying to prevent their deployment, these technologies are adopted rapidly and widely, so the challenge to interoperation is not just the result of resistance to change.

A second explanation is that the main reason that U.S. electronic health record systems do not in general support interoperation today is the historic alignment of incentives. Simply put, few caregivers or caregiving institutions in the United States get paid to reuse information from a remote system unless the remote system is in an affiliated institution, and maybe not even then. To be fair, caregivers equated redoing lab tests, translating and re-entering medication lists, history retaking and the like, as part of high-quality care—what caregivers do for their patients. An important exception to this observation is the role of problem lists. Even though the latter serve a variety of such objectives as reimbursement, every caregiver we've ever spoken to on the subject wants to see any problem list associated with a patient they are seeing for the first time. This is particularly true when the patient crosses a boundary between levels of care.

Currently, the Veterans Affairs (VA) electronic health record does an excellent job of retrieving the records of veterans treated previously in their system. Kaiser Permanente and a short list of other providers and regions have related objectives, as discussed in the National eHealth collaborative's April 2012 *Health Information Exchange Roadmap* report.[30] Some regions, Indianapolis and Memphis, for example, have working information exchanges that operate in support of emergency departments. But as of this writing, these are exceptions; pervasive interoperation awaits the success of Meaningful Use.

Applying our turn-it-into-a-question rubric, *"If an EHR is the answer, what was the question?"* Until recently, the answer was, for many institutions, "How can we stay in business?" And that answer determined much of the functionality of the systems now deployed. Put differently, the chief financial officer (CFO) of the institution was the customer and capturing reimbursable events was the objective. Sometimes capturing these events was associated with improving the quality of care, and sometimes it was workflow streamlining. Only recently are caregiving institutions starting to compete on the basis of EHR functionality supporting quality of care. Sometimes they compete on the basis of their support for PHRs (personal health records). We are waiting, however, to see an EHR system tout its ability to accept a "foreign" patient history in electronic form. Obviously, some EHRs can do this; it's just a capability that does not seem to be featured prominently. To be fair, there are many practical challenges associated with external input to EHRs. For one thing, displays need to clearly indicate the provenance of the information, something that is not currently part of any standard. Then what if the record is 100 pages or longer? Is the receiving caregiver responsible for reading it all? As implied above, this issue is especially challenging across levels of care. Once again, the VA and selected other care enterprises are gaining experience with these tradeoffs. For some time now, the Health Information Management Systems Society (HIMSS) annual meeting has sponsored demonstrations of interoperation by heterogeneous vendors. So once again, in contrast to the economic barriers, the technical barriers to interoperation continue to be reduced or eliminated.

An additional reason for the observed lack of interoperation is that each EHR tends to treat the information it contains idiosyncratically. Thus to fully utilize the information in one system in another system may be somewhere between very hard and impossible. Because of the aforementioned misalignment of incentives, even progress on the simple parts of this problem has been nearly nonexistent. In contrast, whole software engineering disciplines have emerged to handle this challenge in other domains. That is, in certain non-healthcare domains—finance in particular—when the incentives are aligned, there are ways to get some benefit from simple interoperation while at the same time working on the more difficult part of the challenge. As implied, in general this progress has not happened in health care. Another example of the rapid emergence of information technology solutions, even in health care when incentives are aligned, is the ability physicians now have to order medications from their ersonal digital assistant (PDA), also known as a mobile phone or tablet. This development, along with the aforementioned rapid adoption of new imaging technologies, shows that it's possible for health care to adopt new information technology rapidly; and therefore, that the problem is not intrinsic.

So what should you do in the face of this situation? It is proposed that you establish progress from both ends of the scale. At one end, with assistance from the staff that manages your institution's data repository, you formulate a script that generates a daily e-mail to you and your CMO. This e-mail contains a simple report on an increasingly sophisticated set of counts.

The first number in the report is the total number of patients, dead or alive, in the catchment to which you have access. The catchment might be an evolving target, as more sophisticated ambulatory EHR systems come on line, and that's the good news. Refinements of this number will have important uses later. A lower bound on this number is certainly known to and used by the financial side of your institution, but you need direct access to the project catchment and its associated dates, independent of reimbursement. You will need to be prepared for the possibility that the CMO will want a visualization showing how many patients are known to be alive or dead at any given time and how current that information is.

The second number in the report is the count of patients who have a code in their record indicating that someone asserted that they had (and possibly or probably have) metabolic syndrome. As your CMO knows, this will be a very small number relative to the presumed prevalence. You will find a large variety of codes for one or more of hypertension, diabetes, hyperlipidemia, obesity, and the like but not necessarily for metabolic syndrome. These two numbers, crude though they may be, are important bounds on your task. Given these two numbers, you have the first step toward a "dashboard" that would provide your CMO with information that is as close to real time as is practical.

At the other end of the scale, you find someone in medical records or a metabolic syndrome researcher who can find you a single record, paper or electronic, of a patient with metabolic syndrome—whether coded that way or not. You explain the query is not for the perfect record, the largest record, or the simplest record, just a qualitatively representative record. You study this record carefully. Armed with this experience, you ask for nine more such records to make an informal sample of ten. You study these carefully. While the advice seems not to get published, all leading gurus in machine learning advise those starting out on a project to spend several weeks familiarizing themselves with their data. This advice is in direct opposition to those who argue that new methods require only software and computing resources to get useful results.

Based on what you have learned, you formulate a set of criteria by which to expand your sample to a total of 100 records. The criteria include sample repertoires of diagnostic codes, lab tests, and medications. Your CMO will remind you that the medications listed in the EHR are related only to what the patient is or is not taking. You will explain that the EHR medication list represents intent on the part of a caregiver, and that's enough for the moment. The fact that it may not be what was dispensed; if the order ever was dispensed; or is not what the patient is actually taking is a challenge for another day. More generally, as you start to get results you should prepare yourself for arguments that "raw" information from electronic health records is unsuitable for research.[31,32] These observations will remind you that your end goal is usefully identifying a subpopulation at risk of metabolic syndrome.

The objective of your next set of criteria is to retrieve a sample of records describing, to adapt police parlance, "patients of interest." The objective of the sample of 100 is to see what information and what terminology is actually there as opposed to what you think should be there.

Your institution's Information Technology department wants to be helpful, but inevitably, they will abuse your criteria in their effort to implement it. They must struggle with the constraints of their query system and the limitations of the content within, and the fact that it's all a moving target. They will retrieve the most recent 100 patients that fit your criteria, postponing the need to deal with what will surely be many temporal effects.

Nevertheless, you now have 100 records carefully encrypted (protected) on your laptop. You are like a dog finally catching the car it is chasing. You wake up the next morning and decide you need help. Armed with research results from another class, you call in all your favors and assemble a small interdisciplinary team.

Scholarly research suggests that the best problem-solving doesn't come from a group of the best individual problem-solvers, but from a diverse team whose members complement each other. That's an argument for leadership that is varied in every way—in gender, race, economic background and ideology.[33]

Your team's objective is to understand, based on the sample, what terminology and other units of information may be present in whatever form in the records of patients who may have metabolic syndrome, or who have something related to metabolic syndrome. You fulfill this objective by using a mixture of manual and tool-supported efforts. The result is a collection of diagnostic codes, lab test names and results, medication names—drug, dose, and route, noun phrases, procedure codes, and such nonterminologic values as a BMI. To your surprise, this sample exhibits unexpected diversity and a lack of central tendency. For one thing, the number of comorbidities you observe seems to grow alarmingly. Your CMO reminds you privately that your sample will contain practice variations, reimbursement-driven testing and interventions, and instances of missing data; you accept these problems as part of the challenge.

What part of the problem does standard terminology fix, and what else needs to be done . . .?

First, the portion of electronic health records you examine that contain standard terminology is hugely helpful. While there's no guarantee that the information so encoded will be of higher quality or more useful than the preceding nonstandard units of information, it's nevertheless a step forward; *otherwise, you'd need to spend time inventing your own standards and your own reference model.* Now the computer scientist on your team may argue that standard terminology is a distraction and waste of time, and that all he or she needs is "the bits"—or maybe the characters or the words. But, as has been argued from the beginning of this chapter, terminology, especially standard terminology, is about scalable communication: between humans, between computers, and between humans and computers—something that's not possible with bit signatures, word signatures, or text clusters, interesting though they may be.

Second, you now have the beginnings of the best of all possible worlds. Even though you have only 100 records, you have an empirical overlay on the normative standards—the beginnings of a metabolic syndrome reference model. You have a start toward understanding which diagnoses are recorded, which lab test results are recorded, and which medication orders are recorded, instead of the very large repertoire that gets named in the standards. Put differently, *these standards strive for completeness of coverage, and not relevance of coverage.* You are interested in the relevant coverage, obviously. "Relevance" proves to be a difficult concept for computers, and relatively easy for humans. Fortunately, the availability of inexpensive computing resources helps to overcome this challenge. A theory as to why relevance is hard for computers is described by Blois.[34] The combination of the normative view and the beginnings of an empirical view gives you a powerful way to start communicating what you discovered to your CMO and his colleagues. Given this view, an important and nonstandard dimension—time—can be assessed. Absolute time helps you order observations and associated terminology regarding a single patient, but when you want to aggregate such observations across a population, it's less clear how to represent time. Such simple questions as whether to adjust for the age of the patient prove to less straightforward than they might seem. You propose to postpone the harder questions until you're ready for predictive analytics efforts (below).

Third, inevitably you'll have collected some units of information that are not named or named well in standards. The good news is that the extant standards give you the opportunity to focus effort on the process of creating and maintaining your own names for key novel concepts. Resign yourself to the fact that you're not going to get them right the first time, and that's okay. You should try anyway, using the Understandable, Reproducible, and Useful (URU) desideratum.* What you're creating is the MetSyn Terminology Model—something that is mostly constructed from standard terminologies but enhanced in a data-driven way by what you find in your samples. Because you read this chapter, you maintain a clear distinction between external (standard) and internal (your team) authorities. You may find it useful to revisit Elkin (see **References**) regarding the composition of standard terms so as to construct compound terms of use in your context. For one thing, representing more complicated things as compounds of standard terms supports comparability in a way that information models do not.

Fourth and finally, because of your central reliance on standards it is easier to communicate what you're doing both within and beyond your institution. By this time you're aware that your computer science and machine learning team members are correct; you need more records. While extra-institutional comparability will be a journey, your use of standards will make it easier to

---

* First articulated by Keith E. Campbell, MD, PhD, and now used worldwide by terminology creators and maintainers.

understand other attempts to use your reference model to count patients. Without prompting from you, your CMO is already at work trying to find a collaborating institution in which to test your model.

Current Terminology Standards

One source of descriptions of standard terminology is the UMLS Web page titled "UMLS Source Release Documentation."[35] We'll rely on those descriptions in this section—for one thing, while we hope this book gets revised at some point in the future, the UMLS documentation gets updated every time it contains a new version of a source.

Examine the documentation there as a model of one of the things you will need to do with your metabolic syndrome reference model. Prior to doing what the UMLS did, the notion that terminologies as different as those for diseases, lab tests, medications, procedures, and many other things could be put into a homogeneous representation was thought by many to be impossible. Others thought that it could be done but that it would not be useful to do so. The tip of this iceberg is the source descriptions, presented in a homogeneous way. You will want to do the same thing with your metabolic syndrome reference model. That is, you will have a collection of standard names of diagnoses, lab test results, medications, procedures, terms, compositions of terms, and information models. This collection must be actionable on two fronts. First, it must be implementable; it must be able to accept any encounter record and produce a "metabolic syndrome" score (discussed below). Second, it must be explainable—to humans, especially to those humans whose help you will need. Overcoming this challenge—namely, representing heterogeneous things in a homogeneous way—will not be easy, so use the UMLS Source Documentation as one model of how to proceed. The UMLS source pages and Wikipedia pages provide significant cognitive benefit simply by virtue of their homogeneous formats. And a homogeneous format for humans is one step closer to a computer-empowering format, such as RDF (cited above).

One thing not covered by the UMLS source documentation is how to think about each source. Simplifying things even further, one can ask *"Why does a term get added to each source?"* For some sources the answer to this question is obvious but for other sources less so.

As described above, ***ICD*** has sought to classify diseases, historically for the purposes of counting the dead and causes of death, and more recently for health statistics and for reimbursement. Because of its history, it contains, for instance, very fine-grained and numerous classes for tuberculosis—a public health challenge even to this day—but only a single code for prostate cancer. (As you will discover if the data take you there, the coding of cancers and related diseases follows its own set of conventions.)*,36 As implied previously, your project will likely need to deal with codes from several (annual) versions of ICD-9-CM and from ICD-10-CM. **ICD-9-CM** (14,567 disease codes in a recent version[37]) has received relatively few updates lately as efforts have gone into getting **ICD-10-CM** (69,833 "diseases") ready for use. ICD-10-CM has broadened the definition of disease, obviously. Many of the "new" diseases, relative to ICD-9-CM, are what were formerly classified as injuries and poisonings.[38]

SNOMED CT (300,486 concepts, including 66,837 disorders[39]) grew out of pathologists' need to name what they observed. Originally, diseases were named and then described in multiple dimensions—abnormal anatomy, abnormal function, abnormal morphology, etc. Over time, SNOMED was expanded to cover "all" of health care. Diseases are still "defined" where possible through membership in single or multiple classes—"infectious pneumonia" IS_A "pneumonia" and IS_A "infectious disease"—and through relationships to nondisease concepts—"viral pneumonia" has Causative_agent "virus." Some of these details are covered in the Wikipedia entry,[40] but a better way to understand them is by using a SNOMED browser. Several are available on the Web. The NLM SNOMED CT browser requires a license (free to individuals in the United States).[41] This approach to naming means that SNOMED CT and ICD differ in detail, although to a good approximation they cover the same domain. Specifically as of 2013, 38 percent of ICD-9-CM's diseases are named synonymously by SNOMED CT, leaving 62 percent that are not so named.[37] As would be expected, there are about 58,000 diseases named by SNOMED CT that are not synonymously named by ICD-9-CM or ICD-10-CM. As you can surmise, there are some definitional challenges here, but you get the idea.

LOINC "provides formal names and standardized codes for laboratory and other clinical observations."[42] Each of the 67,000+ current names has six parts:

> - *Component: what is measured, evaluated, or observed (example: urea)*
> - *Kind of property: characteristics of what is measured, such as length, mass, volume, time stamp and so on*
> - *Time aspect: interval of time over which the observation or measurement was made*

---

* ICD-O (... Oncology) is now included in SNOMED CT, evidence of terminology convergence.

> *- System: context or specimen type within which the observation was made (example: blood, urine)*
> *- Type of scale: the scale of measure. The scale may be quantitative, ordinal, nominal or narrative*
> *- Type of method: procedure used to make the measurement or observation*[43]

Without LOINC, lab tests from different sites are incomparable. But, while LOINC is a stellar example of formalization,[16,*] it does not typically represent why we might care about the test. For example, one of your colleagues wants to see whether probiotics affect metabolic syndrome; but then she discovers that some of the patients you've identified have ulcers, and then she wants to know how many of the patients were tested for the ulcer-causing bacterium *H. pylori*. There is no localization in LOINC for this concept; instead LOINC represents the fact that there are many different tests for the bacterium—for the antigen, for the antibody, and then its presence in blood, saliva, etc., using many different methods—and the codes for these tests must be collected manually from different neighborhoods in LOINC. The good news is that such collections are then reusable and comparable. Here's an example of a fully-specified LOINC name, a colon (":")–delimited construction of the six parts described above, followed by the expanded version:

> *49898-0*
> *Fully-specified name: Metabolic syndrome: ACnc: Pt:Ser/Plas: Ord*
> *Component: Metabolic syndrome [Presence] in Serum or Plasma*
>
> *Metabolic syndrome: Arbitrary Concentration: Point in time: Serum/Plasma: Ordinal*

Intrigued by this test, you discover that as far as you can tell, it's never been ordered at your institution. One reason may be that it is the component of a lipoprotein panel. It does not report whether lipoprotein is present; instead it reports a probability of metabolic syndrome. It is a probability that is computed from the panel.

RxNorm is another triumph of formalization. It "provides standard names for clinical drugs (active ingredient + strength + dose form) and for dose forms as administered to a patient. It provides links from clinical drugs, both branded

---

[*] See this article for a theory that explains why lab tests are easier to formalize than diseases. Blois, MS. Medicine and the nature of vertical reasoning. *N Engl J Med.* 1988;318(13):847-51.

and generic, to their active ingredients; drug components (active ingredient + strength); and related brand names."[44] Unless you have experience with clinical pharmaceuticals you will be unprepared for the multitude of, say, hypertension medications. *With RxNorm you can aggregate medications by active ingredient.* Again, if RxNorm didn't exist you would have to invent the portions of it related to metabolic syndrome. For example, the FDA assigns each packaging of each medication an NDC (National Drug Code)[45]—codes that you may find in EHR records. RxNorm collects and aggregates these values appropriately *and updates them weekly.*[46]

For example, a medication such as a statin may be used to treat components of metabolic syndrome. A common ingredient is atorvastatin, which RxNorm indicates is present in the branded drugs Lipitor, Caduet, and Liptruzet.

Current Procedural Terminology (CPT) is a product of the American Medical Association (AMA). CPT codes are used by health care professionals for billing of medical services and procedures to public and private health insurance programs.[47] In its traditional form, CPT is an organized list of billing codes with each procedure represented by a 5-digit code. To understand its hierarchy, a CPT user needs to browse the book (or a computer artifact of the book). The printed volume is helpfully arranged in color-coded sections with finger tabs and an alphabetical index for aid in navigation. The CPT code structure, however, makes it difficult to reorganize or make any changes to the hierarchy. To address this problem, the AMA has resequenced codes: for example, code 33262 was moved so that it falls under "33202-33249," which results in a code order that is confusing to humans even in the print world for which CPT was designed.

More recently, the AMA has made available a Developers Toolkit (DTK). This set of data files includes formal representation of an "IS_A" hierarchy, which will facilitate analysis and aggregation of data. In addition, the structure allows for formal connections to SNOMED CT concepts, including associated findings, anatomic sites, and specimens. As the DTK matures, additional explicit relationships within CPT and to other terminologies are being added, supporting additional manipulation of CPT-coded records.

Although there is no procedure to treat metabolic syndrome directly, the presence of certain CPT codes in a patient's EMR may prove useful in constructing your computable definition of metabolic syndrome.[*] For example, codes 43770–43775 represent laparoscopic gastric surgery procedures. As represented in DTK, the hierarchy appears as follows:

Surgery
    Surgical Procedures on the Digestive System
        Surgical Procedures on the Stomach
            Bariatric Surgery Procedures
                Laparoscopy, surgical, gastric restrictive procedures
                Laparoscopy, surgical, gastric restrictive procedure; placement of adjustable gastric restrictive device (eg, gastric band and subcutaneous port components) (43770)
                Laparoscopy, surgical, gastric restrictive procedure; revision of adjustable gastric restrictive device component only (43771)
                Laparoscopy, surgical, gastric restrictive procedure; removal of adjustable gastric restrictive device component only (43772)
                Laparoscopy, surgical, gastric restrictive procedure; removal and replacement of adjustable gastric restrictive device component only (43773)
                Laparoscopy, surgical, gastric restrictive procedure; removal of adjustable gastric restrictive device and subcutaneous port components (43774)
                Laparoscopy, surgical, gastric restrictive procedure; longitudinal gastrectomy (ie, sleeve gastrectomy) (43775)

At its core, CPT is a billing system; it has not traditionally provided terminology suitable for clinical description and analysis. Recently, however, the AMA started releasing consumer and clinician forms of descriptions. For the above example, the simplified versions include:

---

[*] See Question 7.

Consumer forms:
Insertion of adjustable stomach reduction device using an endoscope (43770);
Revision of stomach reduction device using an endoscope (43771);
Removal of stomach reduction device using an endoscope (43772);
Replacement of stomach reduction device using an endoscope (43773);
Removal of stomach reduction device and port beneath the skin using an endoscope (43774);
Stomach reduction procedure with partial removal of stomach using an endoscope (43775).

Clinician forms:
Surgical laparoscopy with placement of adjustable gastric restrictive device component (43770);
Surgical laparoscopy with revision of adjustable gastric restrictive device component (43771);
Surgical laparoscopy with removal of adjustable gastric restrictive device component (43772);
Surgical laparoscopy with removal and replacement of adjustable gastric restrictive device component (43773);
Surgical laparoscopy with removal of adjustable gastric restrictive device and subcutaneous port components (43774);
Surgical laparoscopy with longitudinal gastrectomy (43775).

Of the 9,707 CPT codes in 2013, only 19 percent have been determined to have synonymous meanings with the 57,000+ SNOMED CT procedures. This difference in granularity, along with the lack of structure in the traditional CPT file format, has contributed to CPT's lack of connectedness with other standards.

Finally, *all terminology standards specified by Meaningful Use are found in the UMLS.*

The following table summarizes the examples of terminology standards related to metabolic syndrome.

Table 11-1. Summary of Standard Terminology Terms for Metabolic Syndrome

Concept	Category Related Terms	Source of Standard Terms	12/2013 Version Term	Code	Comment
Metabolic syndrome					A syndrome is a group of symptoms that consistently occur together.
	Disease	ICD-9-CM	Dysmetabolic syndrome X	277.7	Soon to be obsolete but necessary for retrospective analysis.
		ICD-10-CM	Metabolic syndrome	E88.81	Mandated for Q4, 2014.

Concept	Category Related Terms	Source of Standard Terms	12/2013 Version Term	Code	Comment
		SNOMED CT	Metabolic syndrome X	237602007	Earlier code was DB-61052.
	Laboratory Test	LOINC	Metabolic syndrome: ACnc: Pt: Ser/Plas: Ord	49898-0	Reports a probability that lipoprotein panel indicates presence of metabolic syndrome.
	Medication	RxNorm	Atorvastatin	C0286651	Ingredient in Lipitor, Caudet, et al.
	Procedure	CPT	Insertion of adjustable stomach reduction device using an endoscope	43770	Term shown is "Consumer Form."

Predictive Analytics—Why and How?

As you'll remember from earlier in this chapter, you must understand and be able to use terminology and standard terminology as a way to try to identify patients in your population who are metabolic syndrome candidates, or who have metabolic syndrome. Now that you have records of patients containing standard disease, procedure, and medication terms, you can take advantage of a profound paradigm shift in data analysis to develop your phenotype algorithmically. Existing efforts using this approach can be found in the Phenotype KnowledgeBase (PheKB), "a knowledge base for discovering phenotypes from electronic medical records," which "provides a collaborative environment of building and validating electronic phenotype algorithms."[48] Also potentially useful is the related Electronic Record and Genomics (eMerge) Network.[49] Driven by advances in genomics, each of these projects has advanced the notion of algorithmically generated phenotypes. As of this writing there is no record of the projects taking on the metabolic syndrome phenotype, but there is a considerable body of practical advice on how to do this on the PheKB website. Specifically, the phenotype algorithms represented there can be viewed by codes: ICD, CPT, laboratory results, medications, and by vital signs and the results of natural language processing.[*] In addition, methods are described for validating the algorithmic phenotypes so developed.[50]

As part of your graduate training in public health you've studied statistics; you understand, for instance, how to sample a population and estimate

---

[*] Personal conversation, Betsy Humphreys, MLIS, on November 19, 2013.

properties of the population from which you took the sample. Machine learning, specifically current best practices in predictive analytics, takes a different approach. For one thing, it is less concerned with samples and more concerned with using all available data. It's hard to appreciate the differences between the approaches used by classical statistics and that used by machine learning intuitively, so it's best to appreciate these differences experientially. As of this writing there are several online courses—so-called massive open online courses (MOOCs)—devoted to data analysis with example data sets, using an open source statistical package called **R** that you can download and install on your laptop.[51]

One way to proceed is to have your team, using data exploration tools as appropriate, manually categorize your sample of 100 records relative to the degree that the patients seem to have or do not have metabolic syndrome. You could do this categorization by placing them in bins: "not metabolic syndrome," "maybe metabolic syndrome," or "probably metabolic syndrome"; or you could give them a "metabolic syndrome score," say from 0 to 7. The point is to create the beginnings of a so-called gold standard or training set.[*] Simply put, supervised learning algorithms will try to use whatever observables you supply to predict the outcome—your manual assignment—for each record. Your manually created values supply the supervision. One challenge you will face is what to do about missing data. **R** has a way of representing missing data, and this capacity will allow you to explore ways of dealing with it.

While you should not expect magic, because metabolic syndrome is an elusive concept for a reason, you should expect to learn a lot from doing this exercise. One way to proceed is to work from the bottom up and turn every element of your metabolic syndrome reference model into an observable.[†] This may make you uncomfortable—correctly—because you may have more than

---

[*] Two excellent paper and online references are: Hastie T, Tibshirani R, Friedman J. *Elements of statistical learning: data mining, inference and prediction.* 2nd Edition. New York, N.Y.: Springer; 2009. http://www-stat.stanford.edu/~tibs/ElemStatLearn/. Accessed online December 19, 2013. Hastie et al., provides useful and initially sufficient information in Chapter 2. Overview of supervised Learning— 2.3 Two simple approaches to prediction. A related and more elementary reference is James G, Witten D, Hastie T, Tibshirani, R. ; 2013. http://www-bcf.usc.edu/~gareth/ISL/ISLR%20First%20Printing.pdf. Accessed January 17, 2014.

[†] We've learned from text processing, in which every unique word is an observable, that given enough data, this approach can produce surprising results. See for example Segaran T. *Programming collective intelligence: building smart Web 2.0 applications.* Sebastopol, Calif.: O'Reilly Media; 2007.

100 observables being tested on 100 records, but even this *over-fitting* challenge can be overcome by looking at the prediction for each record as you take that record out of the dataset. That is, using what is called *single-value deletion*, you use 99 records to make a model and use that model to predict the "outcome" of the hundredth record; and then you do this 100 times, once for each record, and keep track of the results. You'll be interested in how the 100 models differ from one another, and which records if any break the corresponding model.

At the same time, you can work from the top down and aggregate your observables into the obvious categories—circulatory, lipid, glucose, body weight—and use those categories as new predictors, using the single-value deletion tactic if appropriate. You hope that your top-down aggregations emerge from the bottom-up analysis; to the degree that they do not, you have an opportunity for consultation with experts, being careful to acknowledge the preliminary nature of your results.

Because you can perform these tasks on a laptop computer, you can explore your reference model systematically. One thing you can do is treat the fact that a lab test was ordered as separate from the resulting value and almost certainly conclude that you want both observables. In addition, the sources cited above can help you with *regularization*[52] of lab test values.

You can also make one-observable models, whether based on the bottom-up or top-down observables, and then sort them by the degree that they predict your categorization of the records. Again, if your training in classical statistics makes you worried that some of these models might be good by chance, use the single-value deletion approach to make sure your models are not over-fitting.

Then you can repeat the exercise for all the pairs of observables. Forgetting what this process means formally, it will give you a better feeling for the way in which the elements of standard terminologies relate to one another and to your metabolic syndrome categorization. Just as your sample of one record, 10 records, and 100 records helped you understand which elements of the various standards are relevant to your task, predictive analytics will help you sort out their relative relevance even further.

Part of this paradigm is that you just continue this process as you acquire more records: a combination of "bootstrapping" and "continuous quality improvement." You use the model generated using your gold standard to start examining "unknown" records. If the model "thinks" the record might be a metabolic syndrome patient, or if the record has an explicit metabolic syndrome code, you examine the record for potential inclusion in your training set. In this way you can continue to improve your metabolic syndrome reference model. A little study on your part reveals that there are successful examples of 10,000 or 100,000 observable models, but your CMO's eyes glaze over when you mention this datum, and you decide to continue exploratory analysis of your growing data set. You can warn him that the genotype-to-phenotype models looking at metabolic syndrome will be of this magnitude.

Eventually, you can switch to unsupervised learning,[53] which used to be called clustering. This is the real test of the metabolic syndrome hypothesis: is there a "cluster" of patients that deserves to be examined together in spite of their seeming heterogeneity? And can you find a subset of observables that identify this population? As your sample of records grows in size, you can experiment with the representation of time, using whatever information about time is available in the records, and fold this into your clustering analysis. Your hope is that time-related aggregations will emerge from the data. There is no accepted ontology of time, so create one that serves some purpose in your project.

At some point you and your CMO decide to take on the next phase; namely, to use standards to work backward through the records you have processed to see what predicts what across time, given that you can usefully identify metabolic syndrome patients in the present with your reference model. The next steps are beyond the scope of this chapter, but you can expect that standard terminology, and as appropriate, your terminology, will solve part of the problem and clarify the remaining portion of the challenge. If you can provide your CMO with a "dashboard" that allows him to explore the subpopulation you've identified, then he may think of hypotheses that you have not thought of. In addition, you can try out various "magic boxes"; that is, domain-blind approaches, to see whether these methods can detect anything novel. Some things these methods should detect are the known demographic predictors of metabolic syndrome.

Policy Implications

If Meaningful Use achieves its objectives, you should be ready to try to scale what you've accomplished across ever larger and larger repertoires of records. While technical barriers will continue to be overcome, many clinical "science" problems will remain, but the later will not suffer from lack of information, at least initially. The biggest remaining challenge will be the public policy aspects of privacy and security. Ultimately, patients may need to "opt in" to your study.

Moreover, it will dawn on you that you are part of a large ongoing natural experiment. That is, each level of care will be trying to deal with metabolic syndrome, whatever it is called, in its own way, and with whatever interventions are available, including patient and caregiver education. Any results you obtain will be part of this experiment and may influence the result; and that is a good thing, or so you hope.

Conclusion

The title of this chapter is "Using Terminology and Terminology Standards to Count the Healthy and the Sick." There is no technical reason why metabolic syndrome, and other public health problems, cannot be studied in the entire U.S. population by using extensions of the methods described here. Ironically, health care is the envy of other fields trying work on the semantic web, because to outsiders, health care has ontologies and standard vocabularies, something that almost every other domain lacks. The paradox is that other domains have made progress on interoperation, often without overcoming the interoperation-by-meaning challenge. This chapter has explored what it means to exploit anticipated progress on interoperation, however slow in coming, and observed progress on terminology standards, however imperfect. Last, there is no intrinsic reason why this progress cannot be exploited on behalf of the health of the nation and the world.

CHAPTER 11 DISCUSSION QUESTIONS

Discussion questions are provided for team building or class exercises. Answers for all questions are provided in Appendix C.

Question Number	Question
1	Select terms in the terminology terminology section of this chapter that seem important to you. Arrange them in a graph or table in a way that helps you remember and think about them. Add any terms you think are important that do not appear there. See whether your classmates agree or disagree, and whether you can reach a kind of consensus on how the terms should be clustered and relate to one another.
2	Using metabolic syndrome as the "center," work with your classmates to explain the details of standard terminologies to one another, using one entry from each terminology—one disease, one lab test, one drug, etc. Explore the connections, or lack of them, among these entries.
3	Your CMO gives you a journal submission he has been assigned to review. The submission describes a population in which 90 percent of patients develop metabolic syndrome, and a statistical model that predicts which patients in this population will develop it that is 85 percent accurate. Who, if anyone, is confused?
4	Why does a thesaurus have both a table of contents and an index, and a dictionary has neither?
5	In a dictionary, meaning is defined in a narrative definition. Where and how is meaning defined in a thesaurus?
6	A recent paper asserted that a predictor of a terminology quality problem—inconsistency—is the length, in number of words, of a term. Speculate on why this might be so. See the 2013 American Medical Informatics Association (AMIA) Distinguished Paper Award nominee: Agrawal A et al. "Identifying inconsistencies in SNOMED CT problem lists using structural indicators."
7	Find CPT "procedures" that might suggest a diagnosis of metabolic syndrome.
8	Given what you know about health care and health status, divide

Question Number	Question
	observations with which you are familiar into those that use a reference model and those that use inspection. What can you conclude?

CHAPTER 11 SUMMARY

- Terminology is critical to the advancement of health care.

- Standard terminology enables the study of populations.

- Computers enable predictive analytic methods that can be applied to these populations.

- Standard terminology and these methods help us understand what we know about some population health challenges.

CHAPTER 11 REFERENCES

1. Churchman CW. *The design of inquiring systems: basic concepts of systems and organizations.* New York, N.Y.: Basic Books;1971.

2. Blois MS. *Information and medicine: the nature of medical descriptions.* Berkeley, Calif.: University of California Press;1984.

3. Kleinsorge R, Willis J, Emrick S. *UMLS overview.* AMIA Tutorial 2007;2007.

4. Centers for Medicare and Medicaid Services. Eligible professional's guide to stage 2 of the EHR incentives program. September 2013; http://www.cms.gov/Regulations-and-Guidance/Legislation/EHRIncentivePrograms/Downloads/Stage2_Guide_EPs_9_23_13.pdf. Accessed November 15, 2013.

5. U.S. National Library of Medicine. Unified Medical Language System.® http://www.nlm.nih.gov/research/umls/. Accessed November 16, 2013.

6. Ogden CK, Richards IA. *The meaning of meaning.* Orlando, Fla.: Harcourt Brace Jovanovich Publishers;1923 (1989).

7. Wikipedia contributors. The Meaning of Meaning. Wikipedia, The Free Encyclopedia. June 16, 2013, 02:48 UTC. 2013; http://en.wikipedia.org/w/index.php?title=The_Meaning_of_Meaning&oldid=560100454. Accessed December 18, 2013.

8. Wikipedia contributors. Gerald Reaven. Wikipedia, The Free Encyclopedia. December 5, 2012, 01:52 UTC. 2013; http://en.wikipedia.org/w/index.php?title=Gerald_Reaven&oldid=526444002. Accessed December 18, 2013.

9. Wikipedia contributors. George E. P. Box. Wikipedia, The Free Encyclopedia. September 30, 2013, 14:12 UTC. 2013; http://en.wikipedia.org/w/index.php?title=George_E._P._Box&oldid=575141969. Accessed December 18, 2013.

10. Wikipedia contributors. Reference model. Wikipedia, The Free Encyclopedia. October 17, 2013, 11:34 UTC. 2013; http://en.wikipedia.org/w/index.php?title=Reference_model&oldid=577558540. Accessed December 18, 2013.

11. Wikipedia contributors. Resource description framework. Wikipedia, The Free Encyclopedia. November 22, 2013, 11:51 UTC. 2013; http://en.wikipedia.org/w/index.php?title=Resource_Description_Framework&oldid=582805724. Accessed December 18, 2013.

12. Elkin, PL. *Terminology and terminologic systems.* New York, N.Y.: Springer;2012.

13. Wikipedia contributors. Rofecoxib. Wikipedia, The Free Encyclopedia. October 17, 2013, 23:35 UTC. 2013; http://en.wikipedia.org/w/index.php?title=Rofecoxib&oldid=577642091. Accessed December 18, 2013.

14. Wikipedia contributors. Nosology. Wikipedia, The Free Encyclopedia. June 19, 2013, 14:49 UTC. 2013;

http://en.wikipedia.org/w/index.php?title=Nosology&oldid=560613758. Accessed December 18, 2013.

15. Koerth-Baker M. The not-so-hidden cause behind the A.D.H.D. epidemic. *New York Times Magazine*, October 15, 2013. http://www.nytimes.com/2013/10/20/magazine/the-not-so-hidden-cause-behind-the-adhd-epidemic.html. Accessed December 18, 2013.

16. Blois MS. Medicine and the nature of vertical reasoning. *N Engl J Med.* 1988;318(13):847-851.

17. Wikipedia contributors. International Statistical Classification of Diseases and Related Health Problems. Wikipedia, The Free Encyclopedia. November 15, 2013, 09:33 UTC. 2013; http://en.wikipedia.org/w/index.php?title=International_Statistical_Classification_of_Diseases_and_Related_Health_Problems&oldid=581746616. Accessed December 18, 2013.

18. Chute CG, Ustun B. ICD-11 preview. In: Giannagelo K, ed. *Healthcare code sets, clinical terminologies, and classification systems.* 3rd ed. Chicago, Ill.: AHIMA;2014.

19. Wikipedia contributors. Taxonomy (biology). Wikipedia, The Free Encyclopedia. December 3, 2013, 20:49 UTC. 2013; http://en.wikipedia.org/w/index.php?title=Taxonomy_(biology)&oldid=584421315. Accessed December 18, 2013.

20. Wikipedia contributors. Nomenclature. Wikipedia, The Free Encyclopedia. September 4, 2013, 06:46 UTC. 2013; http://en.wikipedia.org/w/index.php?title=Nomenclature&oldid=571476902. Accessed December 19, 2013.

21. Wikipedia contributors. Nomenclature code. Wikipedia, The Free Encyclopedia. October 14, 2013, 15:43 UTC. 2013; http://en.wikipedia.org/w/index.php?title=Nomenclature_code&oldid=577146218. Accessed December 19, 2013.

22. Wikipedia contributors. Terminology. Wikipedia, The Free Encyclopedia. November 20, 2013, 13:58 UTC. 2013; http://en.wikipedia.org/w/index.php?title=Terminology&oldid=582524863. Accessed November 20, 2013.

23. Wikipedia contributors. Terminology (artifact). Wikipedia, The Free Encyclopedia. October 20, 2013, 16:15 UTC. 2013; http://en.wikipedia.org/w/index.php?title=Terminology_(artifact)&oldid=577991257. Accessed December 19, 2013.

24. Wikipedia contributors. Controlled vocabulary. Wikipedia, The Free Encyclopedia. October 18, 2013, 09:00 UTC. 2013; http://en.wikipedia.org/w/index.php?title=Controlled_vocabulary&oldid=577687575. Accessed December 19, 2013.

25. Wikipedia contributors. Provenance. Wikipedia, The Free Encyclopedia. December 19, 2013, 01:21 UTC. 2013;

http://en.wikipedia.org/w/index.php?title=Provenance&oldid=586722524. Accessed December 19, 2013.

26. U.S. National Library of Medicine. UMLS® Reference Manual [Internet] 2. Metathesaurus. Bethesda, Md.: U.S. National Library of Medicine;2009.

27. Centers for Medicare and Medicaid Services. Clinical quality measures for EHR incentive programs. http://www.cms.gov/Regulations-and-Guidance/Legislation/EHRIncentivePrograms/ClinicalQualityMeasures.html. Accessed December 18, 2013.

28. Wikipedia contributors. Medical classification. Wikipedia, The Free Encyclopedia. October 25, 2013, 06:28 UTC. 2013; http://en.wikipedia.org/w/index.php?title=Medical_classification&oldid=5786 55801. Accessed December 19, 2013.

29. Randal A. One line of working code is worth 500 of specifications. In: Monson-Haefel R, ed. *97 things every software architect should know*. Sebastopol, Calif.: O'Reilly Media, Inc.;2009:22-23.

30. National eHealth Collaborative (NeHC). Health information exchange roadmap. the landscape and a path forward. Washington, D.C.: NeHC;2012. http://www.nationalehealth.org/hie-roadmap. Accessed December 18, 2013.

31. Hersh WR, Weiner MG, Embi PJ, et al. Caveats for the use of operational electronic health record data in comparative effectiveness research. *Medical Care.* 2013;51:S30-S37.

32. Hersh WR, Cimino J, Payne PR, et al. Recommendations for the use of operational electronic health record data in comparative effectiveness research. *eGEMs (Generating Evidence and Methods to improve patient outcomes).* 2013;1(1):14.

33. Kristof ND. Twitter, women, and power. *New York Times.* October 23, 2013. http://www.nytimes.com/2013/10/24/opinion/kristof-twitter-women-power.html. Accessed June 11, 2014.

34. Blois MS. Clinical judgment and computers. *N Engl J Med.* 1980;303(4):192-197.

35. U.S. National Library of Medicine. UMLS source release documentation list. http://www.nlm.nih.gov/research/umls/sourcereleasedocs/index.html. Accessed December 18, 2013.

36. Wikipedia contributors. International Classification of Diseases for Oncology. Wikipedia, The Free Encyclopedia. May 11, 2013, 07:59 UTC. 2013; http://en.wikipedia.org/w/index.php?title=International_Classification_of_Dise ases_for_Oncology&oldid=554560975. Accessed December 19, 2013.

37. U.S. National Library of Medicine. 2012AB ICD-9-CM source information. http://www.nlm.nih.gov/research/umls/sourcereleasedocs/current/ICD9CM. Accessed December 18, 2013.

38. U.S. National Library of Medicine. 2012AA International Classification of Diseases, 10th edition, clinical information. http://www.nlm.nih.gov/research/umls/sourcereleasedocs/current/ICD10CM /index.html. Accessed December 18, 2013.

39.   U.S. National Library of Medicine. 2012AB SNOMED CT source information. http://www.nlm.nih.gov/research/umls/sourcereleasedocs/current/SNOMED CT/termtypes.html. Accessed December 18, 2013.

40.   Wikipedia contributors. SNOMED CT. Wikipedia, The Free Encyclopedia. November 26, 2013, 08:37 UTC. 2013; http://en.wikipedia.org/w/index.php?title=SNOMED_CT&oldid=583358771. Accessed December 19, 2013.

41.   U.S. National Library of Medicine. How to license and access the Unified Medical Language System® (UMLS®) data. http://www.nlm.nih.gov/databases/umls.html#license_request. Accessed December 18, 2013.

42.   U.S. National Library of Medicine. 2012AB LOINC source information. http://www.nlm.nih.gov/research/umls/sourcereleasedocs/current/LNC/. Accessed December 18, 2013.

43.   Wikipedia contributors. LOINC. Wikipedia, The Free Encyclopedia. September 9, 2013, 13:58 UTC. 2013; http://en.wikipedia.org/w/index.php?title=LOINC&oldid=572192112. Accessed December 19, 2013.

44.   U.S. National Library of Medicine. 2012AB RxNorm source information. http://www.nlm.nih.gov/research/umls/sourcereleasedocs/current/RXNORM /. Accessed December 18, 2013.

45.   U.S. Food and Drug Administration. National drug code directory. http://www.fda.gov/drugs/informationondrugs/ucm142438.htm. Accessed December 19, 2013.

46.   U.S. National Library of Medicine. RxNorm technical information. http://www.nlm.nih.gov/research/umls/rxnorm/docs/2013/rxnorm_doco_full _2013-3.html. Accessed December 18, 2013.

47.   U.S. National Library of Medicine. 2012AA Current Procedural Terminology source information. http://www.nlm.nih.gov/research/umls/sourcereleasedocs/current/CPT/. Accessed December 19, 2013.

48.   Vanderbilt University. What is the phenotype knowledgebase? http://phekb.org/. Accessed December 19, 2013.

49.   National Institutes of Health. National Human Genome Research Institute. Electronic medical records and genomics (eMERGE) network. http://www.genome.gov/27540473. Accessed December 19, 2013.

50.   Newton KM, Peissig PL, Kho AN, et al. Validation of electronic medical record-based phenotyping algorithms: results and lessons learned from the eMERGE network. *J Am Med Inform Assoc.* June 2013;20(e1):e147-154.

51.   The R Project for Statistical Computing. http://www.r-project.org. Accessed December 19, 2013.

52.   Wikipedia contributors. Regularization (mathematics). Wikipedia, The Free Encyclopedia. July 29, 2013, 06:24 UTC. 2013; http://en.wikipedia.org/w/index.php?title=Regularization_(mathematics)&oldid=566248211. Accessed December 19, 2013.

53.   Wikipedia contributors. Unsupervised learning. Wikipedia, The Free Encyclopedia. October 22, 2013, 10:05 UTC. 2013; http://en.wikipedia.org/w/index.php?title=Unsupervised_learning&oldid=578239512. Accessed December 19, 2013.

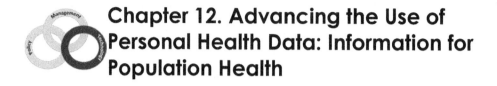

Chapter 12. Advancing the Use of Personal Health Data: Information for Population Health

William Yasnoff, MD, PhD, FACMI

"If you cannot measure it, you cannot improve it."

William Thomson, Lord Kelvin
1824–1907

Chapter 12 Learning Objectives

- Understand privacy concerns associated with the use of personal health data.

- Give examples of the uses of personal health data in population health initiatives.

- Understand the differences between institution-centric and patient-centric Health Information Infrastructure (HII) architectures.

- Identify three types of funding that could support HII systems.

- Recognize that there are policy (health and social) implications with the use of personal health data.

- Know what a health record bank is and how it can serve as the basis of a viable longitudinal patient health record system.

Introduction

Health care data from individual patients are essential to the management and improvement of population health. Traditionally, information about populations has been derived from specialized surveys. For example, since the 1960s the National Health and Nutrition Examination Survey (NHANES)[1] has conducted interviews and physical examinations of a carefully selected sample of Americans. The information obtained, including demographic, socioeconomic, dietary, and health status data, is used extensively by researchers and policy makers. Much of what we know about the prevalence of diseases and health trends (e.g., cancer, high blood pressure) is derived from NHANES information.

NHANES reports, however, are typically not available until several years after the original data are collected. As a result, much of the information we depend on to understand and monitor our nation's health is outdated and unreliable. Even vital statistics of births and deaths, arguably the most complete population health data, are long delayed. A good example of this time lag is the widely publicized announcement in 2007 that cancer deaths in the United States (U.S.) had decreased two years in a row.[2] The latest data available in this report, published in October 2007, were the preliminary mortality data from 2004, nearly three full years earlier. Such multiyear delays in the availability of critical information clearly preclude the possibility of timely interventions.

Ongoing public health agency monitoring of population health also involves processes that have been largely separate and independent from medical recordkeeping. For example, clinicians are required to report certain diseases and conditions to their local public health agencies. These reports are then compiled and transmitted to state and federal public health officials. Such reporting is neither timely nor complete.[3] Until recently, however, such reporting systems were the only mechanisms available for obtaining this information.

As the usage of electronic health records (EHRs) increases, it is increasingly feasible for them to be a source of more timely and complete population health information. In 2013, the Department of Health and Human Services (DHHS) Office of the National Coordinator for Health Information Technology (ONC) reported that over 50 percent of health care providers were using EHRs,[4] a substantial increase over just a few years. While this report is quite encouraging, there is much work left before we have a fully electronic health information system that can provide effective real-time population health monitoring. EHRs alone are not sufficient; there must also be mechanisms to aggregate the information for each person into a coherent whole and then combine that information into a population view. So far, such health information exchange (HIE) efforts have been problematic, with only isolated partial successes.[5]

There are a number of difficult issues that must be addressed in order to successfully develop a health information infrastructure (HII) that makes comprehensive electronic patient information available when and where needed, for both patient care and population health. Among these issues are privacy, information completeness, sustainability, standards, and architecture. We will address each of these issues in detail throughout this chapter along with the central themes of innovative technologies and relevant aspects impacting Health in All Policies (HiAP). First, let's look at how personal data are used for population health.

Use of Personal Health Data in Population Health

Surveillance

Perhaps the most important role for personal health data in population health is surveillance. Public health surveillance is defined as "the ongoing, systematic collection, analysis, and interpretation of outcome-specific data for use in the planning, implementation, and evaluation of public health practice."[6] Its primary purpose is to detect outbreaks of such important infectious diseases as influenza, shigellosis, or salmonella infection. In order for public health officials to intervene with measures to control such diseases, they must be aware of clusters of new cases at the earliest possible time. The current method, which relies on reporting of cases by physicians (typically via the U.S. Mail to local health departments) is slow and unreliable. Clearly, automatic reports to public health based on electronic patient records of individuals could provide more consistent, timely, and complete information to support public health action.

Assessment and Tracking of Population Health

Comprehensive health record information would be extremely helpful for tracking the incidence and prevalence of such chronic diseases as asthma and diabetes. For example, such key indicators as the rate of emergency department visits by asthma patients or the average HbA1c levels in diabetics (indicative of long-term blood sugar control) could be monitored on an ongoing basis. It would also be possible to assess the immunization status of populations and use this information to plan targeted interventions.

Monitoring Effectiveness of Interventions

Population health efforts often involve such specific interventions as screening programs. Evaluation of these efforts is typically expensive and time-consuming, with results typically taking so long that they can be helpful only in guiding the next intervention rather than the current one. The availability of near real-time health records for the population could enable "just-in-time" feedback for population health programs. This improvement in speed would allow adjustments and changes to be made as the interventions proceed, greatly increasing efficiency and effectiveness. Successful efforts could be rapidly expanded while activities that do not produce the desired results could be ended quickly.

Need for Comprehensive HII

To accomplish these objectives, an HII system is needed to provide anywhere, anytime comprehensive electronic patient records. Each individual's records must be accessible in compiled form for health care purposes, and must also be searchable via queries for population monitoring. As we will see in the following sections, such a system can be implemented through a network of health record banks (HRBs), which are community repositories of health records with access controlled by patients. By having health records for each person in one place (although not everyone's health records in the same place) and allowing patients to control access, the difficult interrelated problems of privacy, incomplete information, financial sustainability, standards, and architecture can all be successfully addressed.

Privacy

Importance

Privacy is of central importance when dealing with health records, which may include extremely sensitive personal information. Most people prefer to keep their medical information private, not only to avoid embarrassment but also to prevent possible employment or financial discrimination. Furthermore, failure to assure health record privacy can lead to patients being reluctant to disclose key medical details to their providers or even to avoid seeking medical care in the first place. Even the mere existence of certain records (e.g., a visit to a clinic specializing in sexually transmitted diseases) is sensitive even if no additional details are available. While confidential medical information is essential for population health and can produce many benefits, the use of this information must be carefully restricted and controlled to protect patient privacy.

Types of Privacy Concerns

There are at least two major categories of privacy concerns related to medical information. The first of these might be called "traditional privacy" and is related to the potential damage that can be caused by release of medical information, ranging from embarrassment to employment difficulties or other forms of discrimination. Such problems from inappropriate release of medical information have occasionally become national issues. For example, the 1972 vice-presidential candidate of the Democratic Party, Thomas Eagleton, was forced to step aside after it was revealed that he had suffered from depression that required electroshock therapy.[7] While most such violations of medical privacy are not widely reported or well known, these incidents still occur regularly.[8]

A second and perhaps more widely held concern about medical privacy may be termed "uncompensated use." This concern relates to aggregation of the records of many individuals to produce valuable revenue-generating information without asking permission or offering compensation to those whose data are utilized. The affected individuals often describe this pattern of use as being "cheated," and liken it to having their property used or taken without their consent. It is this "appropriation without consent or compensation" of information that is often at the heart of privacy disputes between large online firms (e.g., Facebook, Google, and others) and their users. The Federal Trade Commission has categorized some of these actions as "unfair and deceptive" trade practices.[9]

HIPAA Privacy Rule

With respect to medical records in the United States, the federal Health Insurance Portability and Accountability Act of 1996 (HIPAA) Privacy Rule adopted in 2002[10] eliminated the requirement of patient consent for disclosure and use of medical records for treatment, payment, and health care operations. These treatment, payment, and operations (TPO) exceptions allow organizations holding medical information sole authority to determine whether a proposed disclosure does or does not qualify under the TPO exception—in essence, whether patient consent for the disclosure is needed. While the 2009 Health Information Technology for Economic and Clinical Health (HITECH) Act[11] requires maintenance of audit trails of TPO disclosures, these audit trail records are not typically shared with the subjects of the disclosures. The result is that consumers currently lack control over the dissemination of their medical records, and are not notified if those records are shared outside the organization that created them.

While final modifications were issued to the HIPAA Privacy and Security rules on January 25, 2013, providing some additional protections of personal health information, it remains to be seen whether these new provisions will be sufficient to secure patients' electronic health records. [12] It is widely understood that the availability of electronic patient records for appropriate and authorized purposes also results in their increased availability for unsavory and even illegal purposes. Because of this possibility, there is a clear need for more rigorous protections to prevent misuse of this sensitive information, which the final HIPAA modifications attempt to provide. Ultimately, the issue relates to how decisions are made about the disclosure of individual medical records. Making anyone other than the patient or the patient's representative responsible for this decision is problematic. It is difficult to convince patients that a third party should decide where their medical records are seen and how they are used. Just making this argument erodes trust, because it is difficult to explain to patients how it is that a third party understands their interests better than they do. When patients become aware that the organizations holding their records now make such decisions unilaterally (and without notification to the affected individual) under HIPAA, they are typically quite uncomfortable and often surprised.

These privacy concerns are clearly reflected in consumer attitudes. Surveys show that between 13 percent and 17 percent of consumers admit to using "information hiding" techniques to limit access to their medical information.[13,14] Examples include deliberately obtaining care from an out-of-state provider or using an assumed name for laboratory tests. It seems likely that such surveys underrepresent the concerns because some people are probably unwilling to disclose such activities. Nevertheless, it is clear that a sizable minority of consumers would opt out of an electronic health record system that prevented them from controlling their own records. These consumers also might organize politically to stop the implementation of such a system. While this scenario may seem a bit alarmist, it is important to recall that a very tiny percentage of concerned citizens successfully petitioned Congress to eliminate the national unique medical identifier provision in the original HIPAA legislation because it was a threat to privacy.

Value of Patient Control

Because of these considerations, allowing all decisions about release of patient records to be entrusted to the patient (with such rare exceptions as mental incompetence) becomes a very attractive policy option. Such a policy would be especially helpful in enabling HII, because it would promote the necessary consumer trust in such a system. While patients today may not be sufficiently informed to make such decisions and therefore might control their records in ways that could result in harm, it seems that the negative consequences of delegating this decision making to anyone other than the patient could be much greater. Rather than assign control of records to a third party, which is potentially even more problematic, patient education about the important uses of their health records seems a better way to address this concern. After all, individuals clearly have the right to decide how their own money is spent, even though ill-advised decisions in this regard can result in serious negative consequences.

The concept of patient consent for access to medical records is not new. In fact, it has been only since the 2002 HIPAA Privacy Rule established the TPO exceptions that widespread access to patient records without consent has been legal. Establishing the right medical information privacy policies is critically important to promote the high level of trust that is required to gain widespread consumer support for an effective HII.

Information Completeness

Importance

Health care information must be relatively complete to have value, either for individual patient care or managing population-level health. Missing information may include vital data necessary for safe and effective decision making. For example, consider an online system that contains patient medication profiles that are uniformly only 50 percent complete. Such a system is very unlikely to be used by providers; it has virtually no value because of the missing data. Even with such a system, patients would still need to be questioned about their current medications. A good rule of thumb is that medical information must be at least about 85 percent complete before it has clinical value.[15]

Furthermore, it is complete information that is critical to reducing costs, improving quality, and ensuring usefulness of the information for population health.

How can providers avoid repeating tests and procedures if they do not have the prior results (or are unaware that prior results even exist)?

How can population health researchers assess the effectiveness of a preventive intervention if the data are incomplete?

In fact, it is this lack of comprehensive patient information that is a major cause of the high costs and avoidable medical errors that are now commonly observed. Provider organizations that consistently have more complete information, such as Kaiser and Group Health, demonstrate both higher-quality and lower-cost care. Therefore, ensuring the availability of comprehensive electronic patient information is essential to achieving the potential cost savings and quality improvement from health information systems.

Incentivizing Electronic Information

Today, each patient leaves records behind whenever he or she receives care. If the records are electronic, then it is conceivable that they could be aggregated into a comprehensive whole. If the records are on paper, however, this process is unwieldy and expensive at best. Even if digitized images of all the paper records could be aggregated, it remains the responsibility of the provider to integrate them into a coherent whole. Images of paper records do not facilitate the reorganization of information into logical categories and timelines to allow rapid understanding of the clinical situation (e.g., to create a consolidated problem list with duplicates removed). Only structured and coded electronic medical records can be manipulated in this way.

Therefore, comprehensive patient records require that all the records be electronic—meaning the universal adoption of EHR systems. EHR adoption is problematic, especially for small physician practices. It is estimated that only 11 percent of the economic benefits of an EHR accrue to the physician practice,[16] so the business case for physician EHRs is extremely weak. The federal HITECH incentive program has greatly increased EHR adoption, but as of late 2013, about half of physicians still do not use an EHR. Moreover, many of those using EHRs have extremely basic systems that do not capture sufficient information.[17]

To ensure the widespread adoption of EHRs by physicians, additional incentives are required. These incentives need to be ongoing in order to create a compelling business case. After all, if EHRs could be obtained by physicians at minimal or no cost, the estimated 11 percent of the benefit they receive would then be a strong motivator for adoption. Therefore, the business model for any system to ensure the availability of comprehensive patient records when and where needed should include ongoing physician subsidies to promote universal EHR adoption and use.

HIPAA requires all health care stakeholders to supply medical records on patient request. Furthermore, if electronic information is requested and available, the records must be furnished electronically. Fees may be assessed, however, to cover the costs of this activity. While these costs are admittedly low when electronic information is being supplied, providing modest payments for such information helps encourage stakeholders to cooperate. Accordingly, it makes sense for a system compiling comprehensive patient records to include some funding to all health care stakeholders for provision of their information.

Need for Regional Approach

While health care is often regarded as a national issue, the reality is that the vast majority of care is given in the immediate area where each person lives. Indeed, even if people are injured or become ill when traveling, they will try to return home for care as soon as they are able. The practical consequence of this "locality" of care is that capturing all the medical information in a local area results in nearly comprehensive records for all the residents. This feature is important because it means that a system that provides comprehensive patient records can be local in scope initially yet capture the vast majority of the needed information. As a result, the system needs to connect only to a limited number of providers and system stakeholders (e.g., hospitals, labs, pharmacies, imaging centers, and physician practices).

By having established connections to all the local health care providers, each local person's comprehensive records can be obtained automatically from those sources. Importantly, the individual need not identify exactly which providers have his or her records (although that would certainly be helpful).

Smaller local populations simplify the problem of patient identification because there are fewer similar or identical names or other demographic data. As described in the case study, one of the problems encountered by Google Health (and other such national systems) is the need for each patient to manually identify and connect with each and every source of their medical record information, typically using a complex multistep process to ensure accurate identity matching. This administrative complexity deters patient participation and also results in less complete information.

Another reason for the local or regional focus of health information systems is to assure achieving enrollment of a critical mass of the population. This number is important so that providers will regularly access and utilize the information that such a system can provide. If only 10 percent of the local population is enrolled in a system that provides comprehensive electronic records, providers will be reluctant to change their office procedures to include the steps necessary to access the system regardless of how helpful the information may be. The small percentage of participants means that most of the patients in each office do not have the benefit of the system, so the few that do will require special "extra steps" to access it. Such "process exceptions" are extremely disruptive and time-consuming, particularly in busy physician offices that derive whatever efficiency they can from standardized procedures. It is easy to see that participation rates may need to be as high as the 70–80 percent range before most physician offices will establish routine procedures to access this new source of electronic medical record information. It is extremely challenging for a national system to achieve such a high participation rate in any one community; a local marketing focus is clearly needed. For all these reasons, a local or regional approach to HII is most likely to be successful. Indeed, the few such systems that have been partially successful (e.g., Indianapolis) have had such a local or regional scope.

Finally, it is important to note the movement toward accountable care organizations (ACOs) and underlying clinical integration programs for increasing population enrollment in systems. These organizations are driving physician engagement and alignment with information systems and quality focused initiatives that are integrated regionally.[18] As the nation learns from these new regional models of care delivery, the models are certain to evolve along with the information system capabilities necessary to improve population health.

Sustainability

Importance

Building an information system that has no mechanism for sustainability is an exercise in futility. While this point is quite obvious, many health information system development efforts still utilize a *Field of Dreams* strategy of "build it and they will come," and simply hope that a good-enough system will result somehow in a sustainable financial model. Most of the efforts to build HII using health information exchanges (HIEs) represent an excellent case in point. The belief is that such systems will be valuable because they will improve health care and reduce costs. Since this is the case, there must be some way to leverage those benefits to pay for the infrastructure. Such an approach ignores the hard reality that organizations and individuals will pay only for clear and compelling value received, not vague future benefits. The specific and well-defined mechanisms whereby a health information system will deliver benefits sufficiently valuable to elicit payment needs to be delineated during the design stage.

Sources of Revenue

There are three general sources of revenue that can be used, individually or in combination, to fund an HII system: taxes; recovery of health care cost savings; and leveraging new value from the information collected by the HII.

Taxes

The availability of comprehensive health information is clearly a public good. Not only does it promote the health and safety of the population, it can also reduce health care costs for both individuals and the government. Given these characteristics, a reasonable and perhaps even persuasive argument can be made that HII should be supported through tax revenue like such other infrastructure as roads, which benefit the general population. The relatively low cost of HII compared to the cost of health care (even the very highest estimates of HII costs are < 2 percent, while 0.2 percent is more realistic) makes tax support an attractive option. Indeed, this approach has to some extent been adopted in Vermont through a tax on health insurance claims, and in Maryland, which has imposed an HII tax on hospitals. New taxes are consistently unpopular and politically challenging, however, so this approach has significant limitations.

Recovery of Health Care Cost Savings

The most prevalent proposed approach to funding HII is through recapture of the resultant health care cost savings. It is estimated that a reduction in health care costs of about 8 percent can be expected from a fully functional HII. [19] Because these savings greatly exceed anticipated costs, recapture is an appealing option. Stakeholders should expect that significant savings will require some initial investment and ongoing operational costs. As long as those costs greatly exceed the savings, it should be easy to convince stakeholders to participate.

These theoretical arguments have proved extremely difficult to implement in practice, however. First, the timing and distribution of the savings are not clear. Naturally, stakeholders are extremely reluctant to make commitments today based on unproven savings of unknown size at an unpredictable future time. Second, it is difficult to assure stakeholders that their financial commitment will be used only for their own beneficiaries. As is typical with a community project such as HII, it is very difficult to allocate the costs in a way that is acceptable to everyone. Finally, the experience of hundreds of communities working on HII demonstrates clearly that this approach is problematic. In the most recent survey of such projects, fully three-quarters indicated that financial sustainability is a critical unsolved problem.[20] If this approach to sustainability were working, this high percentage would not be the case.

Leverage New Value of Collected Information

The final, but least explored, approach to HII sustainability is to leverage the new value created as a result of the availability of comprehensive electronic patient information. This information can enable the delivery of a variety of innovative services to patients, providers, and others that are impractical in today's world of scattered medical information. For patients, reminders and alerts can deliver significant value. As an example, when a patient's information is accessed by emergency medical personnel (indicating that emergency care is being given), the patient's loved ones could be notified immediately. Such a "peace of mind" reminder yields a compelling benefit to family members. Another possible patient-directed application is a "prevention advisor," which would give individually customized notices of tests and procedures needed to maintain or monitor health.

Potential services to providers include rapid delivery of lab results with automatic notification of critical values as well as filtering out normal values not requiring clinician attention. Another possibility is automatic notification (with patient permission) to primary care providers when any of their patients receive care elsewhere.

Public health could benefit from automatic notification of reportable conditions and syndromes, which could be nearly real-time. Both public health and medical researchers could benefit from aggregate reports based on queries of the data, allowing ongoing tracking of disease outbreaks as well as assessments of population health trends and the impact of various treatments.

The establishment of an HII with comprehensive electronic patient records opens up massive opportunities in health technology innovation for a variety of creative developers who are already working on health applications in the Health 2.0 community.[21] Many of these innovative applications have thus far been unable to gain widespread market acceptance because of the need for patients to enter and constantly update substantial amounts of medical information. Once this data entry burden is eliminated with an HII, however, consumers are much more likely to adopt and utilize these applications.

By supporting the HII with the new value generated from the information itself, the anticipated health care savings from the system would no longer represent a burden of allocation and capture. Instead, those savings could become yet another incentive for stakeholders to actively participate in the HII, since they would be able to retain any and all financial benefits generated for their health care operations.

Standards

Importance

In order to be effective, an HII must be able to collect standardized, codified health record information from a variety of sources. Clearly, it is not acceptable to combine a patient's records from three providers when the different designations of the same problem (e.g., high blood pressure, hypertension, and elevated blood pressure) result in three separate problems in the integrated record. Therefore, it is essential that all EHR systems feeding the HII utilize similar standards; and when necessary, that the standardized designations in one system are "mapped" to the specific standard used in the HII. Achieving this interoperability between systems from multiple vendors has been a challenging ongoing issue. National efforts to facilitate the identification and implementation of standards for EHRs are being led by the Office of the National Coordinator for Health Information Technology (ONC), with recommendations coming from their Health Information Technology Standards Committee (HITSC). The HITSC convenes industry leaders each month to assess the challenges faced by the nation's health system in relation to needed standards for EHRs, and to support the Centers for Medicare and Medicaid Services' (CMS) Meaningful Use of EHRs program and work toward recommendations for solutions to these challenges.

Mechanisms for Standards Compliance

There are at least three approaches to achieving standards compliance and interoperability: 1) voluntary; 2) incentives; and 3) mandatory.[15] Clearly, a completely voluntary system does not and cannot work. Each vendor's interests are best served by avoiding compatibility with other vendors. This avoidance serves both to discourage existing customers from switching to competitive products, and to encourage new customers to adopt their systems to ensure compatibility with an existing installed base.

The third option, mandatory compliance, can certainly be effective but is politically difficult to implement. Only the government can mandate standards compliance, and government action requires a strong consensus among the stakeholders. Also, there is good evidence that sufficiently powerful financial incentives can accomplish the same goals with much less political angst.

Incentives for standards compliance are currently being applied through the CMS Meaningful Use of EHRs program that was initiated under the HITECH Act. Under this program, providers adopting EHRs and utilizing them to meet the

Meaningful Use criteria are eligible to receive substantial financial benefits over a five-year period. Stage 2 Meaningful Use includes a requirement that patients be able to view, download, and transmit (VDT) their health records using government-designated standards by the beginning of 2014. The strong desire of providers to comply with Meaningful Use to obtain the financial benefits is creating the necessity for all vendors to incorporate standard export functions in their EHR products. An HII could then continue to provide financial incentives for standards compliance to help reinforce the ongoing use and updating of standards over time.

Architecture

As indicated above, population health uses of medical record information require that the data be easily searchable across patients. Since medical records are currently stored wherever they are created, they must be moved or exchanged to compile a complete longitudinal record of an individual.

Institution-centric Architecture

Up to now, the common approach to such health information exchange (HIE) has been institution-centric, leaving patient records stored where they are originally created (Figure 12-1). To avoid the need to query every possible system in the world for a given patient's records, a central index of all sources of information for each patient is maintained. To compile a patient's record when requested, that index generates queries to the various record sources for that patient. The results are then combined (in real time) to yield the patient's comprehensive record. After each patient visit, new medical records are entered into the provider's EHR system and a pointer (to that system) is appended to the index to ensure that those new records are retrieved when that patient's record is next requested, as illustrated in Figure 12-1.

Figure 12-1. Institution-centric HII Architecture

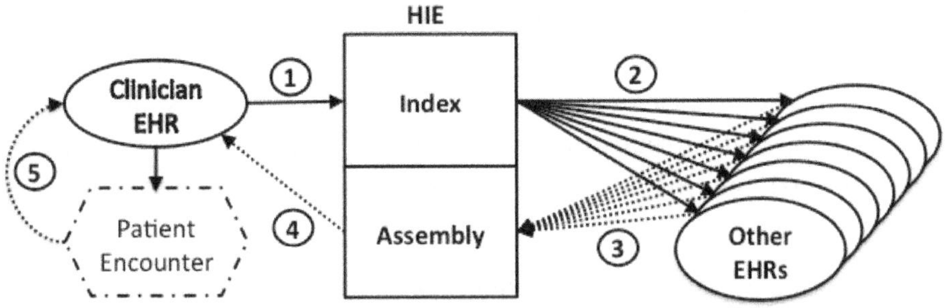

The operational steps of this institution-centric HII architecture are:[22]

1. The clinician EHR requests prior patient records from the HIE; this clinician's EHR is added to the index for future queries for this patient (if not already present).

2. Queries are sent to EHRs at all sites of prior care recorded in the HIE Index.

3. EHRs at each prior site of care return records for that patient to the HIE; the HIE must wait for all responses.

4. The returned records are assembled and sent to the clinician EHR; any inconsistencies or incompatibilities between records must be resolved in real time.

5. After the care episode, the new information is stored in the clinician EHR only.

This architecture allows health care stakeholders to avoid sending records they generate to an outside organization for storage. It does not scale efficiently, however, and is complicated (and thus expensive and error-prone) to operate.[23] Most importantly for population health, such an architecture does not facilitate efficient searching of the data; e.g., to find all patients eligible for pneumovax immunization who have not received it. Such a search would be sequential, requiring the records of every patient to be retrieved one at a time. Such sequential searches have very long completion times that are directly proportional to the size of the population. For example, in a system with 1,000,000 patients, if each patient's records require just two seconds to retrieve and process (a very low estimate), such a search would take at least 24 days (two million seconds).

Even worse, each search requires every connected provider record system to transmit all its information—a massive computing and communications task that also increases the risk of interception or corruption of information. In typical database systems, the long delays inherent in sequential searches are avoided by pre-indexing the records (much like creating an index of a book to allow rapid searching of specific words). Because the resultant indices can be used to reconstruct most of the original data, however, they are in essence equivalent to a central repository and therefore are not consistent with this institution-centric approach that allows retention of data only in its original location.

It is tempting to think that this sequential search problem could be solved by distributing the searches to the provider systems, with the results aggregated to produce a correct response. Distributed searches work properly, however, only if the data in each node are independent. This condition is met only if all of a patient's records are in a single provider system, which is not typically the case. Searches that request more than one patient data item (e.g., patients with asthma who have an emergency room visit), will yield incorrect results unless all the relevant data for a given patient are in just one provider system (i.e., if one system finds a patient with asthma, but without any emergency room visits [which are recorded in another provider's system], that patient will (erroneously) not be counted as meeting the query conditions). Limiting searches to a single item and then combining the results from multiple searches does not eliminate this problem.

Besides this difficult searching problem, response times for retrieving and compiling a single patient record with this architecture can also be very slow. Each time a patient record is requested, the central index indicates those systems where the patient has available records. Each such system is then individually queried, but the final record assembly process cannot be completed until the slowest of the provider systems has responded. As the number of queried provider systems increases, so does the probability of a delayed (or missing) reply from one of them when patient records are requested. Also, more sources of patient information require greater processing time to integrate them all into one combined record. Finally, this retrieval and integration process must be repeated each and every time a patient's records are needed. This process represents a huge computing burden that, as shown in the next section, is completely avoidable.

This institution-centric architecture is also complex to operate. Since the comprehensiveness of records obtained for a given patient depends on the availability of all the provider systems with information about that patient, continuous monitoring of all the provider information systems is necessary. Doing this task requires a 24 x 7 network operations center (NOC) to constantly monitor the operational status of each provider's EHR system. Any problems that are detected would need immediate troubleshooting to correct the problem, meaning that senior IT staff must be available around the clock. The cost of such continuous monitoring is very high, since at least five full-time staff members are needed to cover three shifts seven days a week. The alternative of ignoring this problem would result in sporadic incomplete patient records, which would clearly be unacceptable.

Patient-centric Architecture

Happily, there is a more feasible and efficient alternative architecture for HII: health record banking. This is a patient-centric approach that both addresses the key requirements and can overcome the challenges described above that have stymied current efforts.[5,24] A health record bank (HRB) is defined as "an independent organization that provides a secure electronic repository for storing and maintaining an individual's lifetime health and medical records from multiple sources and assuring that the individual always has complete control over who accesses their information."[25]

Providing patient information for medical care using a community HRB is much simpler than the institution-centric approach (Figure 12-1). Before seeking care (or when care is given in an emergency), the patient records his or her permission for the provider to access his or her HRB account records (either all or part). The authorized provider then retrieves (and downloads, if desired) the patient's records through a secure Internet web portal. Upon completion of the encounter, the provider system uploads new medical records of that visit to the HRB for deposit in the patient's lifetime health record account. The updated records are immediately available for future care episodes, as illustrated in Figure 12-2.

Figure 12-2. Patient-centric HII Architecture

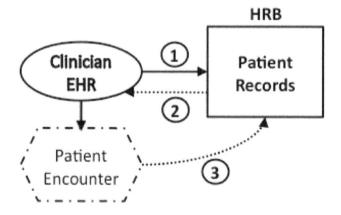

The operational steps of this patient-centric HII architecture are:[22]

1. The clinician EHR requests prior patient records from the HRB.

2. The prior patient records are immediately sent to the clinician EHR.

3. After the care episode, the new information is stored in the clinician EHR and sent to the HRB; any inconsistencies or incompatibilities with prior records in the HRB must be resolved before that patient's records are requested again (but not in real time).

Timeline

The HRB concept was initially proposed as a "Guardian Angel" nearly two decades ago.[26] In the United Kingdom, the term "health information bank" was first used in 1997.[27] A few years later, the HRB concept was termed the "bank of health."[28] In 2006, a policy paper from the Heritage Foundation endorsed health record banking,[29] additional publications described details of HRBs,[30,31] and the nonprofit Health Record Banking Alliance was established to promote the concept.[32] That same year, the State of Washington recommended the HRB approach after a 16-month study,[33] and several large employers collaborated to implement and operate an HRB for their employees via the nonprofit Dossia Consortium.[34] In 2007, the Information Technology and Innovation Foundation recommended the HRB approach for building the U.S. HII,[35] and both Microsoft and Google unveiled patient-controlled medical record repositories (although the Google system, known as Google Health, has since been discontinued; see the case study). Three pilot HRBs were established in the State of Washington in 2009, and one also began operation in Rotterdam, the Netherlands.[36] The concept of patient-controlled record repositories (like HRBs) is now appearing more often in articles discussing the need for comprehensive EHRs.[37-41] In 2011, Australia adopted the HRB approach as national policy, and its "Patient-Centered" EHR system became operational in 2012.[42] Estonia has also implemented a national HRB system.[43]

This historical timeline shows clearly the gradual emergence of a feasible solution for longitudinal patient records management. In relation to this history, the following case study of Google Health provides a glimpse of some of the challenges rooted in the dynamics that exist between the institution-centric vs. the patient-centric architecture approaches to HII.

Case Study: Google Health

Google Health was launched in 2008 as a secure repository in which consumers could deposit all their health information and share it with providers. It was discontinued four years later due to limited customer adoption. According to Google, the product failed to find "a way to translate limited usage into widespread adoption in the daily health routines of millions of people."[44] There has been substantial additional speculation about the reasons for its failure.

Case Study: Google Health

Here we will focus on four key problems:

1. National focus

Because of its national focus, Google Health could not achieve a critical mass of participation in any particular region. In order to get providers to change their office procedures to routinely look at Google Health information, a majority or even a supermajority (perhaps over 70 percent) of patients being seen needed to have Google Health accounts with useful information. It was very unlikely that this high percentage could be achieved in any region without a specific marketing focus there. The national scope also meant that patients were required to undertake multiple steps to link each of their provider information sources to Google Health. In contrast, if there were a focus on a specific region, all the sources in that region could have been connected so that each patient who signed up could automatically be connected to all their information in the area.

2. Incomplete information

Even if Google Health could have been connected to every electronic medical information source in the nation, the information would still have been incomplete because most providers still use paper records. Information from those paper records could not easily be incorporated into Google Health. Furthermore, even if "images" of paper records were stored, the information contained within them could not be readily processed or located automatically. For example, lab results in such a format cannot be used to construct a trend report. To get the full benefit of comprehensive patient records, those records must be electronic and machine-processable, meaning they must be derived from provider EHRs.

There was not, however, a good business case for provider EHR adoption. One study, for example, showed that only 11 percent of the economic benefit of an EHR accrues to the physician in a small practice.[16] While the federal government incentives for EHR adoption under the HITECH Act have greatly increased physician EHR adoption, a large proportion of physicians, particularly in small offices, still use paper records. Google Health did not do anything to address this problem, i.e., further incentivizing EHR adoption for office-based physicians.

3. Trust

It was difficult for consumers to trust Google Health with their sensitive health records. While Google Health ultimately had good privacy policies, they were superseded by Google's overall privacy policy, which does not promise

> **Case Study: Google Health**
>
> individuals full control of all uses of their information. A first step in addressing this problem would have been for Google Health to adopt ironclad privacy policies supporting patient control of their information. It would also have been beneficial for them to advocate for regulation that would make any breaches of their promise of individual control over health records subject to government penalties. Being able to indicate to consumers that promises of information control are backed by government regulation could have helped address the trust problem.
>
> ### 4. No business model
>
> Google Health never had a sustainable business model. The plan was to evolve a model after the system was established. The traditional "eyes on page" business model that Google itself uses to generate revenue with advertising was recognized as problematic in this environment, so Google promised not to allow advertising within Google Health. Of course, Google had the financial capability to operate the service without any source of revenue for a substantial period of time, but users expect that a business will want to profit from its operations. The lack of a business model (or even a vision of a future business model) can be worrisome. The concern is that consumer health information might be used in the future in unanticipated, objectionable ways to support an as-yet-unannounced business model.

The challenges of this case provide key lessons learned to the entire industry. Today, as health information technologies move forward, the issue of personal health records and their relationship to HII is better understood. The importance of sustainable business models along with interoperable architectures that are readily and easily accessible by patients is critical to achieving the long-term benefits that both individuals and the industry need.

Policy Implications

Many new policy issues must be considered in the context of increased adoption and use of EHRs by providers and the creation of HII systems to aggregate comprehensive individual health records from multiple systems.

Privacy

Privacy has already been mentioned as a critical issue for medical records. Some additional policy issues to consider are:

HITECH Changes to HIPAA

One of the most important changes to HIPAA privacy from the HITECH legislation is the requirement for organizations to maintain audit trails of TPO disclosures and make them available on request to patients. Previously, no records were required of TPO disclosures. If an organization determined that a disclosure was covered under TPO, it simply made the disclosure and kept no record. The practical impact was that there was no way to retrospectively determine whether a given TPO disclosure was compliant with the HIPAA Privacy Rule. The HITECH requirement for audit trails has remedied this problem, but there are still serious limitations. Patients must request access to the audit trail information and are still not notified about disclosures. There is also a time limit on retention of the audit trail information. Finally, even if a violation is found, the consumer still has no legal right to redress and the information itself cannot be "undisclosed." Only the HHS Office of Civil Rights and the state attorneys general (the latter added by HITECH) are authorized to take legal action against HIPAA violators.

Potential Future Policy Framework

The limits of the HIPAA policy framework, even as modified by HITECH, are clear. A viable alternative is to return to the policy in place before the 2002 HIPAA Privacy Rule, which was to require patient consent for any and all use of personal health information. This return would also lay the groundwork for ultimately transferring ownership of the medical records to the patient. At present, the provider owns the records, with the patient being entitled to a copy on request. Reversing this policy would help ensure privacy; the provider copy of the records could be restricted to the provider's own use. This change would automatically protect patients from provider disclosure of records without their consent.

Such a major change in how medical information is handled would need to be implemented gradually, however, to avoid disruption of current systems of care. A helpful first step would be to create one or more large-scale demonstration projects to show how patient ownership and control of records can facilitate both better individual health care and improved population health on a regional and national level. Then a gradual transition could be planned over a number of years, allowing for changes in both state and federal law as well as implementation of the new policies in provider health record systems.

> *Patient Education*

In a system in which patients own and control their own information, education and assistance about the decisions to approve or deny access to that information would be critical. The concept of managing personal information is new to most people, so there is likely to be a great deal of confusion about this new responsibility. Just as is now done for patient consent to treatment, systems and policies would need to be established for delegating information access decisions in cases in which patients are unable or unwilling to make their own determinations.

> *Governance and Certification of Compliance*

Rules and procedures must be established for the governance of HII organizations. Because such organizations have authority over sensitive and valuable assets, there is a need for regulation to ensure that their stewardship is both transparent and in the best interest of the stakeholders (primarily patients). Periodic public reporting is essential.

Compliance of organizations handling medical record information should be accomplished through regulation. Organizations should be required to obtain third-party security and privacy audits on a regular basis, just as most organizations are now required to undergo financial audits. These audits would help ensure that information is protected and that policies are in place and enforced to limit access to authorized individuals for allowable purposes.

> *Limits of Patient Control*

Even in a system in which patients own and control their own medical information, the needs of the community may still override individual consent when the justification is compelling. Public health reporting of communicable diseases, for example, has always been done without individual consent because it is necessary to protect the population. Another example is the availability of controlled substance prescription information to providers. It would be dangerous to enable individuals to fraudulently obtain multiple prescriptions for narcotic painkillers by choosing not to allow their providers to access their medication information. In such cases, compromise positions may be needed. For example, should a patient elect to suppress access to controlled substance prescriptions, any provider treating the patient and accessing their medical records could get a message indicating that the patient has so elected (without revealing the actual information). In this way, providers would be alerted to a potential problem, while patients would still have the right not to disclose the information. Additional unanticipated public policy issues requiring a balance between individual rights to information and community interests are likely to arise.

Impact of Meaningful Use and Other HHS Programs

➢ *Increased EHR adoption*

The Meaningful Use of EHRs incentives adopted under the HITECH Act provide substantial financial subsidies for physicians and hospitals adopting and using EHR systems. These subsidies have resulted in a substantial increase in their usage. Recent data indicate that 42 percent of hospitals[45] and over 50 percent of physician offices[17] are now using EHR systems and meeting the Stage 1 Meaningful Use criteria. While Stage 2 has been extended through 2016 and Stage 3 has been delayed until 2017, Stage 2 is under way and starting to be implemented by progressive adopters (both eligible physicians and hospitals) across the U.S. healthcare system.

➢ *Focus on use rather than achieving goals*

On the other hand, the achievement of Meaningful Use by eligible physicians and hospitals does not guarantee the availability of comprehensive electronic patient records when and where needed. To accomplish the latter, an effective HII is needed that performs this function, which requires aggregation of an individual's records from multiple providers.

➢ *View, download, and transmit (VDT) requirement (Stage 2)*

One of the Meaningful Use requirements that is likely to be extremely helpful in facilitating an effective HII is the VDT requirement of Meaningful Use Stage 2 (effective October 2013 for hospitals and January 2014 for office-based providers, with extensions allowed into 2016). All providers are required to offer patients the ability to access and electronically transmit their records to a destination of their choice. All such transmissions must utilize standard formats and coding specified by ONC. To meet this requirement, EHR vendors are working to add this capability to their systems, which is required to maintain compliance with the ONC certification requirements. The overall result is that patients will have the ability to direct their electronic medical records to be sent regularly to a location of their choice so that the records can be compiled over time and made available to subsequent providers.

The VDT capability was first introduced as a concept known as "blue button" by the Veterans Administration in 2010. The idea was that patients would have a "blue button" they could push to download their records. The initial evolution of this process is an "automated blue button" that allows patients to designate a specific destination for new records whenever they are created. This automated blue button is essentially equivalent to the "transmit" portion of the VDT requirement.

> *Query-in, query-out requirement (proposed for Stage 3)*

While the VDT requirement is very positive, at least one of the currently proposed requirements for Stage 3 Meaningful Use is ill-advised and counterproductive. This is the "query-in, query-out" (QIQO) capability that is supposed to be added to EHR systems. The intent is that every EHR be able to query any other EHR for needed data (query out), and also accept and respond with requested data to queries sent by other EHRs (query in).

This capability is an impractical and unworkable requirement. First, there is the authentication problem. Clearly, no EHR should respond to a query unless it is from an authorized source. But how can each EHR determine who is authorized? Would each EHR have a complete directory of users? Would there be a "query clearinghouse" that would check authorization?

Second, there is the issue of system availability and query load. With QIQO, every EHR would need to be available 24 hours a day, seven days a week, to receive queries. These queries would also impose an additional processing load on the system, requiring more communications and processing capacity. This load inevitably would increase the cost of these systems—and their high cost is already a major obstacle to adoption.

Third, how would EHRs know which outside systems to query? Would there be a central clearinghouse with this information? How would it be created and maintained?

Finally, QIQO capabilities would make all EHRs the target of hackers everywhere. Knowing that every EHR is equipped to respond immediately with confidential medical records would make these systems irresistible targets. Medical providers operating EHR systems would need to establish robust firewall and security programs to carefully monitor all incoming traffic—tasks that are very expensive and beyond the capabilities of most office-based physicians.

The proposed QIQO requirement is an effort by ONC to force EHR vendors (through providers) to help implement a key element of the distributed institution-centric HII architecture. This architecture is unwise and impractical (as discussed earlier), so this regulatory attempt to impose it is misguided at best.

> ### *Direct protocol provides useful transmission capability*

The ONC Direct protocol[46] is designed to facilitate movement of standardized, formatted medical record information from one point to another. Although initially envisioned as a provider-to-provider communication mechanism, it can also facilitate transmission of patient information to a location where it is compiled and stored as a longitudinal record. It therefore can be very helpful in facilitating an effective HII.

Impact of Data on Health Policy (individuals and populations)

> ### *Changes can be monitored*

The availability of electronic health records for most individuals is very positive for population health. First, changes in health and trends in care can be measured. For example, medical encounters can be used as a proxy for prevalence of disease, while newly diagnosed cases can be an indicator of incidence.

> ### *More flexibility and experimentation*

Second, the availability of data allows greater flexibility and experimentation with health policy. When it takes years for the impact of a health policy change to be measured (as it does now), there is a natural reluctance to make changes unless there is a compelling reason supported by data confirming the anticipated positive benefits. If population data can be monitored in near real-time, the threshold for policy changes can be lower. Adverse consequences (particularly if unanticipated) can be detected much sooner, before large numbers of people are negatively affected.

Given the interconnectivity that exists across society today, the implications and linkages that affect social policy are also greater as we work toward increased availability of health data. City and state governments can institute policy changes that improve social dynamics related to education, criminal justice, environmental, and housing issues in communities based on improved visibility into the health of its population, which can come only through more timely availability and appropriate use of personal health data. This timeliness underscoreses the importance of a Health in All Policies (HiAP) approach, one of the key themes throughout this book. Personal health data in the twenty-first century will serve as foundational information for decisions that can affect the United States' and global governments' direction in health and social policies that govern the societies within their borders. More accurate and timely information will greatly improve our ability to pinpoint the most important needs of the citizens served and affected by these policy decisions.

➢ *New relationships can be found and studied*

Finally, the availability of population data will allow new and unanticipated relationships of events and activities to be discovered and studied. At present, such studies require the organization and implementation of a clinical trial, an expensive and time-consuming undertaking. But with data readily available, multiple correlations and relationships can be easily tested. It seems likely that many unexpected and useful results will be uncovered from such activities. The complexity of relationships can cross over both health and social policy issues. Identifying and addressing the interconnected challenges that exist will yield newfound progress for the U.S. healthcare system along with other nations as our journey with the evolving use of personal health data continues to unfold.

The Information Economy

As we move into a true information economy, it is increasingly clear that all our personal information (not just health records) has real value, particularly in aggregated form. It seems that continuing our current "Wild West" approach to the management of highly valuable patient information, in which the possessors in general can use it for whatever they wish and keep the economic benefits, is likely to be repeatedly challenged. While it is not possible to predict the results of future policy debates, one clear way to resolve this problem is to declare each individual's personal information his or her property, to be used by others only with permission. Besides the inherent fairness of this straightforward notion, as well as its privacy-protective nature, some observers believe that permission-based use of personal information can also create huge new markets and economic activity.[47] It certainly is clear that health care records have substantial value for both individuals and the population as a whole. It will be interesting to observe the evolution of personal information policy in the years ahead.

Conclusion

The healthcare information of individuals is critical to population health, and the availability of such information on a timely and routine basis can contribute much to the health of our society. Before we can reap the benefits of a health information infrastructure (HII), we must solve the problems of privacy, incomplete information, standards, sustainability, and architecture. Since there is at least one HII approach that addresses these problems (i.e., health record banking), we can anticipate that an effective HII is likely to be implemented in the next few years. It is an alternative approach that can be fully compatible with existing HIEs, as they will likely continue to be part of the national health information technology fabric here in the United States and abroad.[48] Change takes time; and sometimes solving the technical challenges can both precede needed policy innovation and show the way to a needed paradigm shift.

This HII, composed of EHRs and systems to aggregate records from them for each person, will be a critical source of ongoing data for monitoring and improving the health of both individuals and the population in the years ahead.

CHAPTER 12 DISCUSSION QUESTIONS

Discussion questions are provided for team building or class exercises. Answers for all questions are provided in Appendix C.

Question Number	Question
1	Since HII is beneficial to both individuals and healthcare stakeholders, why has it been so difficult to implement?
2	How can an effective HII address concerns about biodefense, the detection of and response to intentional attacks with biological agents?
3	Are public health agencies prepared to take advantage of the capabilities of an effective HII? Why or why not?
4	What public policies need to be adopted to facilitate the more rapid achievement of an effective HII?
5	Describe a feasible and workable HII architecture consisting of a national network of health record banks (HRBs) as an alternative to current HIE approaches using institution-centric architecture. How would patient records be available and get updated for patients needing care outside the region where their HRB operates? How would searches across multiple HRBs for population health purposes be accomplished?

CHAPTER 12 SUMMARY

- Health care information is critical to population health, including surveillance and prevention.

- As health records become primarily electronic, we have an opportunity to create an effective health information infrastructure (HII) that provides anywhere, anytime, comprehensive electronic patient information for both individuals and populations.

- An HII requires solutions to the problems of privacy, incomplete information, financial sustainability, standards, and architecture. At least one proposed approach—health record banking—can address all these problems.

- New public policies are needed to support and accelerate progress towards HII.

- The availability of an effective HII creates many exciting new opportunities for improving population health.

CHAPTER 12 REFERENCES

1.   Centers for Disease Control and Prevention. National Health and Nutrition Examination Survey (NHANES). http://www.cdc.gov/nchs/nhanes.htm. Accessed July 21, 2013.

2.   Espey DK, Wu XC, Swan J, et al. Annual report to the nation on the status of cancer, 1975-2004, featuring cancer in American Indians and Alaska Natives. *Cancer.* 2007;110(10):2119-2152.

3.   Hopkins RS. Design and operation of state and local infectious disease surveillance systems. *J Public Health Manag Pract.* 2005;11(3):184-190.

4.   U.S. Department of Health and Human Services. *Update on the adoption of health information technology and related efforts to facilitate the electronic use and exchange of health information. A report to Congress.* Wasgington, D.C.: HHS Office of the National Coordinator for Health Information Technology;2013.

5.   Yasnoff WA, Sweeney L, Shortliffe EH. Putting health IT on the path to success. *JAMA.* 2013;309(10):989-990.

6.   Thacker SB, Berkelman RL. Public health surveillance in the United States. *Epidemiol Rev.* 1988;10:164-190.

7.   Altman LK. Hasty and ruinous 1972 pick colors today's hunt for no. 2. *New York Times.* July 23, 2012. http://www.nytimes.com/2012/07/24/us/politics/eagleton-pick-in-1972-colors-todays-vice-president-hunt.html. Accessed July 21, 2013.

8.   Health Privacy Project. Medical privacy stories. http://patientprivacyrights.org/media/True_Stories.pdf. Accessed July 21, 2013.

9.   Paul I. Facebook privacy complaint: a complete breakdown. *PC World.* May 6, 2010. http://www.pcworld.com/article/195756/facebook_privacy_complaint.html. Accessed July 21, 2013.

10.   U.S. Department of Health and Human Services. The privacy rule. http://www.hhs.gov/ocr/privacy/hipaa/administrative/privacyrule/index.htm l. Accessed July 21, 2013.

11.   HHS Office of the National Coordinator for Health Information Technology. HITECH Act. http://www.healthit.gov/policy-researchers-implementers/hitech-act-0. Accessed July 21, 2013.

12.   New rule protects patient privacy, secures health information. [press release]. *HHS News.* January 17, 2013. http://www.hhs.gov/news/press/2013pres/01/20130117b.html. Accessed July 21, 2013.

13.   California HealthCare Foundation. National consumer health privacy survey. Sacramento, Calif.;2005. http://www.chcf.org/publications/2005/11/national-consumer-health-privacy-survey-2005. Accessed July 21, 2013.

14. Many U.S. adults are satisfied with use of their personal health records [press release]. Harris Interactive. March 26, 2007.

15. Yasnoff WA. Health information infrastructure. In: Shortliffe EH, Cimino JJ, eds. *Biomedical informatics: computer applications in healthcare and medicine.* 4th ed. New York, N.Y.: Springer-Verlag;2014:423-442.

16. Hersh W. Health care information technology: progress and barriers. *JAMA.* 2004;292(18):2273-2274.

17. Hsiao CJ, Jha AK, King J, Patel V, Furukawa MF, Mostashari F. Office-based physicians are responding to incentives and assistance by adopting and using electronic health records. *Health Aff (Millwood).* 2013;32(8):1470-7.

18. Flareau BF, Yale K, Bohn JM, Konschak C. History and case for action. *Clinical integration: a roadmap to accountable care.* 2nd ed. Virginia Beach, Va.: Convurgent Publishing;2011:3-38.

19. Walker J, Pan E, Johnston D, Adler-Milstein J, Bates DW, Middleton B. The value of health care information exchange and interoperability. *Health Aff (Millwood).* Jan-Jun 2005;Suppl Web Exclusives:W5-10-W15-18. http://content.healthaffairs.org/content/early/2005/01/19/hlthaff.w5.10.long . Accessed July 21, 2013.

20. Adler-Milstein J, Bates DW, Jha AK. Operational health information exchanges show substantial growth, but long-term funding remains a concern. *Health Aff (Millwood).* 2013;32(8):1486-92.

21. Health 2.0. Health 2.0 Home Page. http://www.health2con.com/. Accessed July 21, 2013.

22. Health Record Banking Alliance. *A proposed national infrastructure for HIE using personally controlled records.* Arlington, Va.: Health Record Banking Alliance;2013.

23. Lapsia V, Lamb K, Yasnoff WA. Where should electronic records for patients be stored? *Int J Med Inform.* 2012;81(12):821-827.

24. Yasnoff WA. Health record banking: a practical approach to the national health information infrastructure;2006. http://williamyasnoff.com/?p=26. Accessed July 21, 2013.

25. Health Record Banking Alliance. *Principles and fact sheet.* Arlington, Va.: Health Record Banking Alliance;2008.

26. Szolovits P, Doyle J, Long WJ, Kohane I, Pauker SG. *Guardian angel: patient-centered health information systems.* Cambridge, Mass.: Massachusetts Institute of Technology Laboratory for Computer Science; 1994. http://groups.csail.mit.edu/medg/projects/ga/manifesto/GAtr.html. Accessed July 21, 2013.

27. Dodd B. An independent "health information bank" could solve health data security issues. *British J of Healthcare Computing and Info Management.* 1997;14(8):2.

28. Ramsaroop P, Ball MJ. The "bank of health". A model for more useful patient health records. *MD Comput.* 2000;17(4):45-48.

29. Haislmaier EF. Health care information technology: getting the policy right. June 16, 2006; http://www.heritage.org/Research/Reports/2006/06/Health-Care-Information-Technology-Getting-the-Policy-Right. Accessed July 21, 2013.

30. Ball MJ, Gold J. Banking on health: Personal records and information exchange. *J Healthc Inf Manag.* 2006;20(2):71-83.

31. Shabo A. A global socio-economic-medico-legal model for the sustainability of longitudinal electronic health records - part 2. *Methods Inf Med.* 2006;45(5):498-505.

32. Health Record Banking Alliance. Health Record Banking Alliance Home Page. 2006; http://www.healthbanking.org.

33. State of Washington Health Care Authority. *Washington State health information infrastructure: final report and roadmap for state action.* Olympia, Wash.: Washington State Health Care Authority;2006.

34. Dossia. Dossia Consortium. 2006; http://www.dossia.org. Accessed July 18, 2013.

35. Castro D. *Improving health care: why a dose of IT may be just what the doctor ordered.* Washington, D.C.: Information Technology and Innovation Foundation;2007.

36. Webwereld. Rotterdam start eigen versie elektronisch patiëntendossier. January 14, 2009; http://webwereld.nl/nieuws/54340/rotterdam-start-eigen-versie-elektronisch-pati--ntendossier.html. Accessed July 18, 2013.

37. Steinbrook R. Personally controlled online health data--the next big thing in medical care? *N Engl J Med.* Apr 17 2008;358(16):1653-1656.

38. Mandl KD, Kohane IS. Tectonic shifts in the health information economy. *N Engl J Med.* Apr 17 2008;358(16):1732-1737.

39. Kidd MR. Personal electronic health records: MySpace or HealthSpace? *BMJ.* 2008;336(7652):1029-1030.

40. Miller H, Yasnoff WA, Burde H. *Personal health records: the essential missing element in 21st century healthcare.* Chicago, Ill.: Health Information and Management Systems Society;2009.

41. Krist AH, Woolf SH. A vision for patient-centered health information systems. *JAMA.* 2011;305(3):300-301.

42. Australian Government, Department of Health and Ageing. PCEHR Governance. http://www.yourhealth.gov.au/internet/yourhealth/publishing.nsf/Content/pcehr-governance#.UewpklPEZOQ. Accessed July 21, 2013.

43. Estonia e-Health Foundation. Health information system. http://www.e-tervis.ee/index.php/en/health-information-system. Accessed July 21, 2013.

44. Brown A, Weihl B. An update on Google Health and Google Power Meter. *Google Official Blog.* Vol June 24, 2011:

http://googleblog.blogspot.com/2011/06/update-on-google-health-and-google.html; Accessed July 21, 2013.

45. Desroches CM, Charles D, Furukawa MF, et al. Adoption of electronic health records grows rapidly, but fewer than half of US hospitals had at least a basic system in 2012. *Health Aff (Millwood)*. 2013;32(8):1478-85.

46. Office of the National Coordinator for Health Information Technology. The Direct Project. http://wiki.directproject.org/. Accessed July 21, 2013.

47. Laudon K. Markets and privacy. *Communications of the ACM.* September 1996;39(9):92-104.

48. Yasnoff WA. Comments on advancing interoperability and health information exchange (CMS-0038 NC) (Docket ID CMS-2013-0044). See details about assisting existing HIEs in adopting the HRB approach. (pp. 9-10). April 22, 2013. In: Regulations.gov, ed: http://www.healthbanking.org/pdf/HRBA%20Response%20to%20CMS-ONC%20RFI%20FINAL. Accessed July 26, 2013.

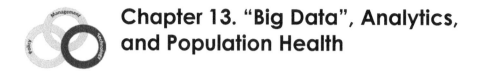

Chapter 13. "Big Data", Analytics, and Population Health

Bert B. Little, PhD

"Facts are stubborn, but statistics are more pliable."

Mark Twain (Samuel Langhorne Clemens, 1835–1910)
American author and humorist

Chapter 13 Learning Objectives

- What is "Big Data" and how is it used in healthcare analytics?
- How is a data warehouse different from a database?
- How is population research important to clinical medical research and vice versa?
- What is the major distinction between an Excel spreadsheet and "Big Data"?
- Name three moral hazards of population health and Big Data.

- Is the *Gattaca* scenario a possible outcome of Big Data in population health? Why or why not?

Introduction

The emergence of "Big Data" in the health industry follows its emergence in other data-intensive industries,[1-3] but lags behind developments in these other industries and areas (e.g., business intelligence, national intelligence services, financial fraud).[4-6] Big Data is a movement that has its own language[7] and is rapidly expanding.[8] The importance of this twenty-first-century technology innovation to the health industry lies in the fact that the health industry is arguably one of the most data-intensive industries in existence, in comparison to such other industries as defense and national security. It also combines sources of data in the convergent life-or-death nature of healthcare. The promise of Big Data is that it allows us to use extremely large data sets to better understand biological and physical processes and patterns. It will enable us to see the entire elephant rather than just the tail or trunk. It will enable us to see the jigsaw piece and where it fits in the whole jigsaw puzzle (a global perspective across time and space) rather than just the neighbors to the single piece (local, regional).[9,10]

What is Big Data?

"Big Data is the term for a collection of data sets so large and complex that it becomes difficult to process using on-hand database management tools or traditional data processing applications."[11]

Big Data is a popular term used to describe the exponential growth and availability of data, both structured and unstructured.[4] Vertical levels of data in healthcare organizations include: person → patient → clinical → patient management → organizational → enterprise level → and extra-organizational (collections of enterprise level data). Horizontal data (e.g., patient demographics, laboratory studies, radiology, surgery, pharmacy, and others) are the multi-industry segment (i.e., that which enables data from multiple health industry segments to be integrated and used across segments and organizational boundaries) wherein the Big Data concept emerges. Big Data differs from "Little Data" because the latter has a larger component of semistructured and unstructured data (e.g., medical dictation, drug/device recall data, etc.), presenting substantial challenges.[12-14]

The phenomenon of this twenty-first-century information tool and asset is simultaneously evolutionary and revolutionary. It comprises all traditional data plus new forms of data (e.g., real-time streaming device data, unstructured text, genetic data, global information systems, etc.) that were effectively incapable of being captured and used for other than highly specialized intended purposes. But the evolution and advancement of computing architectures has ushered in a new era of sense-making out of the complex landscape of previously disconnected information technology systems and data sources.

The insights derived from the Big Data environment related to research can be thought of through multiple categories: biological processes, disease processes, innovation of new devices and information technologies, drugs and therapies and their impacts, etc.[13,15] These new and emergent information technology tools and resources produce value throughout the healthcare system, and ultimately for the individual citizen, whose time as a patient we strive to minimize over the course of his or her life.

A major limiting factor in public health policy and research has traditionally been data, its accuracy, or the lack thereof.[16] Bollier stated, "In U.S. healthcare, arguably, we do not collect any Big Data at all."[17] From 2014 and beyond, the lack of Big Data will become less challenging as systems become more interconnected and analytic tools continue to advance. The clever and motivated public health researcher will exploit Big Data to conduct investigations that involve the universe of data on a topic rather than a sample—this potential will be increasingly ever important for population health-level research. But Bollier[17] is correct because health care and public health data sets are highly disparate in the United States. No single source exists to analyze American health care outcomes or disparities in health care.[16,18] Contemporary problems being addressed include the development of common standards for electronic health records (EHRs), as discussed in earlier chapters of this book. As EHRs progress to a more interoperable stage in their own evolution, they will facilitate stronger Big Data analytics for the healthcare industry and a more engaged patient population.[19] Indeed, population health stands today on the threshold of the era of Big Data.[20,21]

The use of data mining, data warehouses, and data analytics in evidence-based medicine is small compared to its potential. As we shall see later in this chapter, the use of Big Data with the spectrum of related tools and technologies in population health is very small today compared to its future potential. Clearly, this is the dawn of a new era for the use of huge data sets and advanced analytics, which include traditional statistics and epidemiological analysis to support the fields of population health, public health, and clinical medicine, as well as geospatially-rooted multidisciplinary and cross-domain analytics.[22,23]

Clinical quality metrics for population health fall into four broad categories: (1) human biology; (2) health behavior and risk factors; (3) the environment; and (4) healthcare organizations. The Big Data paradigm shift in population health research has as a goal to increase access to genetic data from DNA single-nucleotide polymorphism (SNP) to phenotype, and aggregated up by levels to global data. Information at this level supports the ideal vision for population health research—the inclusion of all relevant data sources. As the industry continues to advance, startling discoveries will be made during this transformational data-driven journey toward improving the health of entire segments of the nation's and world's population.

The purpose of this chapter is to explore the prospects for the growing application of Big Data and advanced analytics in health care. The importance of continued innovation in using Big Data resources to advance population health initiatives has been addressed and will also be emphasized in the final chapter. This chapter concludes by addressing the challenge of reducing complexity in dealing with Big Data analysis along with multisectoral policy (an integral aspect of a Health in All Policies or HiAP approach) to provide strategic governance over massive data sets.[24]

Most large healthcare systems have an EHR (or EMR) system, but they vary in quantity of data and digitized healthcare domains. For example, some EHR systems include data from laboratory tests, radiological findings, and pharmacy transactions. Others do not include these ancillary data sets, and the digitized record is a stand-alone, silo-like record that holds only identifiers, demographics, and diagnostic codes.[25,26] Other approaches push the data, but then the investigator(s) must build their own data warehouse. Universal health care in Canada and the Scandinavian countries has provided the opportunity for record linkage. Numerous important studies have been published using medical record databases from these countries.

> More data may lead to more accurate analyses. More accurate analyses may lead to more confident decision making. Better decisions can mean greater operational efficiencies, cost reductions, and reduced risk.[4]

Large-scale data analytics are in reality based on all preexisting statistical, probabilistic, modeling, and other forms of analyses.[13,14,27,28] Big Data or large-scale data analytics are primarily differentiated from smaller-scale analytics in their ability to operate in parallel computing, large and diverse data environments, and in the ability to handle such nontraditional data sets as freeform text, including computational linguistics, natural language, and text mining processing. Previously, such datasets were too labor-intensive to be useful.

An example of one such data mining and data warehousing project that implements innovative large-scale analytics is the U.S. Department of Agriculture's (USDA) Risk Management Agency's (RMA) crop insurance antifraud research program. The data warehouse contains roughly 19.2 million farm fields that are stored as geo-referenced polygons. The relevant information includes:

- field-level digital soil series;
- digital topographic maps;

- commodity price series;
- daily Moderate-resolution Imaging Spectroradiometer (MODIS) [both Aqua and Terra] satellite data over each field;
- Landsat satellite data bimonthly (each pass);
- daily temperature and precipitation data for each field during the growing season;
- all Doppler radar loops since 2001;
- sub-farm-level data on production;
- insurance liability; and
- indemnity records from 1991 to the present.

The objective of this Big Data system is to improve the integrity of the U.S. crop insurance program that covers American farmers' crops with more than $130 billion of liability.[29-32] The program will approach a petabyte (10^{15} bytes) of information storage by the close of 2014. Pragmatically, one must amalgamate Big Data with large-scale data analytics because neither produces leveraged value by itself. The value of data mining or what has evolved into a Big Data project, as outlined in the USDA example, has generated more than $3.5 billion in cost avoidance for the federal government since 2000, at a cost of approximately $50.6 million.

Slicing and Dicing

Data mining, data warehousing, Big Data, and other such marketing messages or branding efforts are more about the marketing of repackaged technology tools and capabilities than completely new technology. The vast majority of the analytical techniques used in these new technologies remain originally developed tools in statistics, artificial intelligence, and machine learning, as described in Table 13-1.

Table 13-1. Selected Terminology for Big Data

Category	Description
Advanced analytics	Multivariate statistics, machine learning, forecasting techniques, and other complex statistical and artificial intelligence techniques
Data	Values of quantitative or qualitative variables
Database	A collection of data values, usually in electronic form
VLDBs	Very long databases, most commonly 1 terabyte (10^{12} bytes) or larger, or a billion rows
Data warehouse (DW)	A database created from disparate sources that is standardized. Data warehousing usually receives data from outside sources as a data stream or batch update
Data mart (DM)	A selected subset of a data warehouse, or a small data warehouse
Data mining	Techniques of statistical and algorithmic analysis used on large databases, VLDBs, DWs, and DMs
EMR	Electronic medical record
EHR	Electronic health record
GPU	Graphic processing unit
Platform	Combination of (configuration of) operating system software and hardware that supports specific applications

The major difference is sample size, if it is a sample at all. In some instances, the universe of data is being analyzed.[27] Today, sample-based statistical tools used to analyze trillions (terabytes) of observations should be carefully considered because of the underlying assumption that samples are being analyzed; while in the era of Big Data, we are finding more opportunities to examine entire data sets instead of just samples. As analytic capabilities continue to grow for population health-level measures and surveillance, this difference will continue to be an issue of importance.

Data storage and retrieval technology is evolving rapidly; some of the historic trends are noted in Figure 13-1.

Figure 13-1. Brief History of Data Mining, Data Warehousing, and Big Data

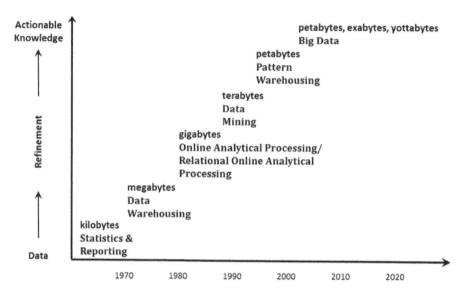

Computing speed, or horsepower, is no longer a significant limiting factor, because it is possible to turn teraflops (trillions of operations per second) in 2014 without a Cray supercomputer. The next generation of processors—the graphic processor units (GPUs)—has emerged. The popular press has characterized the GPU as "a supercomputer on a card" because its computing speed outstrips the conventional central processing unit (CPUs), as illustrated in Figure 13-2.

Figure 13-2. GPU versus CPU Speed Trends[*]

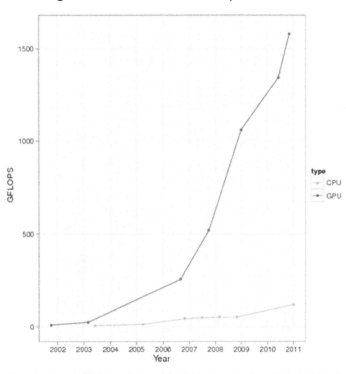

Laptops commonly have in excess of a terabyte of solid-state hard disk storage and graphic processing units (GPUs). These capacities are huge compared to prior eras, as illustrated in Figure 13-1, but today's technologies will be considered antiquated within just a few short years. An important alternative to maintain onsite data storage is cloud computing, which has become standard practice.[33,34] Huge data volumes and high acquisition rates (analog and digital data) mean that Big Data/analytics has evolved rapidly to keep pace with high-speed/high-volume data sources that require advanced processing techniques.

The following are two factual changes that occurred in the past 10–15 years (1999–2014) to allow the evolution of rapid analysis of huge amounts of data:

Horsepower: Contemporary GPU processors can perform trillions of operations per second (teraflops), compared to CPUs, which can perform millions (megabyte scale) or billions (gigabyte scale) of operations per second.

---

[*] Figure developed per R-bloggers News. Gillespie, C. *CPU and GPU trends over time.* Accessed April 26, 2014, at http://www.r-bloggers.com/cpu-and-gpu-trends-over-time.

Storage and retrieval technology: Petabyte (1,000 terabytes)-level storage and retrieval is currently being deployed in the high-end consumer sector, and within two years will be widely used, as illustrated in Table 13-2 below.

Table 13-2. Overview of Digital Storage Scales and Perspectives[*]

Scale	Numeric Definition	Heuristic Example
1 bit	Smallest unit of storage	8 bits make 1 byte
1 byte	One letter of the alphabet	Space for one letter of the alphabet
1 kilobyte	One thousand bytes	Space requirement for a short paragraph
1 megabyte	1 million bytes	Enough space to store a book, 500 pages of plain text
1 gigabyte	1 billion bytes	Storage required for 2012 copies of *War and Peace*
1 terabyte	1 trillion bytes	Digital storage for 2,767 copies of the *Encyclopedia Britannica*
1 petabyte	1 quadrillion bytes	Sufficient storage for approximately 2.8 million copies of the *Encyclopedia Britannica* • 2.5 petabytes: Human brain memory capacity • 98 petabytes: Indexed websites by Google (2013)
1 exabyte	1 quintillion bytes	4.22 exabytes: amount of digital data created in 2008
1 zettabyte	1 sextillion bytes	Digital storage capacity of the world
1 yottabyte	1 septillion bytes	No current example by which to measure this capacity

Because multi-terabyte disks cost less than $150, terabyte storage is becoming commonplace. Cloud computing has brought about a paradigm shift and allows analyses of Big Data without a huge investment in co-located computing infrastructure, because storage and computing can be leased from such entities as Amazon.[13,33] With the continuous decrease in storage cost and

[*]Grant E. The promise of big data. *Harvard School of Public Health, News Magazine.* 2012 Spring/Summer. http://www.hsph.harvard.edu/news/magazine/spr12-big-data-tb-health-costs/. Accessed June 11, 2014.

increase in storage device capacity, unprecedented volumes of data are being acquired and retained. This development requires the data/analytics to not only secure the data, but also to process very-large-volume data sets to provide insights and answers to questions that previously were not feasible to ask (e.g., early warning of national-scale epidemics).

These technological developments, coupled with the exponential increase in digital data and documents, will lead to computing opportunities unparalleled in history; and will support the continued development of population health-level tools and capabilities. Systems that allow the construction of an independent data warehouse are not Big Data. Merged, cleaned, comprehensive data integrated into a parallel processing architecture (e.g., Apache Hadoop, an open-source software framework for storage and large-scale processing of datasets on clusters of commodity hardware) are product characteristics consistent with Big Data.[11,35,36]

Big Data/analytics trajectories have been until now increasingly oriented to analysis of large and/or disparate data sets.[37-39] In 2013, however, there was evidence that some organizations are increasingly unwilling to share their data and instead are keeping it internal for analyses oriented to their own objectives in a competitive environment. While this phenomenon has a significant impact on our ability to analyze multiorganizational or multisource data, practically speaking it has little effect on the architecture of Big Data information technology and systems.[2,40] The analysis of large and disparate data sets requires a dominant technical solution under which a single organization or person may conduct this data analysis.[12,41-43]

The value of Big Data is not intrinsically the data, because its real power as a force multiplier is derived when the data are used in analytics to yield insight, knowledge support, and decision support for a full spectrum of decisions from research to clinical care to business decisions. The exponential increase in the value of data, especially in health care, is achieved when cooperation and sharing of data from multiple organizations enables the transorganizational objectives or individual organizational objectives to be achieved with greater insight and at lower cost—indeed, enabling insights to be developed that would otherwise be impossible to derive.

The Big Data movement is in its infancy for supporting population health and health care, which presents one of the greatest opportunities in the history of the human health sciences. Big Data and population health have an important connection with clinical medicine. At the patient level, Big Data may be used to conduct retrospective studies/trials, and the same data, rolled up to an aggregate level, may be used to analyze population health disparities and needs. Hence, clinical medicine and population health research need the same Big Data resources if inclusion is universal or nearly so. In the vernacular, *the difference lies in how the data are sliced, diced, and aggregated.*

Magnitude of the Big Data, Data Warehouses, and Data Mining in Healthcare

The data residing in data warehouses and different health information technology systems in U.S. healthcare organizations range in quantity and quality, literally from a full paper record to a comprehensive EHR. An interesting perspective on the level of data management, value, and use shows that 25 percent of effort is devoted to data management. Predictive analytics accounted for approximately 19 percent of effort in the healthcare industry, as shown in Figure 13-3, which aligns with efforts in data mining (DM) and data warehousing (DW) operations in general.[27]

Figure 13-3. Types of Data Handling Used by U.S. Healthcare Organizations[*]

US healthcare data apps from top innovators,[1] by data/analytic capability, 2010-12, 100 % =32

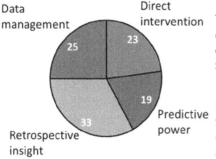

Data management — 25
Direct intervention — 23
Predictive power — 19
Retrospective insight — 33

The apps analyzed cut across all of the US healthcare system's **data-related value at stake**, estimated at **>$300 billion.**[2]

Many use proprietary data generated through such technologies as GPS-enabled devices and mobile apps that capture daily activity or patient-reported outcomes.

[1]Drawn from top 100 submissions to Health Data Initiative Forum, 2010-11, and health technology companies receiving $2 million or more in venture-capital funding, 2011-12; excludes ideas that did not involve big data.
[2]See *Big data: The next frontier for innovation, competition, and productivity*, McKinsey Global Institute (May 2001), on mckinsey.com.
Source: 2010-11 submissions to Health Data Initative Forum; Rock Health, Standard & Poor's Capital IQ; McKinsey analysis

---

[*] Source: Exhibit from "How big data is shaping US health care", May 2013, *McKinsey Quarterly*, www.mckinsey.com/insights/mckinsey quarterly . McKinsey & Company. Reprinted with permission.

Magnitude of the Use of Data Mining in Population Health and Evidence-based Medicine

Important opportunities exist in population health and medicine in the Big Data era. Most of the components of Big Data are already developed in healthcare information systems. The datasets must be processed for accuracy and consistency; joined at the patient level; and engineered to accept data stream updates to ensure that the most recent data are available for analysis. With the nation's goal of working toward universal health insurance coverage of a population, aggregation from the family, neighborhood, community, and broader-level data can provide a multidimensional view that supports population health and health disparity research needs, with substantial financial savings. Figure 13-4 provides a depiction of this concept from multiple dimensions.

Figure 13-4. Geospatial Dimensions of Big Data and Population Health

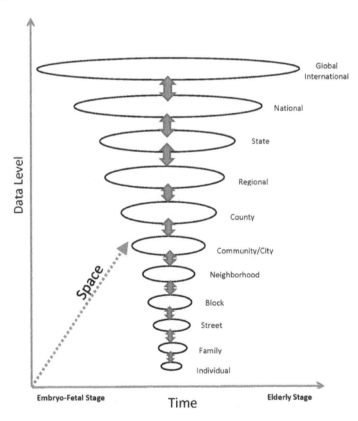

Data Mining and Advanced Analytics

Data mining includes the topical areas known as predictive analytics and advanced analytics. Some people include descriptive spreadsheet reporting (i.e., the old "green bar reports") as data mining, but it is not included here because it is not analytical and lies outside the scope of this chapter. Data mining analysis is largely a collection of techniques in statistics, epidemiology, and artificial intelligence that were established long before the phrase "data mining" was coined in the late 1980s. A graphic classification tree summary of data mining techniques identifies three broad categories: (1) discovery; (2) predictive modeling; and (3) forensic analysis, as illustrated in Figure 13-5.

Figure 13-5. Data Mining Overview[44]

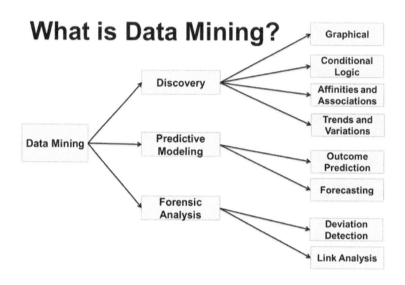

The four techniques to the right of the box labeled "Discovery" are exploratory methods that comprise primarily bivariate-type descriptive statistics, although more than two variables may be explored. The objective of the discovery is to examine univariate and bivariate relationships in the data using graphs, Boolean operators, inter- and intracorrelations, and trends across groups and time.

Predictive modeling is focused on outcome prediction and forecasts. Outcome prediction primarily uses such regression–based approaches as linear and nonlinear multiple regression techniques, and also includes neural networks, polynomial regression, logistic regression, discriminant analysis, and canonical correlation. Forecasting analysis uses the weights that result from regression models, which may be derived from regression-based modeling as above, to extrapolate forward in time. For population health-related modeling and surveillance activities, these analytic tools can be extremely valuable in both research and clinical practice. They can help researchers and practitioners understand the potential impact of new healthcare, economic, or social policy changes on the health of any given segment of the population.

The third category of data mining techniques is forensic analysis. Deviation detection and link analysis are more important than they seem at first glance. Identification and analysis of anomalies may prove more informative than normally behaved data points, simply because there are more differences. Even more information may be gained from linking anomalies and analyzing what the anomalies have in common. Sir Francis Galton (1822–1911), for whom Galton Laboratories in the United Kingdom are named, noted that information is derived from analysis of differences.

While Galton was addressing genetic data, he suggested that the statement, measurement, and analysis of differences (or variance) are the core of traditional statistics.[44] In population health and medicine, true outliers often provide clues in the hunt for associations with and causal links to disease. Linking anomalies to other data (which may or may not be anomalous) has led to discoveries in genetics, population health, clinical medicine, and financial fraud.

Big Data Architecture and Compromises

From the definition of Big Data in the introductory pages of this chapter, one can easily deduce that traditional databases and DW technology cannot adequately manage the vastness of the data in a Big Data scenario.

Which vertical work flow and horizontal distribution of tasking works with Big Data, and how is it different from the traditional DW? How does one attack the problem of processing huge data sets and delivering real-time service?

Examples of Advanced / Predictive Analytics

- Autoregressive Integrated Moving Average (ARIMA)
- Simultaneous Component Analysis (ANOVA)
- Canonical Correlation
- Cluster Analysis
- Discriminant Analysis
- Factor Analysis
- Forecasting
- Genetic Algorithms
- Logistic Regression
- Multivariate Analysis of Variance (MANOVA / MANCOVA)
- Multiple Regression
- Neural Networks
- Regression
- Time Series
- Survival Analysis

The answer: Chop it up and do it in pieces in parallel, then reassemble it for the complete solution.

When the speed of data load and analysis is dragged down by data throughput bottlenecks, the traditional system—a single fast processor with tandem task execution—may no longer meet a project's needs. The solution to the need for speed is moving to a higher order of computing: the parallel processing solution. The computing problem is "cut" into pieces (tasks or blocks) that can be solved or analyzed in parallel, as illustrated in the data architecture and business intelligence graphic in Figure 13-6.

Figure 13-6. Big Data Design vs. Traditional Architecture in Business Intelligence[45,*]

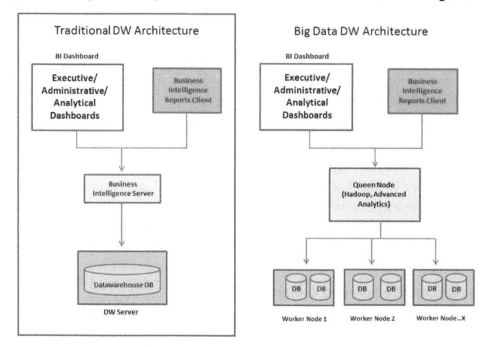

Graphic views like Figure 13-6 illustrate that task execution is not bound by the speed or throughput of a single processor; it is distributed across many (thousands of) processors. At the conclusion of the task, all the solutions can be reassembled into an integrated aggregate solution.

---

* Figure adapted from webpage reference number 45. Khambadkone K. Are you ready for Big Data? 2011. http://www.infogain.com/company/perspective-big-data.jsp. Accessed April 25, 2014.

> **Big Data Benchmarks**
>
> There are four key steps to executing the benchmark:
>
> *1. System setup*: Configure and install the system under test (SUT). This time is not included in the benchmark metric.
>
> *2. Data generation*: Generate the dataset that meets the benchmark specification. This time is not included in the benchmark metric.
>
> *3. Data load*: Load the data into the system. This time *is* included in the benchmark metric.
>
> *4. Execute application workload*: Run the specified big data workload consisting of a set of queries and transactions.

Some vendors market this idea as massive parallelization, which clariifies the mystery of Big Data processing. Flavors of this approach include MapReduce and Hadoop.[11,35] In the Big Data race, the goal is to process more data faster than any prior benchmarked system. An examination of Big Data evaluation criteria may help in understanding what Big Data technology is and the problems it solves. Speed and memory are the endpoints of greatest interest because these are rate-limiting pieces in finding the solution as quickly as possible: (1) load data; and (2) run the job. Data load and run time in turn depend upon input/output (I/O) speed constraints (memory storage) and processing speed (horsepower as measured in executed processor instructions per second). Terabit data transfer and teraflop (trillions of operations per second) are the current technology horizons for which we look to the future. When achieved, petabyte scale will be the next horizon, and so on as noted in Table 13-1. Moore's Law (the doubling of processing power every two years) predicts that technology's rapid-paced increase will make possible in the near future computing problems that were out of reach in recent times.

Some authorities have asserted that Big Data will (1) no longer be able to evaluate causality; and (2) accept quantity over quality, allowing for a certain level of noise just to have a large amount of data.[40] Both premises suggested by Mayer-Schoenberg and Cukier[40] are not acceptable in health care (population health and clinical medicine) because lives and the health of the living are at stake.

Causality and Quantity over Quality: Unacceptable

More data does not necessarily translate to loss of the ability to make causal inferences. For example, the use of VLDBs in medicine has not harmed the ability to examine causality. In the analysis of hundreds of thousands of patients to evaluate a possible causal relationship of dual therapy with clopidogrel (Plavix®) and proton pump inhibitors (PPIs) with myocardial infarctions (MIs) and sudden cardiac death, propensity score analysis in large databases (universe of data) revealed that the hypothesized causal pharmacogenetic relationship was not the apparent cause of MI and sudden cardiac death.[44] Rather it was patient compliance: those patients who were not compliant (i.e., failed to use clopidogrel daily as directed) had the highest risk of untoward outcomes. Such evaluations as this that leverage Big Data assets can be of high value to population health researchers and those professionals in the field of practice.

Some authors suggest that to use Big Data means we must compromise quality for quantity and "accept messiness."[40] In population health research and medical science, it may be categorically stated that the quantity of data cannot offset compromised or low-quality data. It is unimaginable that professionals, consumers, or patients in either of these fields would accept inferior-quality data simply to have more data. No practitioner would trust Big Data results if this tradeoff were the case. It is an absolute necessity to reject the "quantity over quality" paradigm.

Faulty, erroneous, or poor-quality data should not be allowed to drive decisions in population health and medical science. These fields have a mission that affects human health and well-being, quality of life, and ultimately mortality.

Population Health Indicators and Health Data Levels

In the ideal Big Data scenario, prevalence and incidence rates for any public health-reportable entity could be determined from the patient/individual level data because we have the entire numerator and denominator. Any health disparity hypothesis could be investigated; and in this ideal world, even genetic predispositions could be directly evaluated because the data would be available down to the SNP level, as illustrated in Figure 13-7.

Figure 13-7. Human Biology Dimensions in Big Data and Population Health

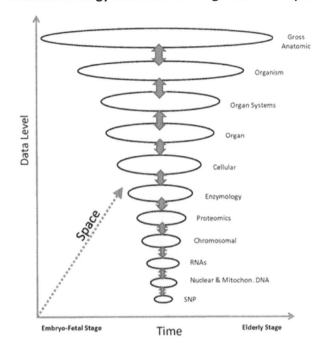

GIS and Environmental Exposures

Geographic information systems (GIS) is a huge field that has great potential for use in population health research and services. Combined with geolocated public health indicators or individual case occurrences, GIS at different levels, as illustrated in Figure 13-4, can aid population health researchers in the discovery of associations (e.g., among data sets and their sources) that may lead to an understanding of relations or causality. One may analyze many population health parameters across space, as shown in Figure 13-4, and time, as shown in Figure 13-7. A very interesting, simple map of the occurrence of coronary artery disease across the continental United States (as illustrated in Figure 13-8) opens an avenue for research.

Figure 13-8. Geographic distribution of mortality due to heart disease, 2000–2004[*]

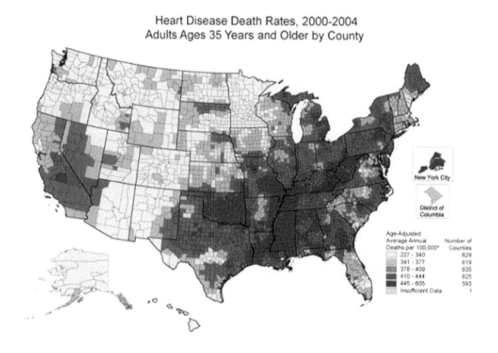

Heart Disease Death Rates, 2000-2004
Adults Ages 35 Years and Older by County

This map illustrates the full spectrum of death rates from heart disease by county across the country. Spatial regression analyses such as this one of such different predictive values as cholesterol levels, genetics, ancestry, or even lifestyles can be very informative and provide insights into this historical trend based on geographic area. For example, note the counties in southeast North Carolina (NC) that are the darkest shade of gray; the National Institute of Health (NIH) has a remote site located in Robeson County to study these associations in heart disease and other disorders.

A simple example of how one might use the Big Data geospatial system to support population health surveillance activities is to track environmental exposures over time for people from such high-risk areas as those who live in areas with lead smelters, other toxic waste sites, or near water pollution caused by certain industrial activities. Using such a system would also aid in detection

---

[*] Source: Centers for Disease Control and Prevention (CDC). Heart disease death rates for total U.S. population. Accessed March 5, 2014, http://www.cdc.gov/dhdsp/maps/national_maps/hd_all.htm

and analysis of disease clusters that may depend on some commonality (intersection) that exists between persons which occurred decades prior. For example, the mean latency for mesothelioma after asbestos exposure is 38–39 years. If Big Data had existed when the asbestos problem started to emerge, preventive research would be far more advanced than it is today.

Regulatory, Ethical, and Genetics Issues

Privacy issues and a host of "use" controversies need to be dealt with properly and as early as possible. Big Data governance is paramount in health care.[47, 48] The misuse of EHR/EMR data could have grave consequences, whether in isolated cases, or as part of an engineered system. An example of misuse of information recently exposed is the use of prescription data by non-healthcare-related insurance companies to set ratings, adjust claims, and deny payments. While many patients may have consented under the Health Insurance Portability and Accountability Act of 1996 (HIPAA) to the release of limited information to allow payment of their medical bills, they did not consent to release the information on an industry-wide basis. Ethical considerations are a higher standard than regulations and are based upon what would be the "right" thing to do.[49] As Big Data resources and governance continue to evolve in the twenty-first century, managing the complexity of privacy and ethics issues will only grow in importance.

Human health and well-being can be improved as Big Data assets for population health services and research continue to grow in adoption and implementation. As Big Data becomes global, the ability to improve the human condition will improve exponentially. Complete data on the human genome (e.g., the intersection of Figures 13-4 and 13-7) will facilitate incredible discoveries, but there are serious vulnerabilities with regard to privacy and improper use.

Historically, adults and children have been rated unfavorably by insurance companies in the United States on the basis of their predispositions to disease, despite the fact that genetic enhancement is not yet available. Consider the Cancer and AIDS Registries;[46] and most recently, the misuse of prescription information by the insurance industry. Effective in 2014, however, insurance companies will no longer be able to discriminate against or deny coverage to any individuals based on any preexisting condition. The U.S. Genetic Information Nondiscrimination Act of 2008 was signed into law, but much more needs to be done and has been put in place on this issue through the Affordable Care Act. As the system continues to be refined, there is still a need to designate an authority to which formal complaints or violations can be reported if discrimination is ever found based upon genotype.[47] Currently, there is no cognizant authority through whom to file a complaint. A major priority for Big Data initiatives in population health research and services and medicine is to provide evidence-based governance that protects human civil liberties.

Core Data Issues for Population Health

A key feature of Big Data and data warehousing is data interoperability. One approach is to physically change the data, and the other extreme is to virtualize any changes to the data, which remain in their native format.[14,48] Nonetheless, enterprise-wide access, integration, and use are the end goal of interoperability.

Regardless of the exact approach used to ensure data interoperability, the data that are ultimately made available for analysis must be standardized (e.g., inches or centimeters, consistent representation). In the same vein, data harmonization makes it possible "to combine data from heterogeneous sources into integrated, consistent, and unambiguous information products in a way that is seamless to the end-user."[49]

Populating the metadata (data about data) in a database system is important for managing Big Data or data warehouse building because this process assures proper matches for volumes of data that would be impractical for humans to examine. Inefficient IT management, however, has led to huge enterprise-level data warehouses without metadata or with unusable metadata. As the Big Data movement advances, more resources will be assigned to retroactively correct such omissions.

Accessing and Using Healthcare Data for Research

A critical path concern for the use of Big Data in health care research is the data flow and what the end-user actually sees and analyzes. Although analysts and analytical types usually have some rudimentary data manipulation skills, they generally need more than minimal assistance in developing the data mart they will use for analysis. Usually a database programmer will be assigned in the data warehouse operation to assist by routinely maintaining an interface for the analysts' use.

Access to health care data entails more than accessing a large database, because it is a collection of more than 100 individual datasets that are joined. Transformation to a form suitable for research is a nontrivial matter. Consider, for example, drug use following a surgical procedure. Many studies report a single point in time as a "yes" or "no" response, usually at discharge, for drug use. The drug use variable (including drug type) must be modeled as a longitudinal time-dependent observation. This is a single example of a much larger problem in health care research, because very few studies have reported prescription drug use as a time-dependent variable.

For researchers to achieve the potential of Big Data, complex transformations from transactional database structures to research database structures like the example above need to be done and integrated into the data warehouse and ready for use in the final served-up product. At this point, IT function hands off the task to an analyst function, usually two different people in separate shops.

Those who analyze health care data must have subject matter expertise because exploratory analyses being conducted with increasing frequency in the Big Data environment require knowledge of the area. The analyst in health care needs knowledge, skills, and abilities different from those of a traditional IT business analyst. Ideally a person educated in a biomedical science is needed, one who also has experience in databases and multivariate statistical analysis to support Big Data-oriented population health research.

WHAT BIG DATA SHOULD BE

Collecting Exposure Assessments in Free-living Populations

Environmental exposures (environmental health) are one of the most interesting and immediate uses of GIS in population health and its potential as the Big Data systems mature and become more comprehensive, ingesting more and more data, increasing numbers of people, and the variables on which data are available. Ultimately, it will be possible to follow a person's medical history longitudinally as it is captured in an EHR/EMR. Coupled with SNP data, the potential for research is beyond our ability to comprehend today. The research paradigm could become a matter of choosing the disease or health disparity and following the signal in the data using the advanced/predictive analytics techniques. If Figures 13-4 and 13-7 were fully realized, it would be possible to determine what caused which disease, and devise an intervention that might be a genetic and environmental "protectant," such that any detrimental protein could be controlled through genetic engineering; environmental toxins could be eliminated rapidly; and their untoward effects minimized through enhanced clearance (excretion and/or metabolism). This determination can also identify and quantify the costs and benefits of attacking the specific toxin or other environmental threat.

Changing the Culture of Population Science Research

"In U.S. healthcare, arguably, we don't collect any Big Data at all."[17]

In a review of PubMed conducted on October 20, 2013, I found 5,478 articles with keywords listed as *data mining* and *medicine*. There were only 147 articles that listed *data mining* and *population health* or *public health*, with the first one having been published in 1998 (see Figure 13-9).

Figure 13-9. Number of Publications in PubMed that included *Data Mining* and *Medicine*

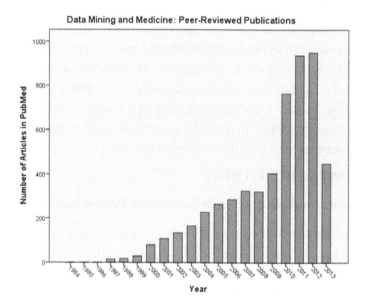

Of 55,128 articles published on *evidence-based medicine* (Figure 13-10), 56 were cross-indexed with the keyword phrase *data mining*.

Figure 13-10. Number of Publications in PubMed with the Phrase *Evidence-based Medicine*

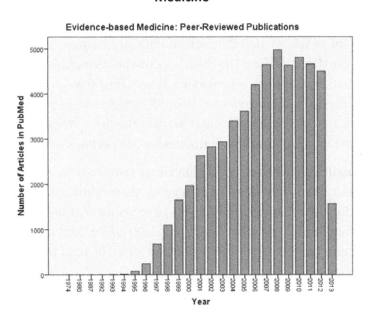

These numbers will change radically as such Big Data resources as data warehouses are integrated into the culture of public health and medicine. As this approach to population health is more widely accepted and employed, a shift may occur in education. A master's in public health degree (MPH) that has an area of concentration in Big Data analytics, either as the terminal degree or as part of a doctoral (MD and/or PhD) program, is appropriate training for future population health researchers. Mainstream media reports suggest that data mining is one of the most promising career paths in the near term.

The Gattaca Scenario and Other Conspiracies: Possible Outcomes

Gattaca Scenario

[A] film [about] a future society driven by liberal eugenics where potential children are selected through preimplantation genetic diagnosis to ensure they possess the best hereditary traits of their parents. A genetic registry database uses biometrics to instantly identify and classify those so created as "valids" while those conceived by traditional means are derisively known as "invalids." While genetic discrimination is forbidden by law, in practice it is easy to profile a person's genotype resulting in the valids qualifying for professional employment while the in-valids—considered more susceptible to disease, educational dysfunction and shorter lifespans—are relegated to menial jobs.

Wikipedia, 2013

In some circles that discuss emergence of the police state or some other authoritarian / totalitarian rule, Big Data is at the core of the conspiracy. The Snowden/National Security Agency affair has revealed the vast scope in volume and breadth of reach of Big Data. How data are acquired and used by the government can directly affect the health, health behaviors, and choices made by consumers, patients, and care providers alike. Conspiracies range from a new era of eugenics based upon universal DNA SNP studies to targeting the 'invalids' whose organs are ripe for harvesting to sustain the life of a 'valid.' Is this the plot for a sequel to Coma, another Robin Cook novel, or perhaps a future society?

These possibilities will garner a chuckle or two from some readers because it does sound rather Orwellian. But ignoring these vulnerabilities may be the opportunity for the emergence of flawed governance.[50] It is important that we remain vigilant and keep the good ship *Big Data* and population health initiatives pointed in the correct direction and guard against their misuse.

The potential misuse of Big Data in health care is a clear and present danger today because it could be used to deny coverage or payments based upon genetic or other information, resulting in federal legislation prohibiting genetic discrimination in health care or employment.[47] All the features that make Big Data such an enormous research resource also represent vulnerabilities to be exploited by those who would use the information for excessive profit, harm, and fraud.[29,30]

Conclusion

One view on Big Data was shared by Harper Reed, chief technology officer for the Obama reelection campaign in 2012.[29,30] Mr. Reed expressed cynical views that what we are calling Big Data is a level of technology that is often not necessary due to the increased power we have achieved in desktop and mobile platforms.

In this chapter we have reviewed the topic of Big Data from a non-technogeek stance and avoided the sales pitch aspect of this technology. The good and the potentially bad and perhaps the ugly aspects are given a balanced consideration because if there is a single certainty, it is that these technological advances will inevitably proceed. For individual health, health care, and the public health industry stakeholders it is up to all of us to try to keep on point with the spirit of the benevolent Big Data era. The power of the tools, technologies, and analytics will continue to bring deeper insights that continue to help identify new ways to improve the health of each population segment. As the United States continues with the expansion and adoption of EHRs/EMRs and the current implementation of ICD-10 or the potential of jumping ahead to the implementation of ICD-11 (or SNOMED CT), the richness of available data will only continue to grow.

Big Data must be properly governed and regulated; otherwise it could evolve into another totalitarian-like state, but with much greater power.[24] The health and wellness of our nation is the greatest asset we have; and the wise use of Big Data resources in the twenty-first century should be for the good and sanctity of preserving and enhancing that which we cherish the most—the health of all segments of the population in the United States.

CHAPTER 13 DISCUSSION QUESTIONS

Discussion questions are provided for team building or class exercises. Answers for all questions are provided in Appendix C.

Question Number	Question
1	The explosion of data use has come to be known as "Big Data." What differentiates Big Data from traditional data analysis?
2	Which digital storage capacity could store all data available in 2013?
3	Name the three major categories of data mining and describe each in a phrase.
4	How does one attack a problem in Big Data that is too massive for CPU-based computing?
5	Are there possibilities for data mining and Big Data in medicine and population health, or have all problems been solved? Elaborate and discuss why. What areas need further research with data mining/Big Data?
6	What is the relationship between patient clinical health information and information used in population health studies?

CHAPTER 13 SUMMARY

- Health care data must be analyzed to become information. These data are vital to population health.

- Health information infrastructure that provides comprehensive electronic patient information for both individuals and populations anywhere, anytime, will be analyzed by Big Data in the future.

- Big Data governance must address privacy, incomplete information, financial sustainability, standards, and architecture.

- Big Data governance policies are needed to assume integrity in data warehousing and analyses.

- The *Gattaca* scenario is science fiction, but is a threat with the emergence of Big Data.

CHAPTER 13 REFERENCES

1. Needham J. *Disruptive possibilities: how big data changes everything.* Sebastopol, Calif.: O'Reilly Media;2013.

2. Kolb J, Kolb J. *The big data revolution.* CreateSpace;2013.

3. Burgess J. *Big data—unabridged guide.* Ruislip, England: Tebbo Publishing;2012.

4. Simon P. *Too big to ignore: the business case for big data.* 1st ed. Hoboken, N.J.: Wiley;2013.

5. Fung K. *Numbersense: How to use big data to your advantage.* 1st ed. Columbus, Ohio: McGraw-Hill; 2013.

6. Provost F, Fawcett T. Data science and its relationship to big data and data driven decision making. *Big Data Journal.* 2013;1(1):51-59.

7. Warden P. *Big data glossary.* Sebastopol, Calif.: O'Reilly Media;2011.

8. Lynch C. How do your data grow? *Nature.* 2008(455):28-29.

9. Ratner B. *Statistical and machine-learning data mining: techniques for better predictive modeling and analysis of big data.* 2nd ed. Boca Raton, Fla.: CRC Press;2011.

10. Smolan R. *The human face of big data.* 1st ed. New York, N.Y.: Against All Odds Productions;2012.

11. White T. *Hadoop: the definitive guide.* Sebastopol, Calif.: O'Reilly Media, Inc.;2012.

12. Schadt EE, Linderman MD, Sorenson J, Lee L, Nolan GP. Computational solutions to large scale data management and analysis. *Nature Rev.* 2010;11:647-657.

13. Little BB, Weideman R, Kelly K, Cryer B. Evidence-based medicine: data mining and pharmacoepidemiology. In: Zanasi A, Temis SA, Brebbia CA, Ebecken NFF, eds. *Data mining VII: data, text and web mining and their business applications.* Billerica, Mass.: WIT Press;2006:307-314.

14. Berman JJ. *Principles of big data: preparing, sharing, and analyzing complex information.* 1st ed. Burlington, Mass.: Morgan Kaufmann;2013.

15. Wu S, Green A. *Projection of chronic illness prevalence and cost inflation.* Washington, D.C.: RAND Health;2000.

16. Lopez AD, Mathers CD, Ezzati M, Jamison DT, Murray CJ. Global and regional burden of disease and risk factors, 2001: systematic analysis of population health data. *Lancet.* 2006;367(9524):1747-1757.

17. Bollier D. *The promise and peril of big data.* Washington, D.C.: The Aspen Institute;2010.

18. Murray CJ, Salomon JA, Mathers C. A critical examination of summary measures of population health. *Bull World Health Organ.* 2000;78(8):981-994.

19. Trifirò G, Pariente A, Coloma PM, et al. Data mining on electronic health record databases for signal detection in pharmacovigilance: which events to monitor? *Pharmacoepidemiol Drug Saf.* 2009;18(12):1176-1184.

20. Koh HC, Tan G. Data mining applications in healthcare. *JHIM.* 2011;19(2):65.

21. Nardon FB, Moura LA. Knowledge sharing and information integration in healthcare using ontologies and deductive databases. *Medinfo.* 2004;11(Pt 1):62-66.

22. Bellazzi R, Zupan B. Predictive data mining in clinical medicine: current issues and guidelines. *Int J Med Inform.* 2008;77(2):81-97.

23. Swan M. Health 2050: the realization of personalized medicine through crowdsourcing, the quantified self, and the participatory biocitizen. *J Pers Med.* 2012;2(3):93-118.

24. Soares S. *Big data governance: an emerging imperative.* 1st ed. Boise, Idaho: MC Press; 2013.

25. McAullay D, Williams G, Chen J, et al. A delivery framework for health data mining and analytics. Paper presented at theproceedings of the twenty-eighth Australasian conference on computer science, Newcastle, New South Wales, Australia, January/February 2005, Volume 382005. http://users.cecs.anu.edu.au/~hdjin/publications/2005/CRPITV38McAullay.iHealthExplorer.pdf. Accessed March 7, 2014.

26. Mullins IM, Siadaty MS, Lyman J, et al. Data mining and clinical data repositories: Insights from a 667,000 patient data set. *Comput Biol Med.* 2006;36(12):1351-1377.

27. Little BB, Shucking ML. Data mining, statistical data analysis, or advanced analytics: Methodology, implementation, and applied techniques. In: Fielding NG, Lee RM, Blank G, eds. *The SAGE handbook of internet and online research methods.* London, England: Sage Publishers;2008:417-449.

28. Little BB. Data mining and research: applied mathematics reborn. In: Hesse-Biber SN, ed. *The handbook of emergent technologies in social research.* New York, N.Y.: Oxford University Press;2011:394-411.

29. Marc P. 'Big data' is bunk, Obama campaign's tech guru tells university leaders. *Chronicle of Higher Education.* October 30, 2013. http://chronicle.com/blogs/wiredcampus/big-data-is-bunk-obama-campaigns-tech-guru-tells-university-leaders/47885. Accessed March 7, 2014.

30. LaLonde H. A new perspective on the health conundrum: a working document. Ottawa, Canada: Government of Canada;1974.

31. Little BB. Testimony on data mining to the United States Senate: TO REVIEW THE AGRICULTURAL RISK PROTECTION ACT OF 2000 AND RELATED CROP INSURANCE ISSUES. COMMITTEE ON AGRICULTURE, NUTRITION, AND FORESTRY. 2005.

32.	Little BB. Review of efforts to eliminate waste, fraud, and abuse in the crop insurance program. Testimony on data mining to the United States House of Representatives. *HOUSE COMMITTEE ON AGRICULTURE.* 2006:23-25.

33.	Jalali A, Olabode OA, Bell CM. Leveraging cloud computing to address public health disparities: an analysis of the SPHPS. *Online J Public Health Inform.* 2012;4(3).

34.	Nielsen L. *The little book of cloud computing, 2013 edition: including coverage of big data tools.* Wickford, R.I.: New Street Communications, LLC;2013.

35.	Holmes A. *Hadoop in practice.* Greenwich, Conn.: Manning Publications Co.;2012.

36.	Nielsen L. *The engine that drives big data* (New Street Executive Summaries). Wickford, R.I.: New Street Communications, LLC;2013.

37.	Baru C, Bhandarkar M, Nambiar R, Poess M, Rabl T. Benchmarking big data systems and the bigdata top100 list. *Big Data.* 2013;1(1):60-64.

38.	Lohr S. The age of big data. *New York Times*, February 11, 2012. http://www.nytimes.com/2012/02/12/sunday-review/big-datas-impact-in-the-world.html/. Accessed March 7, 2014.

39.	Hurwitz J, Nugent A, Halper F, Kaufman M. *Big data for dummies.* Hoboken, N.J.: john Wiley and Sons [For Dummies];2013.

40.	Mayer-Schönberger V, Cukier K. *Big data: A revolution that will transform how we live, work, and think.* Boston, Mass.: Houghton Mifflin Harcourt;2013.

41.	Cohen J, Dolan B, Dunlap M, Hellerstein JM, Welton C. MAD skills: new analysis practices for big data. *Proceedings of the VLDB Endowment.* 2009;2(2):1481-1492.

42.	Liebowitz J. *Big data and business analytics.* Boca Raton, Fla.: CRC Press;2013.

43.	Minelli M, Chambers M, Dhiraj A. *Big data, big analytics: emerging business intelligence and analytic trends for today's businesses.* Hoboken, N.J.: John Wiley and Sons;2012.

44.	Banerjee S, Weideman RA, Weideman MW, et al. Effect of concomitant use of clopidogrel and proton pump inhibitors after percutaneous coronary intervention. *Am J Cardiol.* Mar 15 2011;107(6):871-878.

45.	Khambadkone K. Are you ready for big data? 2011; http://www.infogain.com/company/perspective-big-data.jsp. Accessed April 25, 2014.

46.	National Human Genome Research Institute (NHGRI). Genetic discrimination in health insurance or employment. 2012; http://www.genome.gov/11510227. Accessed January 31, 2014.

47.	Davis K. *Ethics of big data.* Sebastopol, Calif.: O'Reilly Media, Inc.;2012.

48.	Krishnan K. *Data warehousing in the age of big data.* Boston, Mass.: Newnes;2013.

49.   Two Crows Corporation. Introduction to data mining and knowledge discovery. 2005;Third: http://www.twocrows.com/intro-dm.pdf. Accessed January 31, 2014.

50.   Hammergren TC. *Data warehousing for dummies.* Hoboken, N.J.: John Wiley and Sons; 2009.

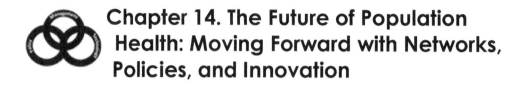

Chapter 14. The Future of Population Health: Moving Forward with Networks, Policies, and Innovation

Richard Wilson, DHSc, MPH

LaQuandra S. Nesbitt, MD, MPH

"Although the linear, isolatable, cause-effect model of scientific problem solving remains as the point of departure for the training of health professionals, practitioners find that the ecological perspectives insinuate themselves into their consciousness; like the photographer's wide-angle shot, they cannot ignore the immensely complex ecological system."[1]

Lawrence Green and Marshall Kreuter,
Health Program Planning: An Educational and Ecological Approach, *2005*

Chapter 14 Learning Objectives

- Recount highlights from previous chapters.

- Gain insights from case studies on technological innovation in the management of asthma; emergency department superutilization; a health and prevention promotion initiative; and a hospital readmission prevention program.

- Gain ideas about what can be done to help improve population health at the level of your community.

- Recognize the importance of innovation in management, policy and technology in improving population health.

The Future of a Healthier America

Throughout this book many authors have contributed their ideas, vision, and evidence on factors that have historically contributed to the current state of the health of our nation's population. While variation exists from one community to another, today we have more highly developed technology, better policy grounded in stronger evidence, and an ability to diffuse new ideas and agendas at an accelerated pace, thanks to advanced information and communication tools. More work is needed, however, to continue improving the health outcomes that we achieve and experience. As Morgan noted in his 1986 management classic *Images of Organizations*:

> As organizations assert their identities they can initiate major transformations in the social ecology to which they belong.[2]

The United States (U.S.) healthcare and public health infrastructure and the communities they serve continue to struggle through a period of major transformation. The cross-industry ecology of healthcare and public health is characterized by a paradigm shift that includes:

- Transition from a volume-driven system of care to a quality-driven system;

- Growth of new types of organizations for delivering care;

- New areas of focus to improve the health and wellness of each community;

- A new generation of healthcare and public health workers with improved tools and practices more grounded in stronger evidence and adaptability to meeting the changing needs of the clients and communities they serve.

Discussing his health care plan during his 2008 presidential campaign, President Barack Obama noted,

> Simply put, in the absence of a radical shift toward prevention and public health, we will not be successful in containing medical costs or improving the health of the American people.[3]

Today we are seeing the beginnings of this shift with new resources and initiatives for advancing improvements in the health of America. The resources, programs, and policy stemming from the 2010 Affordable Care Act (ACA) have been discussed throughout this book. All of these are contributing to this change in the landscape of health care and public health services in America, facilitating the outcomes we hope to achieve in caring for the country's population.

This concluding chapter recapitulates some highlights from the previous chapters of the book; discusses some case studies representative of the transition in American health care, and some concluding thoughts on the future of population health for practitioners, students, policy makers, and leaders in the fields of both health care and public health.

Recapitulation

This book is divided into three sections. The development of each section was overseen by one of the book's executive editors. A summary of the highlights of each section provides an introduction to the conclusion of this book.

Section I of this book discusses a number of key issues related to the management of our nation's health and the accompanying public health infrastructure. Chapter 1 provides an overview of the topic of population health; introduces the social determinants of health concepts; and stresses the importance of moving toward a Health in All Policies (HiAP) approach to integrating health, social, and economic policies, with a focus on overall effects on the health of the population or specific communities. Chapter 2 offers significant fresh insights into the topic of network leadership and the need to adopt this approach to leading our nation's healthcare and public health systems. Due to the growing interconnectivity among organizations as they have evolved to this point in the twenty-first century, and the complexity of public health problems in community contexts, cross-society collaboration will be more and more imperative. Chapter 3 discusses the importance of health impact assessments, a tool and philosophy initiated well over a decade ago in European countries that has been applied in the United States—as exemplified by its adoption as a strategic tool by the San Francisco Department of Public Health. It is gradually gaining wider adoption across the United States. Chapter 4 provides insights from demographic patterns on a global, national, and local level, and how they are likely to impact the public's health in the coming decades. Chapter 5 discusses in detail on a philosophical level the underpinnings of the core differences between the traditional medical care model and the population health model, along with a global perspective on a socio-cultural-ecological construct in the evolving dynamics of health care and public health organizations.

Section II opens with Chapter 6, which describes a model for increasing the impact of population health improvement initiatives and policy changes. These changes are producing new opportunities to promote prevention and wellness, along with highlighting the importance of the *Healthy People 2020* goals for achieving population health outcomes for the nation. Chapter 7 discusses the impact of chronic disease on the nation and the application of the Chronic Care Model. It also covers the organizational evolution in health care, with the emergence of accountable care organizations, patient-centered medical homes, clinically integrated networks, and new opportunities to continue the battle against chronic disease. Chapter 8 covers the important need for a renewed focus in this country on mental and behavioral health services, given the societal transformation we are all undergoing, along with new technology for use in treatment and policy issues that affect the delivery and provision of these types of services. Chapter 9 provides fresh insights into the field of care for the elderly across our nation with subject matter expertise drawn from leaders in the field of elder care.

Section III begins with Chapter 10, which takes us on a journey through the complex initiatives of health information exchanges with an elaborate case study. The authors use the case study to illustrate the inherent and emergent challenges in managing large-scale governance activities to drive regional and national initiatives that affect the health of a population. Chapter 11 provides a novel set of insights on health information terminology and terminology standards, concluding with a description of their relevance to population health initiatives. The author of Chapter 12 offers an alternative approach to health information exchanges through the use of health record banks as a different means of managing and using personal health data along with historical and prospective policy implications. Chapter 13 covers the emergent field of Big Data and population health analytics: a topic that will continue to grow in importance in the twenty-first century with the increasing integration of health and other data assets to manage the health of each community's population.

Influencing Future Direction

As the nation moves forward toward improved disease prevention, health promotion, and health delivery services,[*] what will help the nation adopt the changes that are proposed? In Malcolm Gladwell's book *The Tipping Point. How Little Things Can Make a Big Difference*, he notes,

> . . . there are relatively simple changes in the presentation and structuring of information that can make a big difference in how much of an impact it makes.[4]

---

[*] "Health delivery services" include both health care and public health services.

If we think about the changes we are trying to make in keeping America healthier, the ways and speed with which we can communicate new initiatives, protocols, evidence, and ideas have accelerated greatly just in the last decade. As we create new policies, initiate new interventions, and measure new outcomes, we acquire vital information that can be used to help influence positive healthy behavioral choices across all demographics, cultures, ethnicities, and ages. Making better health choices helps the entire nation. *Healthy People 2020* provides the nation with a set of goals to strive for over the remainder of this decade. Many will be reached and surpassed while others will continue to be addressed in future decades. The Institute of Medicine, in its first workshop on population health improvement in 2013, highlighted a number of examples from around the country of innovative programs that are demonstrating positive effects on their respective communities' population health.[5]

This final chapter presents five concluding case studies that relate to national issues affecting the health and wellness of entire population segments. Critical topics will include the chronic condition of asthma; emergency department super-utilizers; a novel health and prevention promotion initiative; and an innovative community-driven hospital readmission reduction program. The purpose of these case studies is not only to demonstrate a population health approach to specific problems, but also to stimulate the reader's critical thinking as to how program initiatives might be mounted in his or her own community. These case studies are followed by a section on strategic implications for health promotion and education in supporting improvement of population health in the twenty-first century; recommendations for future leaders; then a set of concluding thoughts on this first edition of *Population Health: Management, Policy, and Technology*. But first, let us consider the importance of data in driving health promotion initiatives that benefit entire segments of the population.

Data-Driven Population Health Promotion

Strategies and outcome priorities of population health promotion must be based on data. The question is "What data should be considered?" Traditional public health practice sets priorities by weighing death and disease and the number of people affected by individual health problems. This approach is typified by examining data for the leading causes of death, shown in the table below. The logic of this approach devotes programming and services to those problems that take the greatest toll in lives. Health problems that are less frequent killers as we move down the list of leading causes become defined as relatively trivial concerns unworthy of priority attention.

In fairness, this approach has brought about significant improvements in health status across the United States over the last 50 years. Data from a key report from the Centers for Disease Control and Prevention's National Center for Vital Statistics in 2013 published by Murphy, Xu, and colleagues provide insights into a number of key issues and historical trends that serve as foundational analytic datapoints.[6] Table 14-1 lists the 15 leading causes of death in 2010.

Table 14-1. 15 Leading Causes of Death in 2010[6]

Rank	Causes of Death (per ICD-10, 2004)	Deaths in 2010
1	Heart disease	597,689
2	Malignant neoplasms (cancer)	574,743
3	Chronic lower respiratory diseases	138,080
4	Cerebrovascular diseases	128,476
5	Unintentional injuries (accidents)	120,859
6	Alzheimer's disease	83,494
7	Diabetes mellitus	69,071
8	Nephritis, rephrotic syndrome, and nephrosis	50,476
9	Influenza and pneumonia	50,097
10	Self-harm (suicide)	38,364
11	Septicemia	34,812
12	Chronic liver disease and cirrhosis	31,903
13	Essential hypertension and hypertensive renal disease	26,634
14	Parkinson's disease	22,032
15	Pneumonitis due to solids and liquids	17,011
	All other causes	483,694

Rank	Causes of Death (per ICD-10, 2004)	Deaths in 2010
	Total deaths in 2010 from all causes	2,468,435

Figure 14-1. Percentages of Causes of Death in 2010[6]

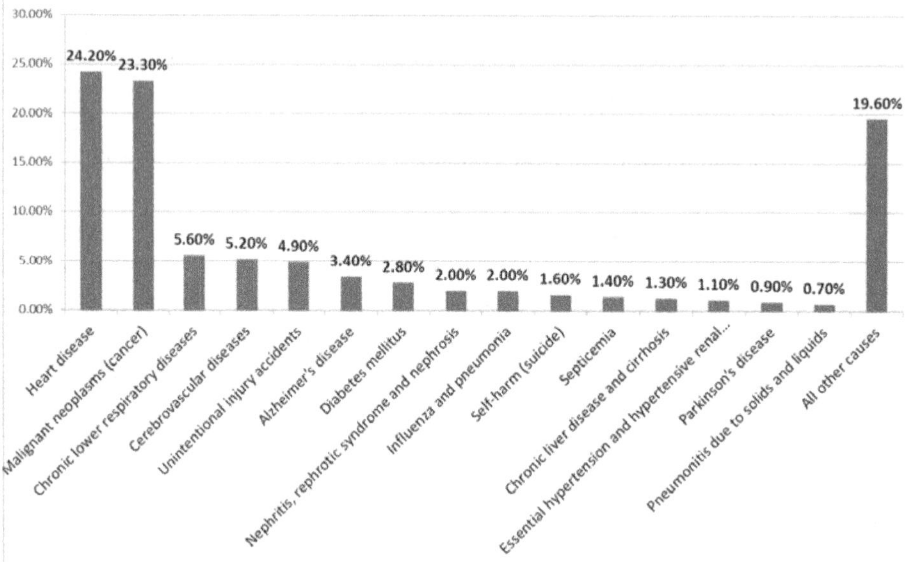

Figure 14-1 is a simple illustration of the impact of each categorical cause of death, especially those with the greatest impact on the nation and its people.

These data identify the most significant causes of death in the United States as of 2010. The CDC report also provided insights into the 50-year decline in death rates from cardiovascular disease, brought about by such direct approaches to disease prevention as population health education, early diagnosis, and improved treatment of heart disease. In addition, the federal anti-tobacco and smoking prevention campaigns of the last half century have helped bring about a steady decline in smoking across many segments of the population—a significant result of such health policy legislation as the 1965 Federal Cigarette Labelling and Advertising Act[7] and the 2009 Family Smoking Prevention and Tobacco Control Act.[8] Both of these acts increased consumer knowledge of the harmful effects of tobacco use and contributed to its declining rate of consumption over the years. While tobacco use is not coded as a cause of death by ICD-9, it was noted in 2012 as the cause of death of 440,000 Americans each year.[9]

These are worthy accomplishments; people are alive today who would not be except for the many disease-oriented prevention programs. While there has been progress in achieving *Healthy People* program objectives over the years, sometimes the outcomes are low-hanging fruit. Health status improvement has tended to occur in those segments of society not significantly affected by health inequities. The typical traditional health promotion effort tends to leave behind the disadvantaged and hard-to-reach.

This disconnect in values had the unintended effect of enhancing the subliminal mistrust that is common in low-income neighborhoods. The so-called experts from health care, academia, and the government came in to fix things, but they rarely consulted the neighborhood or made it an equal partner. Traditional public health practice can take credit for improving the health of individuals and communities, but there are some disadvantages to that way of doing business, as noted above.

The approach advocated here is that priorities are driven by quality of life consequences, not just morbidity and mortality. In most communities in the United States, heart disease and cancer are the leading causes of death, accounting for 47 percent of all mortality.[6] Loss of life by necessity also means loss of quality of life for the victims; however, a population health perspective looks at the community context and the long-term impact of such underlying problems as social determinant factors. Rather than stopping with mortality and morbidity data in setting priorities, it is at least as important for researchers to seek to understand the quality-of-life deficits in communities, and how those deficits interact with health problems. As illustrated in Figure 14-2 below, quality of life can influence and is influenced by health status.

Figure 14-2. Health Status in Relation to Quality of Life

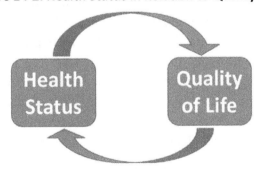

Quality of life is, however, a more "upstream" concern, and therefore should have a greater overall population effect. The data collection needed here is to inventory the nature and extent of quality-of-life deficits, and to determine which health problems contribute to them. Rather than seeking out morbidity and mortality, incidence and prevalence, or even behavioral risk data from the typical public health sources, we should be seeking data from such social research sources as the Census Bureau and the American Community Survey as well as direct input from community stakeholders. As the population health movement grows, it will be increasingly necessary to apply data systems to quality-of-life data in addition to the quantitative epidemiological data. At the present, epidemiological data are readily available with a few computer clicks; for example, from the CDC's National Center for Health Statistics, the Robert Wood Johnson Foundation County Health Rankings, or perhaps even electronic health record systems. In contrast, community quality-of-life data are not so easily accessible: they are scattered through different resources. Moreover, we lack such user-friendly technologies for qualitative data as what would be gathered from focus groups. Quality-of-life data are by definition qualitative, but that doesn't mean the collection and synthesis of these data cannot be more completely automated. Digital and mobile technology will undoubtedly emerge to make this automation possible.

In actuality, this approach to quality of life and focusing on community-driven intervention goes back at least as far as the 1970s, with the publication of the PRECEDE Model (later the PRECEDE-PROCEED Model) that was discussed by Steiner and Wainscott in Chapter 5.[10] Unfortunately, the PRECEDE model never found wide application outside academic circles. The model (especially in its later iterations) blazed a trail for the population health movement, but public health practitioners never welcomed the model—particularly the concept of starting with the community and its quality of life.

One other twist here is that in the population health approach, we not only seek information about a community's deficits, but also about its assets and strengths. This dual approach helps not only with prioritizing intervention targets, but also informs policy makers and federal/state/local health program managers about existing resources and opportunities that can contribute to community health improvement. In Green and Kreuter's 2005 book on health program planning, they discussed McKnight and Kretzmanm's concept of asset maps.[11,12] Asset maps typically include:

- community-based institutions and agencies;

- formal and informal community leadership;
- health care and mental health service providers;
- resources for healthy food and active lifestyles;
- major employers;
- education and training opportunities; and
- advantages afforded by the community's location or other unique features.

Asset mapping considers resources in both the public and private sectors, along with resources in both individual and organizational dimensions.[12] One of the key benefits of asset mapping in support of population health is its value to health program planning. Understanding the landscape of the political, socioeconomic, and built environment in terms of available (or absent) resources can better enable policy makers, researchers, and public health practitioners to create and implement targeted health programs that effectively meet the needs of a community's population.

Little in Chapter 13 addressed many issues regarding Big Data and the future of analytics that have and will help feed the need for data-driven population health initiatives. Our first case study highlights the importance of technological innovation and health education to support the needs of an underserved population in Louisville, Kentucky, dealing with the chronic condition of asthma.

Case Study: Advancing Community Health through Asthma Control

This first case study concerns an effort to decrease the morbidity and mortality of child and adolescent asthma in a section of Louisville, Kentucky, as a population-centric example. Before unpacking the details, we should take a brief backward glance at Chapter 5's discussion of the concept of positive health. Making a chronic health problem the starting point for program planning is inherently a negative approach. In other words, rather than starting with a health problem in order to "solve" population health challenges, one could instead focus on all the factors that would enhance and sustain good health. Historically, the public health enterprise has taken this negative approach to tracking population health measures. For example, it is clear that the *Healthy People 2020* project[13] is mostly about solving health problems directly rather than improving the environmental conditions in which wellness and health equity can improve.

We begin with two observations: 1) society does not yet fully support an exclusively positive health focus on the part of official public health agencies, though progress is being made; and 2) positive and negative approaches to population health promotion do not have to be mutually exclusive. There will always be a need for both. These two points are for the reader to consider throughout this first case and the balance of the chapter.

Background: The Louisville Community and Importance of Positive Health

Louisville, Kentucky, was founded in 1778 and named for King Louis XVI of France.[14] Since that time it has undergone tremendous growth, with a total consolidated population of over 740,000 as of 2010 and an associated demographic transformation, along with slow evolution of residential and occupational conditions, neighborhood development, maturity and decline, and even a change of leadership dynamics and governance.

Certain sections of the city are dramatically deficient in the structures of opportunity. The area most widely recognized as having this environmental and socioeconomic characteristic is called West Louisville. This part of the present city is in fact the birthplace of the community, the first location of residence and commerce when Louisville was in its formative years. Since that time, West Louisville has been left behind and is now characterized by a predominantly minority population; widespread poverty; substandard housing; lower levels of educational attainment; higher rates of unemployment accompanied by low-wage jobs; inordinate exposure to environmental contaminants in the air, water, soil, and the built environment; high rates of crime and violence; and a generalized milieu of hopelessness compared to the rest of Louisville.[15] Figure 14-3 illustrates the concentration of poverty in West Louisville.

Figure 14-3. Percent of Adults (18–64 years) in Louisville Living below Poverty

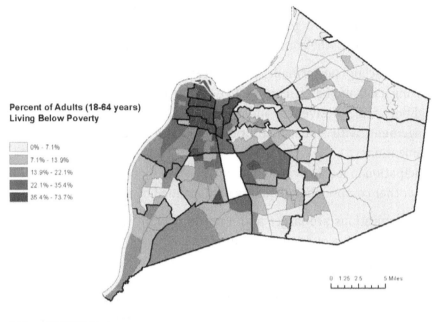

Percent of Adults (18-64 years)
Living Below Poverty

☐	0% - 7.1%
	7.1% - 13.9%
	13.9% - 22.1%
	22.1% - 35.4%
	35.4% - 73.7%

0 1.25 2.5   5 Miles

Data Source: 2007-2011 ACS Estimates

It is not surprising that on the basis of the characteristics shown in Figures 14-3, health status in West Louisville is not good. Some descriptive data are actually available by neighborhood, while other data are available by race and ethnicity only for the city as a whole. The largest minority group in Louisville is African American, making up about 23 percent of the population.[16] Some neighborhoods in West Louisville are greater than 90 percent African American. The evidence indicates that people in West Louisville live shorter lives, compared to residents in other parts of the city, and the gap may be more than 10 years by neighborhood.[17] The burden of chronic disease is proportionately greater and the mortality rate is almost three times higher in parts of West Louisville, compared to other Louisville neighborhoods. Infectious diseases (e.g., HIV) are more common and infant mortality is twice as high as in the city as a whole.

The traditional approach to working to improve the health status of individuals living in West Louisville is to selectively target each of the health problems, especially those most severe and most common, and try to slowly decrease the morbidity and mortality rates. For the most part, that is what the public health enterprise is organized to do, starting with the federal health agencies all the way down to local health departments. In contrast, the authors of this chapter started to think about it in a different way.

Health can be framed as an intermediate outcome, a means to an end. We don't protect and promote health for its own sake, but because health is a great enabler of a set of human goods that are grouped into the general category of quality of life. Some of the common components of quality of life include:

- improved school performance and educational attainment;
- securing a job and being a productive employee;
- neighborhood cohesiveness and pride;
- engagement with such institutions as faith-based groups and service organizations;
- participation in local government; and
- many other components of quality of life valued by society.

Those aspirations are larger and more important than health, even though health may be the sine qua non of quality living.

The Asthma Case Study

A search of the literature has determined that the overall schoolwide impact of asthma on school performance is minimal.[18] The strongest link with asthma is absenteeism. Such other effects as dropout rates or specific school performance are cited, but the evidence is not as strong.[19] The effect becomes more pronounced when children are disadvantaged in other ways[19] (such as by poverty, substandard housing, or tobacco smoke in the home); for children whose asthma causes frequent sleep disturbances;[20] and for children whose asthma is not well managed.[21,22]

Another important literature finding is in the conclusions stated in the Community Guide to Preventive Services regarding asthma.[23] This presentation of evidence-based practice recommends a focus on the home, including assessment of risks; changing the home environment to decrease exposure to asthma triggers; and education regarding environmental hazards and self-management of asthma. The Community Guide also mentions "social services and support," and "coordinated care." There is no specific mention of school-based interventions or services, though they may be implied under social services and coordinated care. This lack of specificity represents a gap in the public health practice evidence, which in turn brings us to the important topic of evidence as such.

Case Study: Solving the Asthma Challenge for Urban Youth

This case study describes a population health intervention designed by the University of Louisville School of Public Health and Information Sciences as a demonstration project in collaboration with the Louisville Metro Department of Public Health and Wellness.

Recently there has been circulated a widely recognized monograph on the topic of health factors, such as asthma, that affect success in school.[24]

Asthma was selected as a focus because:

1) asthma has a distinct causative impact on school performance, particularly among students from disadvantaged backgrounds—most of the children from West Louisville;

2) asthma prevalence is large (> 20 million people total in the United States, > 6 million children < 18 years old); and its incidence (rate of new cases) is growing;[25]

3) asthma's selection as a priority problem by *Healthy People 2020*, specifically to reduce the proportion of children with asthma missing school days;

4) asthma's association with low-income and minority populations;[25]

5) asthma's identification as a priority health problem by the Louisville Metro Department of Public Health and Wellness, because the prevalence of asthma is higher than the rates for Kentucky and the nation as a whole;[26] and

6) Kentucky has a much higher-than-average rate of smoking compared to other states; smoking is recognized as an irritant for children with asthma exposed to secondhand smoke in the home.[27]

Health Promotion and Education Plan

Based on the evidence for intervention with asthma reported in the Community Guide to Preventive Services (see Appendix D), a plan to screen children for asthma was the next step. Preliminary data collection at a middle school in Louisville indicated that there are many children with undiagnosed asthma. This underdiagnosis exists because some children do not receive routine and thorough medical care. It is unknown whether access to health care for these children will improve with the beginning of the ACA provisions because children were already covered by the Children's Health Insurance Program (CHIP). Children will be screened in the schools they attend. Because the consequences of asthma are substantially worse for children of low income and other family disadvantages, and because Louisville's school assignment (busing) plan means that children in each school may be from residences outside the neighborhood of the school, schools with the most disproportionate indicators of disadvantage (e.g., percent of students eligible for free or reduced-price

---

Case Study: Solving the Asthma Challenge for Urban Youth

lunches) will be selected.

Once children screening positive for asthma are identified, they will be defined as a treatment group; for evaluation purposes, a similar set of students with a negative screen will be designated a control group. Both groups will be asked to give permission for medical record monitoring and access to academic achievement data, specifically grade-point averages, standardized test scores, and attendance records. We are relying on personnel in the school system research office to provide deidentified data to track academic measures.

Going forward, children screening positive will be offered a home visit, at which time residences will be inspected for the presence of triggers and irritants. These might include excessive dust from poorly maintained heating and air conditioning systems; cigarette smoke from smokers in the home; the presence of dust mites and cockroaches, dogs or cats in the home; feather pillows; and floor carpeting that traps dust and irritants.

Future Challenges

- **Stigmatization**: Community listening indicated some parents do not want their children "labeled" with an asthma diagnosis because they believe that stigma sets them up for different treatment that is not in the best interests of the child. Parental meetings will be held to establish trust; explain the intent of the study; ameliorate any fears about participation; and set follow-up expectations.

- **Informed consent**: It will be necessary to obtain informed consent from the parents of all students who will be screened in the candidate schools because their children are minors.

- **Access to future medical and academic records:** Obtaining such access will require soliciting ideas for implementation and recruiting parents to serve on a project advisory committee.

- **Home abatement workforce needs:** The school system, health care providers, and managed care organizations do not have personnel trained and available to perform home abatement inspections. Therefore, as part of the demonstration project, the university will recruit, train, and supervise university students to do this work. The students' engagement in this intervention will also establish them as role models for the children with asthma, promoting their buy-in for disease management compliance. Community health workers or peer advisors in the public health workforce may be well suited to fill this role as well.

Case Study: Solving the Asthma Challenge for Urban Youth

The logistics of this demonstration project are quite challenging. In the future, population health promotion would be facilitated by improved linkages between health care providers and school data systems.

In Louisville disadvantaged children who have asthma are covered by the Kentucky Children's Health Insurance Program, which is managed by the Passport Health Plan (Passport), a local nonprofit community-based health plan administering Kentucky Medicaid benefits. By identifying which children need controller medications for their asthma, a significant cost savings can be realized by reducing the number of ER visits and hospitalizations for acute episodes of asthma. It will be necessary to determine how much savings can be realized by identifying those children with asthma managed by Passport who need controller medications, thereby realizing better control and reduction in such expensive health care utilization services as ER visits and hospitalization.

Public schools in Kentucky are paid for daily attendance by the Kentucky Department of Education. In Louisville, the school system receives about $25 per day for each child attending. Because asthma is a significant cause of absenteeism, it is responsible for lost revenue. The school system is therefore incentivized to invest in asthma abatement to boost state funding. It will be necessary to determine how much the school system can invest in abatement within the constraint of state daily attendance funding. Population health promotion initiatives pay attention to population impact, including cost/benefit analyses. This is an important aspect of population health promotion: when possible, policy makers should link usual medical costs with potential cost savings from prevention strategies.

The take-home message for population health promotion is that in a real community setting, collaboration and active engagement by multisectoral stakeholders is essential for project success.

Figure 14-4 highlights the desired outcomes of the demonstration project. The vision of the demonstration is to have a systematic impact on short and long-term aspects of population health.

Figure 14-4. Outcomes of the Asthma Project as Population Health[*]

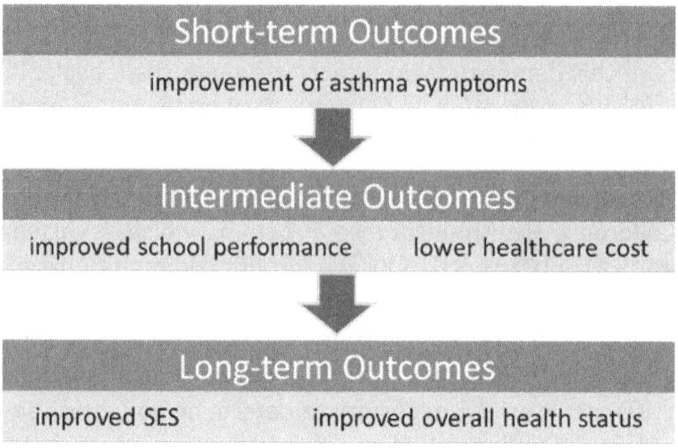

Air Quality and Technology Innovations for Asthma Patients

The Louisville Metro Government identified asthma as a serious concern for the city, and decided to take a data-driven approach to tackling the asthma problem. They created the Louisville Asthma Data Innovation Project, which sought to better understand what is behind the city's high rates of asthma. The project was selected to be part of the IBM Smarter Cities grant program. The IBM team gave Louisville specific recommendations regarding their data management and sharing. The recent Data Informed article stated,

> . . . one of the recommendations was to mine public schools for asthma information, work more closely with school districts, and share the information with constituents as a whole. None of this was data Louisville had used to inform public health research in the past.[28]

Sharing and analyzing data in new ways is increasing the depth of our understanding of public health challenges.[29]

The Louisville Asthma Data Initiative pilot project was implemented in June 2012 with an intervention including data collection and feedback to patients and care teams for 12 months, led by Propeller Health (formerly Asthmapolis). Propeller Health developed a system of sensors and apps that record when and where patients use their inhalers.[30] The data captured may then help physicians make more informed clinical interventions and help patients track and manage

---

[*] SES is an acronym for socioeconomic status (see Chapter 5).

their condition.[31] Health care providers historically have had inadequate tools to understand the severity of patients' asthma, chronic obstructive pulmonary disease (COPD), and other chronic respiratory disease, which limits the providers' ability to predict and prevent serious and costly uncontrolled episodes. Although the data are preliminary as of early 2014, promising improvements in asthma control occurred over the course of the study. There were reductions in health care service utilization, which will be evaluated with claims data in the future. Not unexpectedly, several asthma hotspots were found. They were influenced by proximity to air pollution, industry, and urbanization. This pilot study is an excellent example of technological innovation that addresses such population health problems as air quality and asthma across the community. In future expansions of the program, enrollment will focus on achieving a representative sample across Louisville, including children in West Louisville.

Evidence for Population Practice

For many years, traditional public health practice was somewhat routinized, meaning that workers did what they always did without much consideration of evaluation results or theory. There was not a lot of careful thought, especially at the action level, regarding why traditional public health practitioners took certain actions and what outcomes were achieved. Public health was considered one of the helping professions, and it certainly seemed like that's what we did.

The game has changed. Evaluation, evidence, and science-based practice are the new imperatives for public health, and this change is certainly resonating with the development of population health concepts. Going forward, practitioners, supervisors, funders, and external stakeholders are going to lean on sources of evidence to guide strategic program planning and implementation. Evaluation will be essential for those problems lacking a decisive set of evidence. Practice that is not evidence-based will be permitted one time, but with conscientious evaluation, that practice will be shown to be effective or it will be discarded. Knowing how slowly the public health enterprise evolves, this prediction is overly optimistic, but every indication is that we are moving in this direction.

Appendix D contains a list of organizations that maintain clearinghouses for the evidence of practice. Some of the listings are broad and generic while others focus on a narrow range of practice. For each item there is a Web link for the body of evidence as well as a description of the specific purpose of the evidence website.

Case Study: Emergency Department Super-utilizers

Emergency departments (EDs) across the country have seen excessive usage over the years by ED super-utilizers. The following case study from Camden, New Jersey, highlights some of the challenges and successes in dealing with these patients in 2011.

Case Study: ED Super-utilizers and the Camden, New Jersey, Project

As hospitals look to minimize the most expensive aspects of their organization, emergency department (ED) super-utilizers gain immediate attention. These patients are known as "frequent fliers," and often have such serious chronic conditions as heart failure, diabetes, kidney disease, or psychiatric problems, according to KHN/Post.[32] Super-utilizers typically fall into one of three categories:

- Medicare beneficiaries who have difficulty affording the medicines they need to control their conditions;

- So-called dual eligibles, who qualify for Medicaid and Medicare and tend to shift between EDs for treatment for medical conditions tied to substance misuse or homelessness; or

- Individuals with private insurance.[33]

These patients fall within one percent of the costliest group battling multiple diagnoses, and they are estimated to use 21 percent of the $1.3 trillion spent on health care in 2010.[32] According to a study conducted by the University of Iowa, super-utilizers are more likely to be insured through Medicaid than by private insurance.[34] Because the issue of super-utilizers has become so widespread, the federal government is taking steps to address the problem at the most fundamental level. The Care Transitions program, which has been adopted by CMS, "takes into account a patients' medical and mental health needs and focuses on social barriers that might trigger unnecessary readmissions."[33]

Super-utilizers often present such significant challenges to the health care system as chronic conditions, homelessness, substance abuse, physical disability, dental disease, mental health problems, and physical disability.[34] Due to social factors, many super-utilizers have trouble keeping their appointments and demonstrating the literacy necessary to navigate the healthcare system. Furthermore, they may have experienced negative encounters with primary care providers in the past and therefore continue to use the ED.[35]

The high costs of super-utilizers may be better understood when looked at through the lens of an individual healthcare system. One pioneering case example in this area is from Camden, New Jersey, where early work was

Case Study: ED Super-utilizers and the Camden, New Jersey, Project

conducted on the needs of super-utilizers and ways to reduce their costs.[36] Researchers on this project found that two expensive city blocks accounted for four thousand hospital visits for nine hundred people in six-and-a-half years, totaling $200 million in health care bills.[34] One patient in the study had three hundred and twenty-four admissions in five years, and the most expensive patient cost insurers $3.5 million. This study also found that one percent of the 100,000 persons who used Camden's medical facilities were responsible for 30 percent of the costs.[36]

Fortunately, a multi-functional team in Camden started looking for answers to help the super-utilizers receive the care they need. Dr. Jeffrey Brenner, leader of this team, began his approach by looking for the most difficult patients in the system. The first individual they found was a gentleman with severe congestive heart failure, chronic asthma, uncontrolled diabetes, hypothyroidism, gout, and a history of smoking and alcohol abuse.[36] This individual weighed 560 pounds and had spent as much time in the hospital system as out of it in the previous three years. He was also in the intensive care unit with a tracheotomy, a feeding tube, and septic shock from a gallbladder infection. Dr. Brenner visited with him daily in search of answers to explain how someone can become a super-utilizer, and proposing possible solutions to helping this population.

Dr. Brenner learned that his sample super-utilizer was once a productive member of society but was plagued by decades of poor health and social problems that compounded over time. The patient had a history of alcoholism and drug addiction that interfered with his employment, his health insurance, his housing, and the ability to have a consistent set of doctors. The patient at one time had had an active social network, including family ties, a church, and Alcoholics Anonymous. Brenner's patient's many complex health problems made it difficult to keep his many medications filled and taken on schedule.

After two months in the intensive care unit, the patient recovered enough to be discharged from the hospital. As outlined above, however, without help in navigating the health and social environments, the patient will likely return to the hospital. Dr. Brenner double-checked the plans from the specialists to ensure that the medications and protocols fit together in a way that was helpful to the patient's overall health. When the plans didn't seem to make sense, Brenner telephoned specialists to sort out the questions. Dr. Brenner partnered with an LPN and coordinated home visits to educate the patient on healthy eating, monitoring blood sugar levels, and ensuring he was taking his required medications.

To truly help the patient, Dr. Brenner had to go beyond the ordinary measures a doctor usually takes. A social worker was called in to help the patient apply for disability insurance. This income helped him to move out of welfare motels and

Case Study: ED Super-utilizers and the Camden, New Jersey, Project

obtain a consistent set of health care providers. After a few years of these types of intensive health and social interventions, this 'worst of the worst patient' showed dramatic improvement.

> The team pushed him to find sources of stability and value in his life. They got him to return to Alcoholics Anonymous, and urged him to return to church. He has gone without alcohol for a year, cocaine for two years, and smoking for three years. He lives with his girlfriend in a safer neighborhood, goes to church, and weathers family crises. He now cooks his own meals. His diabetes and congestive heart failure are under much better control. He's lost two hundred and twenty pounds, which means, among other things, that if he falls he can pick himself up, rather than having to call for an ambulance.[36]

After seeing the success of the initial patient, Dr. Brenner began to receive many referrals for similar patients. In order to sustain his practice financially, he applied for small grants from the Merck Foundation and the Robert Wood Johnson Foundation. The Camden Coalition didn't have money for a clinic, so their approach relied mostly on grassroots tactics of home visits and phone calls. Over the phone, they inquired about prescription refills, medication adherence, housing issues, and other social factors that could be affecting their patients' health. By visiting the super-utilizers in their homes, the team could more quickly determine whether their pill bottles were full, empty, easily located, or in some cases, buried under food remains and newspapers. In a specific case, the Camden team helped a patient move to housing where his medication adherence could be much better.

Work like this can be all-consuming, but Dr. Brenner and his team are making a big difference for the super-utilizers they are helping. The first 36 super-utilizers averaged 62 hospital visits per month before joining the program and 37 visits after joining the program. This change represents a 42 percent reduction, and hospital bills that dropped from $1.2 million per month to around $500,000 afterward—a 56 percent reduction in hospital cost.

Solving the medical care-related population health challenges in the twenty-first century will require continued work like that of Dr. Brenner described in the New Jersey example above. These are systemic problems rooted in social, economic, cultural, and health issues that have arisen not only in the United States but also abroad. Since the 1986 enactment of the Emergency Medical Treatment and Active Labor Act (EMTALA), the financial and moral responsibility[37] shifted to acute care facilities that provide emergency department services. To achieve improved population health, finding solutions like those described in this case example will be essential. While super-utilization is centrally a clinical care issue, it also lies on the frontier between medical care and the population health system, going beyond the experience of individual super-utilizers.

In light of the widespread impact of super-utilization on communities and the health of the population served by healthcare and public health systems nationwide, a second case study is provided on the way in which a Louisville-based multisectoral team approached this national challenge on the local level, starting in 2012.

Case Study: Louisville Metro Super-utilizers Network

In 2012, city officials and healthcare leaders in Louisville, Kentucky, were faced with increasing concerns about the stability of the city's safety net system and the impact of the changing dynamics of the healthcare system. With growing health care expenses in the local correctional facility, a historical financial commitment to the local safety net hospital, and a longstanding financial relationship with one of the city's federally qualified health centers, as well as a highly anticipated decision from the Supreme Court regarding the legalities of the individual mandate for health insurance, city leaders sought to identify better ways to manage the health care of the city's indigent population.

A small group of key stakeholders convened and decided to focus on high utilizers of health care in inappropriate care settings. The initial project led to a focus on the top 50 patients with the highest number of emergency department (ED) visits to the city's safety net hospital, the University of Louisville Hospital (ULH). This list was then refined to focus on the patients who used the emergency department for nonemergent conditions.

The ULH Population Health Committee convened a Community-wide Complex Case Treatment Planning Conference to discuss six of the aforementioned patients with representatives of:

- Seven Counties Services, the local community mental health provider: Chief Medical Officer, Director of Case Management, Director of Emergency Psychiatry

- Phoenix Healthcare Center for the Homeless, federally qualified health center: Executive Director, Director of Nursing, Supervisor of Homeless

> ## Case Study: Louisville Metro Super-utilizers Network
>
> Health Services, Hospital Liaison, Case Manager
>
> - University of Louisville School of Medicine: Emergency Medicine faculty member, Emergency Medicine resident and Internal Medicine Gastroenterology fellow
>
> - University of Louisville Kent School of Social Work: Two faculty members who specialize in addiction
>
> - University of Louisville School of Nursing: faculty
>
> - University of Louisville Hospital: Director of Emergency Department Nursing, Director of Care Coordination, Director of Admissions, Director of Management Engineering, ED Case Manager, Social Worker, Manager of Outpatient Pharmacy, and Financial Counseling Supervisor
>
> For each patient, University Hospital's experience with the patient was presented, including number of ED visits; inpatient admissions; medications history, including the Kentucky All Schedule Prescription Electronic Reporting (KASPER) report (Kentucky's prescription drug monitoring program); psychosocial history; family history; and U of L Physicians provider history.
>
> Key outcomes and lessons learned to date include:
>
> - The city needed to use a person-centered rather than an organization-centered approach to care for these community members. The Emergency Department provided care while the patient was in the department but did not have a way to systematically link the patient to community resources.
>
> - The Emergency Department staff needed to sign a narcotics medication management contract with several patients. The ED staff needed to develop a way to make the contract available to ED staff when the community member presented for the next ED visit.
>
> - A population health flag (PHF) was developed for the hospital information system. A PHF is added to each identified patient at the medical record level. Each time a patient account is created for an identified patient, the PHF appears in the header section of the Emergency Department's electronic health record system. Also, a report that lists all patients who had an account created the prior day with any type of PHF is generated as part of day-end processing and e-mailed to members of the ULH Population Health Committee. If a community member's primary care

Case Study: Louisville Metro Super-utilizers Network

quarterback works for another organization, the name of the organization is added as the PHF.

- The community-wide team is both learning about the programs available in Louisville and providing input into these programs. For example, the team has learned a great deal about the Housing First model (an approach to the problem of homelessness) and permanent supportive housing case management, and provided input into the hours when case managers are available. The ULH ED staff recommends that case managers work later into the evening based on the time of day that ED super-utilizers usually present to the ED.

The community-wide case conference continues to convene monthly. The annualized healthcare savings are estimated at approximately $694,000 and the number of ED encounters decreased by over 50 percent. Of great importance is that the number of stakeholders with an interest in participating in the case conference and joining the Metro Super-utilizers Network continues to grow and includes representatives from health care (medical, dental, mental health), substance abuse treatment, supportive housing, and criminal justice. As a way to bring the work of the ULH Population Health Management Complex Treatment Care Conference to scale and to make it sustainable, the network has identified five critical success factors:

- A **common needs-assessment instrument** should be used by all community partners so that every person in the community will be directed to the appropriate services regardless of their point of entry in the system;

- A **standard release of information** should be created and used by all community partners to address concerns related to HIPAA and the sharing of behavioral health information (issues addressed in Chapter 8);

- A **community-wide treatment plan** should exist to avoid duplication of services and allow for better coordination of services;

- **Standardized outcome measures** are needed to align the work of all partners; and

- **Single complex case management software** should be used by all community partners.

Emergency department overutilization is a chronic problem with systemic challenges in communities across America. The homeless population of each community is often a demographic group that experiences "disproportionately high rates of chronic and acute health conditions and traumatic injuries," which leads to the need for excessive use of safety-net acute care emergency services.[38] The Camden, New Jersey, case study and the Louisville Metro Super-utilizers Network both provide examples of where the nation is attempting to meet this challenge driven by socioeconomic, cultural, and access to care implications. Multisectoral partnerships are and will continue to be essential to solving this population health challenge in each community level with engagement from public, private, and nonprofit stakeholders.

Case Study: The National Challenge to Reduce Hospital Readmissions

The passage of the ACA in 2010 included the Hospital Readmission Reduction Program (HRRP); a number of studies since that time have indicated the importance of targeted interventions, improving care coordination between primary care and inpatient providers, and strengthening patient education.[39] The HRRP started on October 1, 2012. White and colleagues noted in a 2014 *Journal of Family Practice* article that there are several patient factors which increase the potential for readmission; they include

> 1) feeling unprepared for discharge; 2) difficulty performing activities of daily living; 3) trouble adhering to discharge medications; 4) difficulty accessing discharge medications; and 5) lack of social support.[40]

Hospital readmission is recognized as a high-priority issue in population health for every community across the country. We present here a third case study of a public-nonprofit partnership that has made progress in meeting this national challenge on the local level.

Case Study: Reducing 30-day Readmissions
Jewish Hospital and Louisville Metro Public Health and Wellness

In 2012, Jewish Hospital, a member hospital of the KentuckyOne Health system, partnered with the local health department, Louisville Metro Public Health and Wellness, to address issues related to health equity in Louisville, Kentucky. One of the initiatives in the "Upstream to Equity" project was designed to decrease hospital readmission rates among high-risk patients who live in targeted zip codes.

Case Study: Reducing 30-day Readmissions
Jewish Hospital and Louisville Metro Public Health and Wellness

Reducing the rate of hospital readmissions for certain health conditions has been identified as an important way to lower health care costs and improve quality of life for patients. The reasons for hospital readmissions are often related to many of the social concepts discussed in Chapter 5. Building increased social capacity and self-efficacy in patients has led to improved health outcomes. Hospital staff members are well trained and highly skilled in managing patients in the hospital setting and to prepare them to return home, where their care will presumably be handed off to a provider in the outpatient setting. Similarly, outpatient providers are highly skilled and able to manage patients when they arrive in the office. The challenge in avoiding readmissions is to monitor what happens to the patient in the time and space between the two sets of providers. Jewish Hospital and Louisville Metro Public Health and Wellness set out to understand and solve this problem.

During a nine-month period, patients who met the following criteria were considered eligible for participation in the Transitions of Care program: admitted to the hospital on a 30-day readmission; lived in a targeted zip code; insured by Medicaid or uninsured; and discharged to home with or without home health care. Those who were eligible for the program received a nurse bedside visit and were offered post-discharge support from a community care navigator (CCN) that consisted of weekly phone calls. A subset of participants was assigned to a lay community health worker (CHW) who made weekly home visits.

Preliminary findings[*] for this pilot project suggest that patients who received only the bedside nurse visit had a 30-day readmission rate of approximately 41 percent as compared to a 30-day readmission rate of 23 percent for the group that received post-discharge support. Those who received the most intense support from the CCN and CHW had even lower readmission rates. Qualitative feedback from the CCNs and CHWs was also informative. CCNs and CHWs reported that their patients often lacked money to purchase medications; lacked support at home; had no access to paid medical care or insurance; and were overwhelmed with family issues.

This case study provides an example of how health systems can partner with

---

[*] Preliminary evaluation conducted by REACH Evaluation.

> ### Case Study: Reducing 30-day Readmissions
> ### Jewish Hospital and Louisville Metro Public Health and Wellness
>
> local health departments to facilitate collaboration between clinical medicine and public health to advance the goals of population health. Even as health systems leaders become increasingly aware of the impact that the social context in which patients live has on their ability to manage their health conditions, the health system's ability to affect those conditions *directly* is limited. The only way to have a direct influence on those conditions is through effective public policy. CHWs can, however, help patients who have low health literacy, limited access to transportation, and other penetrable barriers to the healthcare system become better utilizers of the system and subsequently improve their intermediate health outcomes.
>
> Local health departments have used their workforce (nurses, peer advisors, and paraprofessionals) to conduct home visits to improve maternal and child health outcomes for decades. Local, state, and federal policymakers should explore ways to develop appropriate reimbursement schemes that will allow the expansion of the public health workforce to provide home visitations for patients with chronic health conditions.

This Louisville-based case study provided further evidence of the complicated patient-centered factors noted by White and colleagues. The core issues to improve patient engagement on the population level in regard to this national dilemma extend beyond the scope of acute care providers and will require multisectoral partnering to help patients reduce their risk of readmission.

Case Study: Health and Prevention Promotion Initiative

A fourth case study, originated by William Yasnoff, a national leader in health informatics and the author of Chapter 12, provides a compelling and meaningful case for sustainable community population health organizations enabling comprehensive electronic patient records through the use of health record banks (HRBs).

Case Study: Health and Prevention Promotion Initiative (HAPPI)

Helping individuals maintain their health and avoid unnecessary medical care is an increasingly important priority. The transition of our nation's medical payment system from "pay for volume" to "pay for value" reflects this new emphasis. Moreover, the Affordable Care Act incentivizes prevention and population health through such innovations as accountable care organizations (ACOs), in which medical care savings are shared with providers.

In the past, provider organizations have not generally been involved in prevention and population health. To address this new priority, they must engage new types of staff and establish new processes. Shortell has observed that competing medical care delivery organizations in communities that are implementing population health and prevention activities would enjoy increased efficiency and effectiveness if they were to collaborate to create a single community organization for these purposes.[41,42] Such a Population Health Organization (PHO) could address all the prevention, care coordination, and health management needs of the entire community with a single staff that could achieve economies of scale from dealing with all the residents at once instead of multiple subsets. In addition, a community PHO would have financial incentives to address long-term prevention initiatives, because all the stakeholders would still benefit despite the predictable shifts of members over time among the competing medical care organizations.

To maximize effectiveness, a PHO must have access to comprehensive electronic patient records for all community residents. This access allows individually targeted, accurate reminders based on the specific medical conditions and needs of each person. Without this resource, substantial time, energy, and expense must be devoted to identifying persons needing particular services or interventions, which detract from the resources available for service delivery. It can also potentially result in erroneous interventions; for example, a reminder for a colonoscopy might be sent to a patient who, unknown to the PHO, just had the procedure.

Health record banks (HRBs), or community repositories of comprehensive electronic patient records,[43-46] are ideally suited to the needs of a PHO. HRBs put patients in charge of a comprehensive copy of all their personal private health information, including both medical records and additional personal data that can be added by the patient. HRBs might also include community-wide human services, housing, and environmental health data. The patient explicitly controls who may access which parts of the information in his or her individual account.[47] When patients seek care, they give permission for their health care providers to access some or all of their up-to-date health records. When care is complete, the new records from that visit or hospitalization are securely deposited at the patient's request into the HRB and made available for future use.

Case Study: Health and Prevention Promotion Initiative (HAPPI)

This approach solves the problems of 1) privacy (through patient control); 2) stakeholder cooperation (because the patients request their own records, the HIPAA regulations require every stakeholder to provide them electronically if they are available in that form); and 3) financial sustainability (with revenue from optional applications, or "apps," for use by patients as well as use of their data for research purposes, but only with their permission). The copies of records in the HRB do not replace the original records, which remain in the medical care institutions where they were created.

In addition, HRBs can generate revenue well in excess of their operational costs from apps, advertising, and fees for access (with permission) to research data. For example, a "peace of mind" app that automatically notifies loved ones when an emergency physician accesses HRB records (meaning that the person is undergoing emergency treatment) is a compelling value to consumers and their families for which they would likely be willing to pay a modest fee, e.g., $20/year. With consumer permission, HRBs could identify patients eligible for clinical trials as well as produce aggregate anonymized reports of great value to researchers and policy makers.

By sharing part of the revenue generated from these research applications on a pro rata basis with consumers who are account holders, they would have an incentive to allow their data to be used for these purposes. Earnings could be used not only for HRB operations but also for supporting and expanding community-wide prevention and population health activities. HRBs can also promote electronic information by providing ongoing permanent subsidies of electronic health records (EHRs) for outpatient physicians, thereby assuring much higher levels of adoption, resulting in more complete information for each patient.

Combining a PHO and HRB into what we call a health and prevention promotion initiative (HAPPI) results in a financially self-sustaining entity that can deliver population health and prevention services as well as comprehensive electronic patient records for the community. The PHO organizes and executes prevention and population health activities, while the associated HRB provides the necessary patient record information. The revenue generated by the HRB can support both HRB operations and the prevention and care coordination initiatives of the PHO. Therefore, once it has been started, a HAPPI can be internally self-sufficient without the need for additional reimbursement or outside funding.

Why are HAPPIs important?

Ten years after the creation of the Office of the National Coordinator for Health

Case Study: Health and Prevention Promotion Initiative (HAPPI)

IT (ONC), we have not yet identified a feasible and sustainable path to ensuring the universal availability of comprehensive electronic medical records—the goal set forth in the executive order that established the ONC. While much progress has been made in the adoption of electronic health records (EHR), efforts by health information exchanges (HIEs) to integrate the scattered records of individuals have been plagued by problems of privacy, stakeholder cooperation, public trust, and the lack of a model for sustainability. The HAPPI concept provides a new and compelling approach to creating community organizations focused on population health and prevention (now a critical priority for medical care delivery organizations), supported by the availability of comprehensive electronic medical records for all residents. A HAPPI need be capitalized only once, after which it is financially sustainable and provides substantial benefits to all health care stakeholders. Establishment of HAPPI organizations is a feasible path to developing our nation's health information infrastructure.

The fourth case study is an example of a way to address the challenge of healthcare reform and traditional public health on a community-wide health promotion level by thinking about a future community-wide population health organization (PHO) that could address all the prevention, care coordination, and health management needs of the entire community with a single staff that could achieve economies of scale by dealing with all the residents at once instead of multiple subsets. This type of organization, potentially a new community health value alliance combined with HRBs, or community repositories of comprehensive electronic patient records for all residents of the community, is ideally suited for the needs of a PHO, as discussed by Yasnoff.

While this case study presents a scenario for improving population health, it also implicitly advocates (and would be supported by) changes in policy. First, health information about each individual should be controlled by that individual. This stipulation would not only recognize the inherent interest of each person in the privacy of his or her own health information, but also reinforce the necessity of engaging the targets of health interventions—in this case by always requiring their consent for the use of their information. While such a policy is consistent with Fair Information Practices,[46] it would be much more privacy-protective than the existing HIPAA Privacy Rule (discussed in Chapter 12), which allows use without consent of patient records for treatment, payment, and health care operations (as determined by the holder of the information, which can clearly result in biased decisions about disclosure). Second, establishing sensible state and/or federal regulations governing the operation of HRBs (e.g., requiring periodic publicly disclosed independent audits to assess the robustness of their privacy and security practices) would help to promote the necessary trust in these new organizational custodians of sensitive health care information. These suggested policy initiatives again demonstrate the important influence of policy on population health.

Population health, like patient care, depends on accurate and complete information about the health of individuals. Therefore, frameworks that assess the availability of comprehensive health information for everyone in the community should be included as key indicators of population health in communities.[49] While such measures are indirect, it is difficult to envision how a community could achieve its maximum health potential without comprehensive information about individuals.

Health Promotion and Education: A Necessity for Improving Population Health

In the twenty-first century, the population of any given community in the United States or around the globe typically comprises a diverse array of people from different cultures, ethnic backgrounds, and socioeconomic statuses (SES). As we move forward as students, researchers, policy makers, and practitioners involved in the delivery and assessment of health services, we must remember the role and value of health promotion programs and education of consumers in every community. The health behaviors of individuals and segments of any population may be changed over time through increased consumer knowledge, incentives, and penalties[50] enacted through local, state, and federal policy— especially focused through Health in All Policies (HiAP) approaches. Some targeted health communication campaigns and federal acts, as noted earlier in this chapter regarding the United States' efforts over the past 50 years with anti-tobacco and smoking prevention efforts, serve as a strong example of effectiveness in curbing some unhealthy behaviors. On the other hand, health communication campaigns about the potential dangers of alcohol, drugs, food, and unprotected sexual activity have been rather less successful.

Second, as described by Randolph, Whitaker, and Arellano in an article published in 2012 in *Evaluation and Program Planning*, there are multiple options for health promotion interventions within every environment. Such options may include: a) entertainment education (to educate the public); b) community outreach and advocacy efforts; c) Internet-based education; d) policy changes; and e) the training of health care providers.[49] The reason for noting this spectrum of intervention strategies is that in order to move a nation and any group to take action or make changes in the twenty-first century, there must first be meaningful communication. In the light of technological advancements over the last two decades, our ability to reach individuals and entire populations of consumers and patients is drastically different from what it was in the past. As Green and Kreuter noted, "Health programs do not spring from a social vacuum."[52] Needs for new health programs and health delivery services arise as society evolves; as people relocate from rural to urban areas; and as population demographics shift (e.g., the 'silver tsunami' effect[53] with the aging of the Baby Boomer generation in America).

As the nation moves forward, it requires a new focus that involves the shift to a "culture of health," as noted in the Ottawa Charter and by the World Health Organization's report on the social determinants of health.[54] To participate in this new culture, we all should listen to and engage in health promotion initiatives that can positively influence the lives we live in each of our communities. Adopting the "citizen-centered health promotion" approach introduced by Woolf, Mercedes, and colleagues in a 2011 article offers one path to reach the goal. Citizen-centered health promotion

> . . . refers to a coordinated multisector community effort to bring about a way of life—at home, work, and school—that makes it easier for members of a community to adopt and maintain healthful practices.[55]

Implementing this concept requires meaningful community engagement through focused public-private partnerships with sustained efforts that move people to action. These efforts will serve the purpose of advancing population health in the communities we all live, work, and play in throughout our lives.

Recommendations for Future Leaders

The concepts in this text have provided many theories and practical examples of ways in which future leaders can think about problem identification and development of interventions to improve population health. In order to change our health outcomes, we must change the way we address health-related matters. The critical first step is to recognize that we must treat health as a social good that enables people to live productive lives and contribute actively to our society in meaningful ways. It also means that we must view population health through a different lens. Each leader should consider the following questions:

- **What steps should be taken to implement the concepts in this text?**
- **What is your role as a leader in the era of population health?**

- **Where is your value alliance for the tasks you have to complete as a leader?**

Health system leaders and health care providers may read this text and understand their role as improving population health through better management and the appropriate use of technology. Public health practitioners may see their role in improving population health as better management and policy implementation. Policy makers may view their role as crafting more effective policies; and students in the health professions may be in the formative stage of their career, when they still have the luxury of choosing to be a provider, practitioner, or policy maker. Future leaders will do well to recognize that their role requires proficiency in recognizing the interplay of management, policy, and technology; and the need to form strategic partnerships and alliances (collaborations) that ensure that the three always work together, never in isolation.

The medical care enterprise has adopted a transdisciplinary approach to care provision in which physicians, nurses, dentists, social workers, pharmacists, physical therapists, occupational therapists, and other allied health professionals all work together to address the healthcare and social needs of patients and families. While this approach has demonstrated some improvement in outcomes, it fails to address the social determinants of health and does not reach the people living in the community setting who can benefit from primary prevention strategies. To this end, each leader from the spectrum of participant entities operating in each community, whether public or private, nonprofit or academic, health care or public health, may consider the following checklist of actions as they build their own strategies for their communities and the populations they serve.

Table 14-1. Population Health Leader's Action Checklist

Category	Action
Partnerships	Establish multisectoral partnerships that widen the perspective on what is needed and the possibilities of what can be done to help those in greatest need in each community.
Alliances	Seek out and create value alliances and networks of trust to bridge stakeholder interests with common population-level goals of improving outcomes in health, socioeconomic, and wellness measures.
Complexity Thinking	Manage human interactions from the perspective of their impact on patient engagement, organizational effectiveness, and community-level health improvement and progress.
Social Determinants	Deepen your understanding of the linkages between the social determinants of health and the multigenerational occurrence of chronic conditions that affect various community sectors.
Innovation	Continuously seek innovative interventions in management approaches, policy (e.g., social, health, and economic-oriented), and novel technologies that can be replicated across communities.

In addition to these actions, each of us should remember the critical importance of ensuring that the Health in All Policies (HiAP) concept is embedded in our acceptance of health as a social objective. This policy focus will support the movement toward multisectoral teaming of representatives from public health, public safety, planners and civil engineers, parks and recreation, housing, economic development, transportation, and education. If every sector develops public policies for education, the built environment, criminal justice, and economic development that are equitable, just, and informed by their impact on health, not only will population health be improved by reduction of inequities in health, but health disparities can be diminished in the process.

Conclusion

Nash and colleagues stated in the opening segment of their 2011 book, *Population Health, Creating a Culture of Wellness,*

We are faced with many challenges in health care and the strategies we use to address both existing and emerging challenges will determine the future health of our nation.[56]

Many strategies have been discussed throughout this book, covering the spectrum of management, public policy, and technological dimensions necessary for the student, researcher, policy maker, and practitioner to understand in order to improve the health of the nation's population. The challenges we face in society affect the health of every segment in our population. Our success will be influenced by the social determinants of health and the health inequities that still exist. We can reach many goals by welcoming future technological innovations and their diffusion; collaborative management at the community, state, and national levels; and adoption of a Health in All Policies perspective when developing new social, health, and economic policies. Perhaps our first goal is to leave the nation and the world a healthier place for the generation that follows us.

In closing, we leave you with this consideration. Joseph Jaworski noted in the conclusion of his 1996 book *Synchronicity, The Inner Path of Leadership* that

> . . . we see that the future is not fixed, and we shift from resignation to a sense of possibility. We are creating the future every moment.[57]

We all have the capacity to move into the future and mitigate the health inequities that plague many communities. Improving a nation's health is a multigenerational process. It requires collaborative leadership to drive public-private initiatives—a necessity to improve the environment in which we live, work, and play for every generation that follows. Each of us needs to remember that we have a chance to shape the future. The past is fixed, but we as a nation learn lessons along the way, build new health care programs, teach future practitioners and researchers, and train the future leaders of our nation's healthcare and public health systems.

With this commitment as a calling, the future is bright. Population health can be improved and progress will be made. So let us take the next steps to prepare for, engage, and lead in building a healthier nation.

ACKNOWLEDGMENTS

The authors gratefully acknowledge the contribution of Tom Walton, MS, MDiv, System Director, Healthy Communities and Academic Relation, KentuckyOne Health for development support of the Louisville Metro Super-utilizers Network case study. Also wish to acknowledge Andrew McCart, MBA, Continuing Lecturer, Purdue University, Department of Technology, Leadership, and Innovation (PhD candidate, University of Louisville School of Public Health and Information Systems) for development support on the Camden, New Jersey, ED super-utilizers case study.

CHAPTER 14 DISCUSSION QUESTIONS

Discussion questions are provided for team building or class exercises. Answers for all questions are provided in Appendix C.

Question Number	Question
1	What is the difference discussed in the chapter between traditional public health practice and the concept of population health promotion?
2	What is meant by quality of life, and how does understanding it at the population level aid in health policy development?
3	What is asset assessment and how is it different from needs assessment?
4	What are asset maps and how do they help communities evaluate and improve population health?
5	What are the sources of quantitative and qualitative data, and how can they be merged into a community analysis?
6	In the asthma case study, who were the different stakeholders and what was the importance of their roles in the project?
7	How is the solution to ED super-utilizers in both the Camden, New Jersey, and Louisville, Kentucky, case studies derived from population health concepts rather than clinical medicine?
8	What is the novel policy potential that can emerge with HAPPIs?
9	What is the role of health promotion programs?
10	What are the five categories in the Recommendations for Future Leaders?

CHAPTER 14 SUMMARY

- The U.S. healthcare and public health infrastructure is undergoing a period of major transformation—one that is redefining the 'cross-industry' ecology for which they exist.

- The City of Louisville serves as an instructive example of the impact of health and economic inequities on every community in America.

- Highlights from previous chapters provide a synopsis of key points from Sections I through III.

- The Health and Prevention Promotion Initiative (HAPPI) case study provides a novel case for sustainable population health organizations (PHOs) to be enabled through the creation and use of health record banks.

- The challenges faced in the United States and abroad affect the health of every segment of a nation's population. Success in meeting those challenges depends on the social determinants of health, community-level health inequities, and the strategies and programs that communities put in place.

- For the Louisville children's asthma management program targeted to support children in West Louisville, the health promotion and education plan included: a) screening children for asthma in the schools they attend; b) selecting the schools with the most disproportionate indicators of disadvantage; c) defining children who screen positive for asthma as a treatment group; d) asking parents for permission for medical record monitoring and access to academic achievement data to track concurrent academic progress; and e) offering children who screen positive a home visit to inspect their housing for the presence of triggers and irritants.

- Emergency department (ED) overutilization is a systemic challenge in many communities across America. Two case studies were provided from Camden, New Jersey, and Louisville, Kentucky, that show the importance of multidisciplinary and multisectoral partnering to engage the best available resources to aid the disadvantaged members of the community in reducing ED overutilization.

- Health promotion programs are critical in educating consumers and other stakeholders across communities of the impact of different health behaviors that may be changed over time through increased consumer knowledge, incentives, and penalties enacted through local, state and federal policies. The concept of citizen-centered health promotion emphasizes public-private partnerships and multisectoral engagement in order to improve population health in all our communities.

- Five recommendations were made for future leaders to consider: a)

CHAPTER 14 SUMMARY

partnerships; b) alliances; c) complexity thinking; d) the impact of social determinants; and e) innovation. The most important consideration across these areas is their common link to caring for any community's population and the underlying importance of the concept of Health in All Policies (HiAP).

CHAPTER 14 REFERENCES

1.   Green LW, Kreuter MW. *Health program planning: an educational and ecological approach.* Fourth ed. New York, N.Y.: McGraw-Hill;2005.

2.   Morgan G. Unfolding logics of change: organization as flux and transformation (Toward a new view of organizational evolution and change). *Images of organization.* Newbury Park, Calif.: Sage Publications, Inc.;1986:245.

3.   Fielding JE, Tilson HH, Richland JH. *Medical care reform requires public health reform: expanded role for public health agencies in improving health..* Washington, D.C.: Partnership for Prevention;2008. http://www.prevent.org/data/files/initiatives/medicalcarereformrequirespubl ichealthreform.pdf. Accessed April 24, 2014.

4.   Gladwell M. The three rules of epidemics. *The tipping point: how little things can make a big difference.* New York, N.Y.: Back Bay Books;2000:25.

5.   Institute of Medicine, Board on Population Health and Public Health Practice. Chapter 3. Current models for integrating a population health approach into Implementation of the Affordable Care Act. *Population health implications of the Affordable Care Act, Workshop summary.* Washington, D.C.: The National Academies Press;2013:7-10.

6.   Murphy SI, Xu JQ, Kochanek KD. Deaths: final data for 2010. National vital statistics reports, vol. 61. Hyattsville, Md.: National Center for Health Statistics;2013.

7.   Daynard RA, Gottlieb MA, Sweda EL, Friedman LC, Eriksen MP. Prevention and control of diseases associated with tobacco use through law and policy. In: Goodman RA, Hoffman RE, Lopez W, Matthews GW, Rothstein MA, Foster KL, eds. *Law in public health practice.* New York, N.Y.: Oxford University Press;2007:427-428.

8.   Curfman GD, Morrissey S, Drazen JM. Tobacco, public health, and the FDA. *N Engl J Med.* 2009;361(4):402-403.

9.   Koh HK, Sebelius KG. Ending the tobacco epidemic. *JAMA.* 2012;308(8):767-768.

10.   Green LW, Kreuter MW. A framework for planning. *Health program planning: an educational and ecological approach.* Fourth ed. New York, N.Y.: McGraw-Hill;2005:8.

11.   Green LW, Kreuter MW. Social assessment, participatory planning, and situation analysis. *Health program planning: an educational and ecological approach.* Fourth ed. New York, N.Y.: McGraw-Hill;2005:52-54.

12.   McKnight JL, Krentzmann JP. Mapping community capacity. In: Minkler M, ed. *Community organizing and community building for health.* New Brunswick, N.J.: Rutgers University Press;1997:163, 165.

13.   U.S. Centers for Disease Control and Prevention. *Healthy People 2020.* http://www.cdc.gov/nchs/healthy_people/hp2020.htm. Accessed August 1, 2013.

14. Metro Louisville Government. Louisville Facts & Firsts. http://www.louisvilleky.gov/visitors/louisville+facts+and+firsts.htm. Accessed April 29, 2014.

15. Louisville Metro Department of Public Health and Wellness. *Health equity report, 2011. The social determinants of health in Louisville Metro neighborhoods.* Louisville, Ky.: Louisville Metro Public Health and Wellness;2011.

16. U.S. Census Bureau. State and county quickfacts. Louisville/Jefferson County (balance), Kentucky. 2010; http://quickfacts.census.gov/qfd/states/21/2148006.html. Accessed May 2, 2014.

17. Greater Louisville Project. Place matters. 2013; http://greaterlouisvilleproject.org/wp-content/uploads/2013/11/place_matters.jpg. Accessed May 2, 2014.

18. Moonie S, Sterling DA, Figgs LW, Castro M. The relationship between school absence, academic performance, and asthma status. *J Sch Health.* 2008;78(3):140-148.

19. Bonilla S, Kehl S, Kwong KY, Morphew T, Kachru R, Jones CA. School absenteeism in children with asthma in a Los Angeles inner city school. *J Pediatr.* 2005;147(6):802-806.

20. Diette GB, Markson L, Skinner EA, Nguyen TT, Algatt-Bergstrom P, Wu AW. Nocturnal asthma in children affects school attendance, school performance, and parents' work attendance. *Arch Pediatr Adolesc Med.* 2000;154(9):923-928.

21. Celano MP, Geller RJ. Learning, school performance, and children with asthma: how much at risk? *J Learn Disabil.* 1993;26(1):23-32.

22. Schmier JK, Manjunath R, Halpern MT, Jones ML, Thompson K, Diette GB. The impact of inadequately controlled asthma in urban children on quality of life and productivity. *Ann Allergy Asthma Immunol.* 2007;98(3):245-251.

23. Community Preventive Services Task Force. Asthma control: home-based multi-trigger, multicomponent environmental interventions. Atlanta, Ga.: 2013; www.thecommunityguide.org/asthma/multicomponent.html. Accessed May 2, 2014.

24. Basch CE. Healthier students are better learners: a missing link in school reforms to close the achievement gap. *Research Review No. 6* 2010; http://www.equitycampaign.org/i/a/document/12557_equitymattersvol6_web03082010.pdf. Accessed May 2, 2014.

25. Moorman JE, Rudd RA, Johnson CA, et al. National surveillance for asthma--United States, 1980-2004. *MMWR Surveill Summ.* 2007;56(8):1-14.

26. King B, Dube S, Kaufmann R, Shaw L, Pechacek T. Vital signs: current cigarette smoking among adults aged ≥18 Years—United States, 2005-2010. *MMWR Morb Mortal Wkly Rep.* 2011;60(35):1207-1212.

27. Sippel JM, Pedula KL, Vollmer WM, Buist AS, Osborne ML. Associations of smoking with hospital-based care and quality of life in patients with obstructive airway disease. *Chest.* 1999;115(3):691-696.

28. Villano M. In Louisville, fresh look at health data correlations drives efforts on asthma. 2013; http://data-informed.com/in-louisville-fresh-look-at-health-data-correlations-drives-efforts-on-asthma/. Accessed May 7, 2014, 2014.

29. Marcus J. Leveraging data for public health. 2013; http://propellerhealth.com/2013/02/leveraging-data-for-public-health/. Accessed May 7, 2014.

30. Van Sickle D, Maenner MJ, Barrett MA, Marcus JE. Monitoring and improving compliance and asthma control: mapping inhaler use for feedback to patients, physicians and payers. Paper presented at Respiratory Drug Delivery Europe 2013; May 24, 2013, Berlin, Germany.

31. Van Sickle D, Magzamen S, Truelove S, Morrison T. Remote monitoring of inhaled bronchodilator use and weekly feedback about asthma management: An open-group, short-term pilot study of the impact on asthma control. *PloS One.* 2013;8(2):e55335.

32. Boodman SG. Costliest 1 percent of patients account for 21 percent of U.S. health spending. *Kaiser Health News.* October 7, 2013. http://www.kaiserhealthnews.org/Stories/2013/October/08/one-percent-of-costliest-patients.aspx. Accessed April 24, 2014.

33. California Healthline. Hospitals, insurers focus on ED super-users to help curb costs. October 8, 2013. http://www.californiahealthline.org/articles/2013/10/8/hospitals-insurers-focus-on-ed-superusers-to-help-curb-costs. Accessed April 30, 2014.

34. Stamy CD, MacKinney AC. Emergency department super utilizer programs. Iowa City, Iowa: Center for Rural Health Policy Analysis;2013. http://cph.uiowa.edu/ruralhealthvalue/education/Super%20Utilizers.pdf. Accessed April 24, 2014.

35. Hunt K, Weber E, Showstack J, Colby D, Callaham M. Characteristics of frequent users of emergency departments. *Ann Emerg Med.* 2006;48(1):1-8.

36. Gawande A. The hot spotters: can we lower medical costs by giving the neediest patients better care? *The New Yorker*, January 24, 2011. http://www.newyorker.com/reporting/2011/01/24/110124fa_fact_gawande?currentPage=all. Accessed April 24, 2014.

37. Menzel PT. The cultural moral right to a basic minimum of accessible health care. *Kennedy Inst Ethics J.* 2011;21(1):79-119.

38. Chambers C, Chiu S, Katic M, et al. High utilizers of emergency health services in a population-based cohort of homeless adults. *Am J Public Health.* 2013;103(S2):S302-S310.

39. Williams MV. Where's the beef? progress on reducing readmissions. *J Hosp Med.* 2014;9(4):266-268.

40.   White B, Carney P, Flynn J, Marino M, Fields S. Reducing hospital readmissions through primary care practice transformation. *J Fam Pract*. February 2014 2014;63(2):67-74.

41.   Shortell SM. Bridging the divide between health and health care. *JAMA*. 2013;309(11):1121-1122.

42.   Shortell SM. *A bold proposal for advancing population health.* Discussion Paper, Institute of Medicine, Washington, DC. http://www. iom. edu/Global/Perspectives/2013/BoldProposal;2013. Accessed April 24, 2014.

43.   Dodd B. An independent 'health information bank'could solve data security issues. *BJHC*. 1997;14(8):2.

44.   Ball MJ, Gold J. Banking on health: personal records and information exchange. *JHIM*. 2006;20(2):71-83.

45.   Shabo A. It's time for health record banking! *Methods Inf Med*. 2007;46(5):601-607.

46.   Yasnoff WA, Sweeney L, Shortliffe EH. Putting health IT on the path to success. *JAMA*. 2013;309(10):989-990.

47.   Health Record Banking Alliance. HIE architecture and business model white papers. http://www.healthbanking.org. Accessed March 11, 2014.

48.   Westin A. Records, computers, and the rights of citizens: report of the secretary's advisory committee on automated personal data systems. Washington, D.C.: U.S. Department of Health, Education and Welfare; 1973.

49.   Labkoff SE, Yasnoff WA. A framework for systematic evaluation of health information progress in communities. *J Biomed Inform*. 2007;40(2):100-105.

50.   Riegelman R, Kirkwood B. Social and behavioral sciences and public health. *Public Health 101: Healthy People—Healthy Populations*. Sudbury, Mass.: Jones and Bartlett Learning;2015:82-84.

51.   Randolph KA, Whitaker P, Arellano A. The unique effects of environmental strategies in health promotion campaigns: A review. *Eval Program Plann*. 2012;35:344-353.

52.   Green LW, Kreuter MW. Social assessment, participatory planning, and situation analysis. *Health program planning: an educational and ecological approach*. Fourth ed. New York, N.Y.: McGraw-Hill;2005:30.

53.   Schumpeter. The silver tsunami. *The Economist*, February 4, 2010. http://www.economist.com/node/15450864. Accessed April 24, 2014.

54.   Davies SC, Winpenny E, Ball S, Fowler T, Rubin J, Nolte E. For debate: a new wave in public health improvement *Lancet*. April 4, 2014. doi: 10.1016/S0140-6736(13)62341-7. [Epub ahead of print]

55.   Woolf S.H., Dekker M.M., Byrne F.R., W.D. M. Citizen-centered health promotion: building collaborations to facilitate healthy living. *Am J Prev Med*. 2011;40(1):S38-S47.

56. Pracilio PV, Reinfsnyder J, Nash DB, Fabius RJ. The population health mandate. In: Nash DB, Reinfsnyder J, Nash DB, Fabius RJ, Pracilio PV, eds. *Population health: creating a culture of wellness*. Sudbury, Mass.: Jones & Bartlett Learning, LLC;2011: xlix.

57. Jaworski J. Creating the future. *Synchronicity: the inner path of leadership*. San Francisco, Calif.: Berrett-Koehler Publishers;1996:183.

Appendix A: Glossary

Accountable care organization (ACO): A collaboration between physicians, hospitals, and other providers of clinical services that will be clinically and financially accountable for health care delivery for designated patient populations in a defined geographic market. The ACO is physician-led with a focus on population-based care management and providing services to patients under both public- and private-payer programs.

Activities of daily living (ADLs): Routine self-care activities (feeding, bathing, dressing, and the like) that people perform every day without need of assistance.

Assertive community treatment: Interprofessional teams, including psychiatrists and nurses, which provide community-based intensive psychiatric and rehabilitative services to people with serious mental illness on a 24-hour basis to decrease hospitalization and help reach rehabilitation goals.

Baby Boomers: The largest demographic cohort in the United States, born between 1946 and 1964.

Big Data: The collection of information assets and its sources across industries, requiring innovative processing to generate insights and support decision making.

Chronic Care Model: An evidence-based model created by Wagner in the 1990s that focuses on the delivery of planned, proactive, population-based care rather than acute episodic care for patients with chronic diseases. The six components of this model are illustrated in Figure 7.2.

Chronic disease: A complex illness that persists for an extended period of time and is difficult or impossible to cure completely.

Chronic disease networks: Networks of coordinated health care interventions and communications for populations with these types of diagnoses and conditions in which patient self-care efforts are significant.

Citizen-centered health promotion: A coordinated multisector community effort to bring about a way of life—at home, work, and school—that makes it easier for members of a community to adopt and maintain healthful practices.

Clinically integrated network (CIN): A collection of physicians and hospitals working together as an integrated unit to achieve economies of scale in care delivery; enable joint contracting with insurers; and launch programs designed to increase the quality and coordination of patient care while reducing the cost of that care.

Coalition: A set of individuals or groups in a community cooperating in joint actions for a common cause.

Cognitive behavioral therapy (CBT): A form of psychotherapy developed by Aaron Beck in the 1950s that focuses on the interactions between thoughts, emotions and behavior, and provides interventions that are effective in relieving distress in these areas.

Community coalition action theory: A model for developing and evaluating the effectiveness of community coalitions developed by Butterfoss and Kegler.

Complex adaptive systems: Systems composed of multiple components that display complexity and adaptations to input. These systems consist of self-organized components that display complex dynamics ranging from simple periodicity to chaotic and random patterns showing trends over time.

Complex responsive processes: A theory concerned with the local, largely conversational interactions among people; power relations; ideology as the basis of choice; and the social background of peoples' interactions.

Complexity science: The study of the phenomena that emerge from a collection of interacting objects.

Construct Validity: Extent that an operation measures that which it is intended to measure.[*]

Dual eligible population: The group of persons entitled to Medicare Part A and/or Part B and eligible for some form of Medicaid benefits.

Ecosystem: An economic community supported by a foundation of interacting organizations and individuals. Member organisms also include suppliers, lead producers, competitors, and other stakeholders.

Electronic health record (EHR): Records in electronic format capable of being shared across multiple care settings and organizations. They may include data on each patient's demographics, medical history, medications and allergies, laboratory test results, radiology results, vital signs, and billing information.

Enabling constraints: The paradoxical way in which a social process simultaneously allows its participants to act while limiting the scope of their actions.

Face validity: A phrase used to describe a term whose meaning is understandable without reference to the context of the term in a formal terminology.

Health and Prevention Promotion Initiative (HAPPI): HAPPI is the combination of a Population Health Organization (PHO) and a Health Record

---

[*] Bagozzi, R.P., Youjae, Y., Phillips, L.W. Assessing Construct Validity in Organizational Research. *Admin Sci Quart.*1991;(36)3:421-458.

Bank (HRB) which results in a financially self-sustaining entity that can deliver population health and prevention services as well as comprehensive electronic patient records for a community.

Health in All Policies (HiAP): An approach to policy making that considers the potential effects of all proposed legislation on health, and encourages the adoption of only those regulations which have a positive or neutral effect on health.

Health information infrastructure (HII): A digital technology system (or network of systems) that makes comprehensive electronic patient information available when and where needed for both patient care and population health.

Health information exchange (HIE): As a noun, a third-party nonprofit organization formed to enable the sharing of patient information among multiple healthcare organizations. As a verb, the activity of exchanging patient health records across disparate systems and locations.

Health record bank (HRB): A community repository of health records with access controlled by patients.

Individual health insurance mandate: A provision of the 2010 Patient Protection and Affordable Care Act that requires most adult Americans to purchase health insurance or pay a penalty.

Integrated dual disorders treatment: An intervention model based on the premise that treating either substance abuse or mental illness in someone who has both diagnoses is less effective than treating both simultaneously.

Interorganizational network: A network of three or more organizations working together toward a common purpose; a set of three or more organizations linked to one another.

Meaning triangle: A diagram of a triangle used to explain that the connection between a symbol and a category of patients who have some specific elements in common is a concept. The concept is the apex of the triangle. The symbol and the category of patients are the two other vertices of the triangle. See Figure 11-1.

Medicare Shared Savings Program (MSSP): The Medicare ACO program initiated under Section 3022 of the ACA that provides financial incentives for Medicare ACOs which reduce health care costs while meeting quality performance standards.

Mental health parity: The rule that the financial restrictions (deductibles, co-pays, or visit limits) that a health plan places on behavioral health services may not exceed the restrictions on medical or surgical services.

Metathesaurus: A large multipurpose and multilingual vocabulary database containing biomedical and health-related concepts and the relationships among them.

Network: A set of nodes and links that represent individuals, organizations, computers or any other kind of object.

Network leadership: The group of persons who guide a connected system of organizations and their members to collaboratively address and overcome complex problems.

New Deal: The collective term for a group of new domestic economic programs developed and passed by Congress and President Franklin D. Roosevelt from 1933 to 1936. The programs were aimed to stimulate the nation's economy to bring it out of the Great Depression.

Nomenclature: A collection of names and rules for creating names.

Old-old population: Demographic group (regardless of ethnicity or gender) aged 85 or older.

Ontology: A formal collection of category names with defining relationships among them.

Organizational network: A set of people and organizations who are connected to an organization.

Palliative care: Interventions intended to relieve pain and suffering in patients rather than providing a cure.

Patient navigation: A set of services intended to help individuals seeking care and manage their own health to find their way through the complexities of the health care system.

Patient Protection and Affordable Care Act of 2010 (PPACA or ACA): Landmark federal health care legislation with key policy changes that include expanding health insurance, initial accountable care organization rules, mandates for health insurance exchanges, healthcare workforce programs, community transformation programs, and public health and wellness programs and policies.

Population health: The health outcomes of a group of individuals, including the distribution of such outcomes within the group.

Population health ecosystem: A conceptual model involving four overlapping ellipses that include social policy, individual/consumer health, traditional public health, and heallthcate systems. See Figure 1-2.

Population health management: The technical field that utilizes a variety of individual, organizational, and cultural interventions to help improve the morbidity patterns (i.e., the illness and injury burden) and the health care utilization behavior of defined populations.

Population health organization (PHO): A new health service delivery entity intended to address all the prevention, care coordination, and health management needs of the entire community with a single staff.*

Population health promotion: The communications, educational, and advocacy initiatives employed by multisectoral and comprehensive community stakeholders to influence health behaviors and policy making. This concept pays attention to population impact, cost/benefit analyses, and linking medical costs to prevention strategies.

Population health research networks: Collaborations between multiple parties to measure the incidence and prevalence of disease in given populations, identify the causes of diseases, and develop interventions to reduce the impact on the population.

Population pyramid: An illustration that depicts the distribution of various age, race, ethnicity, gender and other demographic group factors for a defined population, showing the trend for the selected demographic factor as the population ages.

Power dynamics: The study of the formation of power hierarchies in groups or societies; or how power is exercised by some group members and responded to by others.

Public health: The science and art of preventing disease, prolonging life and promoting health through the organized efforts and informed choices of society, organizations, public and private groups, communities, and individuals.

Reference model: A framework of clearly defined concepts used to assess a quality or characteristic of an object or process, typically for purposes of comparing 'what we have' with something 'we don't have.'

Social determinants of health: The living conditions and social circumstances that contribute to differences in health status for individuals and populations.

Social network: A set of people connected to one another.

Terminology maintenance: Keeping up with changes in human understanding of the world and changes in the uses to which humans put their terminology.

Terminology model: An abstraction that makes explicit what can and cannot be represented in a terminology that adheres to that model.

Time travel: The ability to retrieve what an obsolete term or code meant when it was in use, and what if anything has replaced it in present usage.

---

* Population health organizations are defined by Yasnoff in the Chapter 14 case study of the Health and Prevention Program Initiative (HAPPI).

Value alliance: A group of participants with aligned interests pursuing an outcome with value for each of them.

Young-old population: Demographic group (regardless of ethnicity or gender) between 68 and 82 years of age.

Appendix B: Author Biographies

Susan Olson Allen, PhD, has an extensive evaluation background, having served as the evaluation director of the Covington, Kentucky, Independent School District's Safe Schools/Healthy Students Initiative; for the Louisville Metro Health Department's Community-Based Emergency Response Training Program; and as evaluation manager of the Jefferson County, Kentucky Public School District's Safe Schools/Healthy Students Initiative. She also has an extensive background in housing. Allen wrote and administered the Comprehensive Grant Program for the Housing Authority of Louisville (HAL), overseeing new construction and rehabilitation of public housing developments and scattered site units, with budgets ranging from $12 million to $15 million per year. She also served on numerous committees for the Park DuValle Redevelopment Project, a $178 million revitalization of an entire neighborhood in the City of Louisville. Since 2007 she has been assistant professor in the School of Public Health and Information Sciences at the University of Louisville, where she focuses on and teaches courses in health impact assessment and health and the built environment. Allen holds a master's degree in security policy studies from the George Washington University, and a doctorate in urban and public affairs from the University of Louisville.

William Altman, JD, MA, serves as Executive Vice President for Strategy, Policy and Integrated Care for Kindred Healthcare, Inc., the nation's largest provider of diversified postacute and long-term care services. Altman's career has focused on health and long-term-care policy, with special emphasis on improving the quality of care and quality of life for elderly people. Prior to joining Kindred, Altman served in a variety of capacities in the public and private sectors, including the Agency for Healthcare Research and Quality in the U.S. Department of Health and Human Services, and health policy consulting firms and law firms specializing in healthcare issues. Altman is a past president of the Acute Long Term Hospital Association (ALTHA); he previously served on the American Hospital Association's President's Council on Post-Acute Care, and on the Board of the Federation of American Hospitals. He is also the current chair of the Louisville Metro Board of Health and has worked closely with the Louisville Department of Public Health and Wellness on a range of public health initiatives in Louisville. Altman was appointed a delegate to the 2008 White House Conference on Aging. He was the recipient of the Thomas J. Watson Fellowship, pursuant to which he conducted a study on long-term care and aging policy in Sweden, Denmark, and Norway. In addition to a law degree, he holds a master's degree from the Humphrey Institute of Public Affairs and has studied public health policy at the University of Michigan. Altman has testified before Congress, and speaks and writes frequently on Medicare/Medicaid reimbursement, quality of care, and health care reform.

Raymond Austin, PhD, is assistant professor in the Department of Health Management and Systems Sciences in the University of Louisville School of Public Health and Information Sciences. Austin holds a PhD in public administration/public affairs from the University of Illinois. He has served as the director of planning and program development for the Southern West Virginia Regional Health Council and was on the faculty of the University of Illinois in the Department of Community Health. Austin also serves on the Kentucky Health Information Exchange's Coordinating Council's Business Development and Finance Committee.

Catherine Batscha, DNP, PMHCNS-BC, PMHNP-BC, is assistant professor in the University of Louisville School of Nursing. Batscha received a doctor of nursing practice degree from the University of Illinois at Chicago. She has worked as an advanced practice nurse in inpatient, outpatient, and residential settings, serving people with serious mental illnesses for more than thirty years; and has training in both cognitive behavioral therapy and cognitive behavioral therapy for psychosis. She has done research on transitions from inpatient to outpatient settings in people with psychotic disorders, and on metabolic syndrome in people receiving antipsychotic medications. She was a research clinician on an NIMH-funded study investigating the effect of CBT on psychosis in adherence to medications in people experiencing a first episode of psychosis.

H.J. Bohn, Jr., MBA, is a published author, book designer, and editor of contemporary health care books as principal for KMI Communications, LLC. Bohn is also a doctoral candidate in public health at the University of Louisville School of Public Health and Information Sciences (2014). His past published works include:

- Co-author of *Accountable Care: A Roadmap for Success,* 1st ed. (2011);
- Co-author of *Clinical Integration: A Roadmap to Accountable Care,* 2nd ed. (2011);
- Author of *Your Next Steps . . . in Healthcare Transformation* (2011);
- Co-author of *M.D. 2.0.: Physician Leadership for the Information Age* (2012);
- Editor of *mHealth: Opportunities and Challenges* (2013);
- Co-author of *The Six Ps of Physician Leadership: A Primer for Emerging and Developing Leaders* (2013);

Ron Crouch, MA, MSSW, MBA, is director of research and statistics, Kentucky Education and Workforce Development Cabinet, overseeing the development of databases on demographic, social, educational, workforce, and economic issues and trends relating to the state of Kentucky. His office is developing tables, spreadsheets, and ARC/GIS maps looking at national, regional, and local

Kentucky realities. Crouch served as director of the Kentucky State Data Center (KSDC) at the University of Louisville from August 1988 until his retirement at the end of May 2009. He has developed a national database analyzing trends by both census regions and states. He also has developed census profiles for all 50 states, including population pyramids by race and Hispanic origin, a population chart showing population trends by age by race and Hispanic origin, and tables indicating trends on demographic, social, and economic variables. Crouch's vocation is knowledge dissemination. He is a graduate of the University of Louisville with a major in sociology and minors in political science and economics. He holds master's degrees in sociology (MA) and in social work (MSSW) from the University of Louisville, and an MBA from Bellarmine University. He did doctoral work in sociology at the University of Kentucky.

Robert J. Esterhay, MD, has a research interest in network participation theory as it applies to individuals, organizations, and networks. Esterhay has been at the informatics crossroads of individual health, health care, and population health for more than 35 years in his education, work experience, and academic setting. He is associate professor and chair of the Department for Health Management and Systems Sciences in the School of Public Health and Information Sciences at the University of Louisville. His 1969 medical school thesis involved computer-assisted learning utilizing computer-simulated patients for training medical students, medical residents, and medical school faculty. This work was completed prior to personal computers, the Internet, and the World Wide Web. In the mid-1970s, he led an early implementation of an electronic medical record information system at the University of Maryland Cancer Center; and in the mid 1990s, a nationwide implementation of an electronic medical record system in 60 long-term acute care hospitals, and 300 nursing homes for Kindred Healthcare (formerly Vencor). Some of his accomplishments include: taking the ideas and concepts for a cancer information system for the National Cancer Institute (NCI) and creating NCI's PDQ®—a comprehensive cancer database that continues to be used on the Internet today; serving as a member of the Kentucky TeleHealth Network Board; serving as the first co-chair of the Kentucky e-Health Board; analyzing community health information exchanges (HIEs) funded by the Kentucky Science and Engineering Foundation, and using the developed governance model to create the Louisville HIE.

Renee Vannucci Girdler, MD, FAAFP, is associate professor and vice chair of family medicine at the University of Louisville Department of Family and Geriatric Medicine. She received her MD from the University of Kentucky College of Medicine and completed her family medicine residency at the University of Kentucky. Prior to relocating to the University of Louisville in 2004, she was the vice chair of clinical affairs at the University of Kentucky Department of Family and Community Medicine. Girdler's research interests include clinical research in chronic disease management and practice management. She served as the physician champion for the Department of Family and Geriatric Medicine during its participation in the Association of American Medical Colleges' (AAMC) Academic Chronic Care Collaborative from 2005 to 2007. Its participation was based on the chronic care model, which focused on diabetes care. As a system leader, she has expanded this model to numerous chronic conditions in the department. This work provided the framework for an Improving Health Outcomes Program (IHOP) grant to improve outcome measures in patients with diabetes through use of a chronic care coordinator and multidisciplinary team. Other research endeavors include utilization of peer advocates in patients with diabetes to improve self-management, quality of life, and diabetes biomarkers. Girdler teaches students and residents in the clinical setting at the University of Louisville while maintaining her established clinical practice. She was recognized as a TOP DOC in Louisville for excellence in clinical care in 2013.

Scott Hedges, MD, is the senior vice president for medical services with Seven Counties Services, Inc., the regional mental health center for Louisville, Kentucky, and surrounding counties. Hedges is also a clinical faculty member in the Department of Psychiatry and Behavioral Sciences at his alma mater, the University of Louisville School of Medicine. Hedges' community service includes his membership and active participation on the community health committee of the Greater Louisville Medical Society and the committee on community and rural health with the Kentucky Medical Association. He is a 2010 Fellow of the National Council of Community Behavior Health Physician Leadership Program, a 2008 Fellow of the Health Enterprise Network, and recently appointed by the governor to serve on the Kentucky Department of Medicaid Services Pharmacy and Therapeutics committee. Early in his career, Hedges did mission work in Nigeria through his community of faith. He is married and the father of two outgoing teenage boys.

Stephanie Suzanne Lipow, MLIS, is a senior biomedical informatics analyst for Medical Science and Computing, Inc., who has worked on medical terminology projects for more than twenty years. She has primary responsibility for the analysis and transformation of each version of the more than 150 source terminologies included in the National Library of Medicine's Unified Medical Language System (UMLS), and the National Cancer Institute's NCI Thesaurus. After completing her master's degree in library and information services at the University of California, Berkeley, Lipow continued her training in the associate fellowship program at the National Library of Medicine. Her undergraduate degree is from Stanford University. She serves on the board of her local public library foundation.

Bert B. Little, M.A., Ph.D. is Associate Vice President for Academic Research and Professor of Computer Science and Mathematics (Departments of Engineering and of Mathematics) at Tarleton State University in the Texas A&M University System. Since 2000 Little has worked on research projects for the VA in gastrointestinal and cardiology with current assignment in the Medical

Services Division of the VA Medical Center in Dallas. Little worked on lead pollution in Dallas for the past 30 years, efforts that led to an Environmental Protection Agency Superfund cleanup in 1992, and subsequent lowering of child and adult blood lead levels below the national average. He has also studied the effects of lead on human health in Mexico, China, and Poland. Little has been the principal investigator and executive director of a data mining/data warehousing program for the United States Department of Agriculture (USDA) since 2000, assisting in detection of fraud, waste, and abuse in a program that covers more than $125 billion in liability across the United States and has saved approximately 3.5 billion for American taxpayers.

Little and his research center have received national and international awards for data mining, data warehousing, Big Data, and predictive analytics that include:

- 2010 Institute of Electrical and Electronics Engineers (IEEE) Best Data Mining Case Study.
- EPIC Data Mining Award, Teradata Corporation, Washington, D.C., October 2012.
- Ventana Research Data Mining Award, San José, California, November 2012.
- The Data Warehouse Institute (TDWI), Best Practices in Data Warehousing: Implementation of leading-edge solution to a Big Data problem, San Diego, California, 2013.
- Government Computing News (GCN) Award, Innovation in Big Data IT, Washington, D.C., 2013.
- American Council on Technology–Industry Advisory Council (ACT-IAC), Excellence in Enterprise Efficiency in Data Mining and Data Warehousing, March 2014.

LaQuandra S. Nesbitt, MD, MPH, is a board-certified family physician who is the director of the Louisville Metro Department of Public Health and Wellness in Louisville, Kentucky. Nesbitt also serves as assistant professor in the Department of Health Management and Systems Science at the University of Louisville School of Public Health and Information Sciences. Prior to her current role at LMPHW, Nesbitt served separate terms as senior deputy director of the Community Health Administration and senior deputy director of the Center for Policy, Planning, and Evaluation of the District of Columbia Department of Health. Nesbitt has also served as assistant professor in the Department of Family and Community Medicine of the University of Maryland School of Medicine. She received her bachelor of science degree in biochemistry from the University of Michigan-Ann Arbor; her medical degree from Wayne State University School of Medicine; and her master of public health degree in health care management and policy from the Harvard School of Public Health. Nesbitt completed her internship in family medicine at the University Hospitals of Cleveland/Case Western Reserve University and her family medicine residency in the University of Maryland's Department of Family Medicine, where she served as chief resident. She completed her fellowship training with the Commonwealth Fund Harvard University Fellowship in Minority Health Policy.

James G. O'Brien, MD, FRCPI, is the Margaret Dorward Smock Endowed Chair in Geriatrics and director of the Institute for Sustaining Health and Optimal Aging at the University of Louisville. He completed his undergraduate and medical training at University College in Dublin, Ireland; his residency in family medicine at Saginaw Cooperative Hospital in Michigan; and his fellowship in geriatrics at Duke University. He is a member of Alpha Omega Alpha, a fellow of the Gerontological Society of America and the American Geriatrics Society, a recipient of the Champion for the Aging Award by Elderserve, Inc. of Louisville, Kentucky, and an inductee of the Arnold P. Gold Honors Society for Humanism in Medicine. Since 2003, he has served on the Governor's Task Force on Abuse and Neglect of Elderly for the Commonwealth of Kentucky. O'Brien was editor of a 1999 issue of the *Journal of Elder Abuse and Neglect* titled Self-Neglect: Challenges for Helping Professionals; in addition he was the primary author or co-author of three of the articles in that issue. He has over 50 publications in peer-reviewed journals, two textbooks, and 15 textbook chapters; and serves on the editorial board of the *Journal of Elder Abuse and Neglect*. He has given multiple presentations at national and international meetings and was inducted as a fellow of the Royal College of Physicians of Ireland in March 2011.

John P. Reinhart, CPA, MBA, CNA, is the founder and CEO of the International Center for Long Term Care Innovation (InnovateLTC). InnovateLTC is a for-profit talent management and market development firm that focuses on disruptive products, service models, and technologies transforming both the quality of life and care for the global aging population. The firm was formed in collaboration with the University of Louisville's Nucleus Life Science Commercialization Center and Signature Healthcare LLC. Reinhart served previously as chief innovation officer of Signature Healthcare and led their Intra-Preneurship Pillar strategy. Reinhart is a serial entrepreneur specializing in providing strategic services to emerging market segments. From 1999 through 2003, he was the president and chief operating officer of Advanced Imaging Concepts, Inc., an ambulatory sector healthcare software company that was subsequently acquired by Allscripts Healthcare Solutions, Inc., where he then served as executive vice president of the Clinical Solutions Group from 2003 to 2006. He is a licensed certified nursing assistant and completed his MBA in health sector policy and management from the University of Miami. In 2012 he co-authored a chapter in the book titled *ACOs: Bridging the Health Information Technology Divide.*

Marc Rothman, MD, earned his medical degree from the New York University School of Medicine, followed by internship and residency in internal medicine and fellowships in geriatrics and clinical epidemiology at the Yale School of Medicine. At Yale he conducted research in frailty, patient decision making, and postacute care outcomes. He practiced medicine with the Permanente Medical

Group in northern California, and was the director of the postacute medical and palliative care practice of the Kaiser Permanente San Francisco Medical Center. He joined Kindred Healthcare as chief medical officer of the Nursing Center Division in 2011. Rothman is board-certified in internal medicine, geriatric medicine, and hospice and palliative care medicine; and is a member of the American Geriatrics Society, the American Medical Directors Association, the American Academy of Hospice and Palliative Medicine, the American College of Physicians, and the Society of Internal Medicine.

Kathleen Smith, MBA, MPH, is manager of Government Affairs and Public Policy for Kindred Healthcare, Inc. Prior to joining Kindred, Smith worked on postacute and long-term care issues at the consulting firm Avalere Health in Washington, D.C. She also spent over five years in the Office of Management and Budget, working on Medicare regulatory and legislative issues and reviewing demonstration projects. Smith reviewed countless drafts of the Affordable Care Act for policy and budgetary implications, and to ensure alignment with the Administration's policies. She earned her joint master's degree from the University of Illinois, where she studied health policy and administration; and a bachelor's degree in science from McGill University in Canada.

Robert William Prasaad Steiner, MD, MPH, PhD, is professor in the University of Louisville School of Public Health and Information Sciences. Steiner received his medical degree from the University of Louisville, his PhD in epidemiology from the University of North Carolina at Chapel Hill, and his master's degree in public health from the School of Public Health at the University of North Carolina at Chapel Hill. Steiner previously served as associate professor in the Department of Family and Community Medicine of the School of Medicine, University of Louisville; deputy director and liaison for the University of Louisville and the Jefferson County Health Department in Louisville; and director of the Healthy Communities Constanta Partnership for Women's Health in Romania. He is a Fellow of the American Board of Preventive Medicine and the American Academy of Family Physicians.

James H. Taylor, DMan, MBA, MHA, served as president of the University of Louisville Hospital from August 1996 through February 2013. He assumed the role of special advisor to the executive vice president for Health Affairs at the University of Louisville and CEO of University Medical Center in March 2013. Taylor was president of the Medical Center Hospital of Vermont from 1982 through 1994 prior to its evolution into Fletcher Allen Health Care. He held administrative positions at St. Luke's Hospital in Kansas City, Missouri, from 1975 to 1980. Taylor holds a doctorate in management from the University of Hertfordshire in the United Kingdom; a master's degree in hospital administration from the University of Minnesota; and a master's degree in business administration from the University of Hawaii. He received his undergraduate degree from Washington and Jefferson College in Pennsylvania. He is a fellow of the American College of Healthcare Executives and has served on the American Hospital Association board of trustees, the Kentucky Hospital Association board of trustees, and the Vermont Hospital Association board of trustees. He was chair of the American Hospital Association Regional Policy Board I and chair of the Vermont Hospital Association.

Judah Thornewill, PhD, is founder and chief executive officer of GroupPlus, LLC, a consulting firm specializing in networks and collaboration in health and education domains. He is also assistant professor (adjunct) in the School of Public Health and Information Sciences at the University of Louisville. Thornewill earned his PhD in interdisciplinary studies from the University of Louisville in 2011 with a dissertation on factors affecting participation in health information exchange networks. Prior to his work with GroupPlus, he served as director of the Collaborative Communities Research Program in the Department of Health Management and Systems Sciences (DHMSS) at the University of Louisville School of Public Health and Information Sciences from 2003 to 2009. While there, he organized and led the Louisville Health Information Exchange and led multiple research studies in health-related areas. He is a published author and has taught courses at the university, including "Network Leadership: How to Lead and Succeed in a World of Networks," and "Teaching in the Cloud: A Course for Faculty and Administrators."

John H. Tobin, DMan, MPH, retired at the end of 2010 after a 35-year career in hospital management, 23 of those years as CEO of Waterbury Hospital in Connecticut. He received a doctor of management degree from the University of Hertfordshire in England in 2003, and a master of public health degree from Yale University in 1975. He received his undergraduate degree from the University of Connecticut. Throughout his career, Tobin served on boards or committees of numerous community service organizations concerned with social services, education, philanthropy, and economic development. His professional involvements include extensive service to the Connecticut Hospital Association, including a term as chair; and a term on the American Hospital Association's Regional Policy Board I. Tobin currently serves on the boards of a community bank, a large performing arts center, an advocacy group for Medicaid reform, and the advisory board of the Programs in Healthcare Management and Insurance Studies at the University of Connecticut School of Business in Storrs. Tobin has received many service awards, including the T. Steward Hamilton, MD, Distinguished Service Award (Connecticut Hospital Association) in 2004 and the Frederick and Lucy Kellogg Award for Dedicated Service to Your Community in 2006–2007 (United Way of Greater Waterbury) Board of Trustees. Relatively late in his career, he developed an interest in the application of concepts from the complexity sciences to management practice, and plans to use the leisure time that retirement affords to further develop that interest through continued study and writing.

Mark Samuel Tuttle, AB, BE, FACMI, is a computer scientist who has worked on medical terminology projects for more than 30 years. As part of a team at the University of California, San Francisco, he proposed and helped build the prototype of what became the U.S. National Library of Medicine Unified Medical Language System Metathesaurus. At Lexical Technology, later Apelon, he was the lead extramural architect of the Metathesaurus, and worked on terminology projects at the National Cancer Institute, the U.S. Veterans Administration, the Department of Defense, other federal agencies, and Kaiser Healthcare. Tuttle is the author or co-author of more than 100 articles and book chapters on the subject. He was the teaching assistant for the world's largest massive open online course (MOOC): Stanford University's "Introduction to Artificial Intelligence." More recently, he has worked on applications of machine learning to Big Data. Tuttle earned a liberal arts degree and an engineering degree from Dartmouth College and enrolled in the master of science program at the Thayer School of Engineering before transferring to the PhD program in computer science at Harvard. He taught computer science at the University of California, Berkeley, and medical information science at the University of California, San Francisco, for 15 years. He is a Fellow of the American College of Medial Informatics (FACMI). Currently working on software development for data mining, Tuttle also helps coach high school football and lacrosse.

Barry Wainscott, MD, MPH, ABPM, received his MD from the University of Louisville and his MPH from the University of California, Berkeley. He is board-certified in public health and preventive medicine. He served as manager and chief physician with the Communicable Disease Branch of the Kentucky Department of Public Health from 2000 through 2005. His prior public health experiences include: medical consultant to the Kentucky Department of Public Health; deputy director, medical director, and primary care director pf the Jefferson County Health Department in Louisville; director of preventive medical services for the Santa Barbara County health agency in California; and physician health officer developing a district health department with regional programs serving a number of counties in north-central Kentucky. His community health experience also includes the role of physician in preventive medicine with the University of Louisville Student Health Services. Wainscott is currently assistant professor in the Department of Health Management and Systems Sciences of the University of Louisville School of Public Health and Information Sciences. His teaching in public health management, health finance and financial management, human resource management, and various related areas draws on his professional career experiences. With an appreciation of the role of population community and contextual considerations, his interests include communicable disease control; disease prevention and management; and health system efficiency and effectiveness.

Sara E. Walsh, PhD, MPH, is an assistant professor of health administration in the School of Health Sciences at Eastern Michigan University in Ypsilanti. During the development of this text, she was a senior program officer at the Foundation for a Healthy Kentucky, where she coordinated the foundation's data collection and dissemination efforts. She previously served as health program manager for the Kentucky State Data Center and as a cancer control specialist for the Kentucky Cancer Program, both at the University of Louisville. Walsh earned her PhD in the Department of Health Promotion and Behavioral Sciences at the University of Louisville School of Public Health and Information Sciences.

Sandra Wilkniss, PhD, is the former senior legislative assistant for health care in the office of U.S. Senator Jeff Bingaman (2011–2012). She started in Senator Bingaman's office in 2010 as an American Association for the Advancement of Science/American Psychological Association Congressional Fellow, focusing on health and mental health policy. Prior to that, Wilkniss was the director of Thresholds Institute, the research and training arm of Thresholds Psychiatric Rehabilitation Centers in Chicago; and adjunct assistant professor at Dartmouth Medical School, Department of Community and Family Medicine, and the University of Illinois at Chicago Department of Psychiatry. Wilkniss completed her PhD in clinical psychology at the University of Virginia in 2000. She has worked as a scientist-practitioner specializing in serious mental illness in various hospital, university, and community settings in New York, Illinois, and Virginia.

Richard W. Wilson, DHSc, has held academic public health positions at Western Kentucky University and the University of Nebraska, and currently serves as chair and professor in the University of Louisville's Department of Health Promotion and Behavioral Sciences. He teaches students enrolled in the MPH and PhD programs, and over the years has guided hundreds of undergraduate and graduate public health students. Wilson is also a frequent consultant and evaluator for local health departments, state governments, schools, and mental health agencies. He has been very active in tobacco control and drug abuse prevention initiatives. Wilson is the author of numerous publications, is a frequent presenter, and has published a successful textbook titled *Drug Abuse Prevention: A School and Community Partnership*.

William Yasnoff, MD, PhD, FACMI, is a well-known national leader in health informatics. He heads a consulting firm that helps communities and organizations successfully develop health information infrastructure systems and solutions, and enables universities to organize and grow academic informatics programs. He is also CEO of the nonprofit Health Record Banking Alliance, which promotes community repositories of electronic health information under consumer control. Previously, as senior advisor to the National Health Information Infrastructure (NHII) of the U.S. Department of Health and Human Services, he initiated and organized activities leading to the creation of the Office of the National Coordinator for Health Information Technology, establishing the NHII as a widely recognized national goal. Yasnoff earlier implemented the nation's first successful statewide immunization registry (in Oregon); then spent five years at the CDC as a pioneer in the field of public health informatics, organizing the first national consensus agenda-setting conference in 2001 and co-editing the textbook *Public Health Informatics and Information Systems*. He is associate editor of the *Journal of Biomedical Informatics* and professor of informatics at Minnesota, Johns Hopkins, Louisville, and Illinois (Chicago). He was a board member of the American Medical Informatics Association in 2003–2004, and has authored over 300 publications and presentations. Dr. Yasnoff earned his PhD in computer science and MD from Northwestern University, received an honorary doctorate in public health from the University of Louisville in 2006, and was elected a Fellow of the American College of Medical Informatics in 1989.

Anthony M. Zipple, ScD, MBA, is the President and CEO of Seven Counties Services, a regional community mental health center headquartered in Louisville, Kentucky. He received his doctorate in science from Boston University and his master's in business administration from the University of New Hampshire. Zipple, a licensed psychologist, has had a 35-year career in behavioral health. He has worked as an executive in provider organizations, consulted across the United States and in Singapore, and has served in academic settings as a faculty member and senior research associate. Zipple is a Fellow of the Psychiatric Rehabilitation Association and recipient of the Association's John Beard Award for outstanding contributions to the field of psychiatric rehabilitation and the Irving Rutman Award for outstanding leadership as a psychiatric rehabilitation executive.

Appendix C: Answers to Chapter Questions

CHAPTER 1

QUESTION 1: *What is population health—a concept, field of study, or a new discipline of management?*

ANSWER:

Population health can be considered both a concept and a field of study. A population can be defined as the people within a given geographic region and stratified based on their demographics or statistical characteristics. The health of the population can first be broken down on the basis of different subpopulation segments. Thus the health of any population can be affected by a wide range of socioeconomic and demographic factors; and the means of influencing or maintaining the health of any given population segment may vary depending on the health determinants of greatest import to the population.

QUESTION 2: *What are the three central themes to be addressed throughout the following chapters in this book?*

ANSWER:

Three central themes were identified to be addressed by each of the authors throughout the chapters in the book. Those themes are:

- Network leadership

- Health in all policies

- Technological innovation

QUESTION 3: *What are the four ellipses of the total population health ecosystem?*

ANSWER:

Given the different ways of dissecting the population, Figure 1-2 provides a model of the population health ecosystem containing four elements:

- Individual / consumer health

- Healthcare systems

- Traditional public health

- Social policies

QUESTION 4: *What are the factors that contribute to the United States' health disadvantage as noted by the IOM's 2013 report?*

ANSWER:

The five factors identified include:

- Patterns of food consumption shaped by environmental issues;

- Social inequality, unemployment, and lack of health insurance;

- High-stress environments leading to higher prevalence of substance abuse, illness, violence, and criminal activity;

- Greater availability of firearms in the United States compared to peer nations.

QUESTION 5: *In general, what are the police powers granted to local public health officials by the U.S. Constitution?*

ANSWER:

The police powers conveyed to public health officials of each state by the U.S. Constitution predominantly empower and fund them to:

- Regulate individuals to stop or reduce the transmission of communicable disease; and

- Regulate professions and businesses through licensure and maintaining safe and healthy conditions.

CHAPTER 2

QUESTION 1: *What is a collaborative network? Give an example.*

ANSWER:

A collaborative network comprises three or more individuals, organizations, or networks cooperating to achieve a shared goal they can't achieve alone. Examples: Wikipedia; community collaboration to protect the public from the 2009 influenza pandemic.

QUESTION 2: *Why is collaboration increasing in population health? Give an example.*

ANSWER:

Collaborative efforts are increasing because 1) the world is increasingly interconnected; 2) people are increasingly mobile; and 3) the growing use of information technology. Example: the response to the 2009 influenza pandemic.

QUESTION 3: *How is network leadership different from traditional organizational leadership?*

ANSWER:

Organizational leaders can use the power of hierarchy to get things done. Network leaders have to emphasize the building of trust and connections over time.

QUESTION 4: *Why is network leadership important? What difference can it make?*

ANSWER:

In networks, people and organizations can "choose" not to collaborate, but failure to work together can have a major effect on population health. Network leaders make a difference by facilitating collaboration and bringing people and organizations together in ways that improve population health.

QUESTION 5: *What are the three steering mechanisms (i.e., the three-legged stool) that leaders can use to effect change? Give an example of the use of each one in population health.*

ANSWER:

The first mechanism is power (the stick). Example: new legislation requiring sidewalks and bike paths. The second mechanism is money (the carrot). Example: financial incentives for hospitals and physicians to invest in health information technology and exchange. The third mechanism is trust (the network). Example: collaboration between hospitals and physicians in a community to improve patient care across care settings.

QUESTION 6: *How can social capital be measured? Give an example.*

ANSWER:

Social capital is measured through questions like "How much do you trust ___ to do the right thing? Example: a simple survey conducted between community public health officials and community education officials that show the level of trust (social capital) in place.

QUESTION 7: *What is groupthink? Give an example.*

ANSWER:

Groupthink is a phenomenon that occurs when members of a leadership team listen to only one or two voices to make decisions and stifle dissenting opinions in order to reach a consensus without considering other options. An example of groupthink would be the leader of a team who punishes anyone who disagrees with him or her, and blocks team members from communicating with outside parties about the issues under debate.

QUESTION 8: *What is an example of an emerging area of opportunity for network leadership in population health?*

ANSWER:

Population health research networks that include consumer consent for use of data.

CHAPTER 3

QUESTION 1: *Which city public health department in the United States is providing best practices in HIAs?*

ANSWER:

The San Francisco Department of Public Health.

QUESTION 2: *What is DYNAMO-HIA and how can it be used in the United States?*

ANSWER:

DYNAMO-HIA is a Web-based application developed in Europe between 2003 and 2009 to evaluate the impact of new policies on the determinants of health in a community or country. Data sets in the DYNAMO-HIA are from European countries; the application is available free of charge on the Internet at http://www.dynamo-hia.eu.

QUESTION 3: *From the Louisville Loop HIA example, what health determinants were identified as being of most importance to or impact on the community?*

ANSWER:

The four health determinants identified for the Louisville Loop were: 1) access to parks; 2) environmental issues; 3) the need for more physical activity; and 4) safety.

QUESTION 4: *What are the two key components of the San Francisco Public Health Department's Healthy Development Measurement Tool (HDMT)?*

ANSWER:

The two key components of the HDMT are (a) a set of community health indicators; and (b) a checklist of a wide range of issues affecting a population's health.

QUESTION 5: *What is an HIA and what are its five components?*

ANSWER:

An HIA is a health measurement process that should employ both qualitative and quantitative methods of research, and the assessment itself should accordingly be based on both qualitative and quantitative data. Its five steps are: screening, scoping, assessment, evaluation, and reporting.

CHAPTER 4

QUESTION 1: *What are the demographic trends taking place around the world?*

ANSWER:

The world's population has been growing dramatically over the past 200 years, mainly due to high fertility rates in both developed and underdeveloped countries. The fertility rates are now below replacement level in the developed countries and falling in the developing countries. The world population is projected by the United Nations to peak at the end of the twenty-first century and then start declining. Virtually all population growth in the world now is due to longevity rather than fertility.

QUESTION 2: *What are the demographic trends taking place in the United States?*

ANSWER:

The United States now has a fertility rate below replacement level, with immigration and increases in longevity entirely driving our population growth. In addition, most growth under age 45 in the United States is occurring among our minority populations; the non-Hispanic white population is declining not just as a percentage of the population but also in raw numbers. Growing ethnic and racial diversity is changing the face of the United States.

QUESTION 3: *How do these demographic trends vary by region and state?*

ANSWER:

We are experiencing major population differences by region and state. with the Northeast and Midwest experiencing very limited population growth and the South and West having significant population growth. The regions and states with more diverse populations are in the South and West, and diversity is the driver of their population growth. In addition, within regions and states population growth is occurring primarily in the Baby Boomer and older population cohorts.

QUESTION 4: *What are the consequences of diversity and longevity in relation to public health?*

ANSWER:

We have an increasingly diverse population; however, there are many barriers to good health as income, educational attainment, poverty levels, socioeconomic well-being, and access to health care are all greater concerns in minority populations. In addition, longevity is now a major factor in population growth, with limited growth in our working age-population and high growth in our aging population. It is not yet clear who will be the caregivers of our growing aging population. Moreover, as the data indicate, health care expenditures rise significantly with age, so how do we slow the growth of health care expenditures? Can we develop a public health system geared more to a safer, healthier environment and geared less to higher expenditures related to failure to address quality of life issues? "We are all better off, when we are all better off."

QUESTION 5: *Who is right as to whether health care is a right or a privilege?*

ANSWER:

We currently have a polarized society, in which some think that we are our neighbors' keepers and that there is a societal responsibility to take care of everyone's educational, economic, and health care needs for the betterment of society. Others have the attitude that we are all on our own and society bears no responsibility to insure the well-being of our population so that "survival of the fittest" should be the rule of the land. There are also some mediating positions that attempt to strike a balance between the two extremes.

CHAPTER 5

QUESTION 1: *What are the basic differences between the traditional medical care model and the public health or population health model? How are these differences important to a broader comprehension of health?*

ANSWER:

In traditional medical care model, a provider delivers care to an individual with a disease. In the population health model, a community ensures conditions in which people have maximal opportunities to maintain their health. The former involves one-to-one relationships and actions to address disease. The population health model, on the other hand, assumes the existence of complex and contextual interrelationships and resource bases within a community as major contributors to the health of its people.

QUESTION 2: *Why is consideration of the role of social determinants in health essential for assessment and planning for community/population health?*

ANSWER:

Social determinants relate to environmental, economic, educational, cultural, and other factors, influencing not only the health of individuals and aggregates of individuals, but also of the collective communities whose characteristics transcend the sum of their participants' characteristics. These social determinants are critical factors in achieving true community or population health.

QUESTION 3: *What are the implications of the complex interconnections of the health and social domains for policy development within a population?*

ANSWER:

If the health and social domains are interconnected in a complex way, health is affected by and becomes a consideration for virtually all policy development and implementation in all aspects of the population, integral to all policies focused on the improvement of the community's quality of life.

QUESTION 4: *What is the basic social-cultural-ecological construct for health? Why is it important to population health?*

ANSWER:

The social-cultural-ecological construct of health is based on a complex interactive relationship between factors that are not addressed in the traditional medical model. Population health therefore depends on such nonmedical factors in the development of health policy to be effective on a population rather than individual level.

QUESTION 5: *Why is the concept of positive health important as a behavioral and a psych-social mechanism to drive improvement in quality of life?*

ANSWER:

The concept of positive health means that there is a state of personal health that transcends the absence of disease. It recognizes and builds on another dimension related to wellness and positive health beyond the traditional medical model. Therefore the policies, programs, and activities addressing total community or population health must include approaches related to the concept of positive health, not just the absence of disease, in order to truly enhance people's quality of life.

CHAPTER 6

QUESTION 1: *List an example of an intervention for each tier in the Health Impact Pyramid. How much individual effort is necessary for the intervention to succeed?*

ANSWER:

The Health Impact Pyramid can be used to illustrate many different types of population health issues. One example would be interventions to reduce smoking-attributable mortality. At the tip of the pyramid is "counseling and education." One example of this approach might be a telephone quit line to help individual smokers quit. It would take considerable effort from marketers to promote the quit line, counselors to deliver this message effectively to all who needed to hear it, and even more effort on the part of the smokers who need to retain and apply that information whenever they have a craving.

The next tier on the pyramid is "clinical interventions." One example might be physicians intervening with their tobacco-using patients and writing a prescription for a smoking cessation medication. Because many smokers already see a health care provider, less effort is needed to reach the target population with this intervention. The literature tells us that smokers are more likely to quit successfully with a combination of counseling plus medication than with counseling alone. Still, most smokers need multiple cessation attempts before they are able to quit; and relapse is always a concern.

On a third step, we have "long-lasting protective interventions." Some researchers are investigating a nicotine vaccine. The nicotine vaccine is intended to break the cycle of addiction by interfering with the way nicotine binds with receptors in the brain. Although this intervention is still in development, the benefits for a vaccinated individual would persist, making the person less susceptible to relapse. There would be a significant amount of effort required to get individuals vaccinated, but it would not require the same amount of ongoing effort that is needed for traditional cessation and relapse prevention strategies.

The next tier on the pyramid is "changing the context." Interventions on this level might include state and local policies to prohibit smoking in public places. Once these laws are in place, they require very little effort to maintain and enforce, but the potential benefits include limiting the temptations to relapse for those who have successfully quit; limiting the amount of tobacco that current smokers use; reducing others' exposure to secondhand smoke; and changing social norms to discourage others from starting to smoke, especially youth.

The base level of the pyramid is "socioeconomic factors," which refers to addressing the root causes of disease and disparities. Studies have shown that individuals with low educational attainment are more likely to smoke, and are therefore at an increased risk of smoking-attributable mortality. While improving educational attainment in this country will take considerable effort, the potential benefits extend far beyond smoking. Education affects not only smoking rates, but also nutrition, stress, environmental exposures, access to health care services, and many other aspects of health.

QUESTION 2: *What are the five key determinants of health addressed by* Healthy People 2020*? How is this edition different from previous editions in the* Healthy People *series?*

ANSWER:

The five key determinants are:

1. Economic stability
2. Education
3. Social and community contexts
4. Health and health care
5. Neighborhood and the built environment

Previous editions of the *Healthy People* series did not emphasize the importance of these determinants. *Healthy People 2020* is the first to name social determinants of health as a specific topic area.

QUESTION 3: *How did the American Recovery and Reinvestment Act support technology innovation for population health improvement?*

ANSWER:

One of the key ways that ARRA supported technology innovation was through the HITECH Act, which created standards for the "meaningful use" of electronic health records and initiated the proliferation of health information exchanges. While electronic health records already existed, the law brought this technological innovation into widespread use.

QUESTION 4: *A provision of the Affordable Care Act will require chain restaurants to post nutritional information about their menu items. In which tier of the Health Impact Pyramid does this intervention fit? Why?*

ANSWER:

Posting nutritional information at chain restaurants is an example of "changing the context." By providing customers with additional nutrition information at the point of purchase, the information makes it easier to select lower-calorie or more healthful options.

QUESTION 5: *What health information technology infrastructure elements were addressed in the chapter from the 2009 HITECH Act and the 2010 Affordable Care Act?*

ANSWER:

The chapter described a number of infrastructure elements, including new national standards for the collection of demographic data. These standards are a provision of the Affordable Care Act that will affect a wide range of federal data collection efforts, and increase the quantity and quality of information available to population health researchers and practitioners. A major infrastructural development that emerged from the HITECH Act was the creation of meaningful use standards for electronic health records.

CHAPTER 7

QUESTION 1: *List the components of the Chronic Care Model. How is the Expanded Chronic Care Model different from the Chronic Care Model?*

ANSWER:

1) Self-management support; 2) delivery system design; 3) decision support; 4) clinical information; 5) community resources; 6) organization of the health system.

This model incorporates prevention and population health promotion efforts, including health-oriented public policy, creating supportive environments, and strengthening community action.

QUESTION 2: *How can such technology as electronic health records, disease registries, and Web-based portals affect chronic disease outcomes?*

ANSWER:

These advances in technology create new options for access and communication. Smartphone applications are being utilized as a means of delivering behavioral health interventions.

QUESTION 3: *A provision of the Affordable Care Act is to reduce disparities in the United States. How might patient navigators offer a solution in targeting health care disparities?*

ANSWER:

Patient navigators offer a promising solution in targeting health care disparities through facilitating access to health care and improving quality for underserved populations.

QUESTION 4: *What percentage of healthcare costs are expended on chronic disease?*

ANSWER:

a. 30 percent; b. 50 percent; c. 75 percent. C is the correct answer.

QUESTION 5: *What percentage of the population is predicted to have type 2 diabetes mellitus by 2050?*

ANSWER:

a. 15 percent; b. 25 percent; c. 33 percent; d.45 percent. C is the correct answer.

CHAPTER 8

QUESTION 1: *Why has behavioral health care parity taken so long to be identified as an issue and why is it still not fully realized?*

ANSWER:

a. Behavioral health may be undervalued by the broader healthcare system.

b. Financial margins in behavioral health tend to be low relative to other specialties, decreasing the health system's interest in advocating or negotiating for expansion.

c. The efficacy of contemporary behavioral health interventions is often understated, particularly in the case of serious mental illness.

d. A broad understanding of the biological underpinnings of behavioral health conditions developed only slowly and relatively recently.

e. Research on the impact that behavioral health conditions have on medical illnesses and treatment costs is relatively new.

f. Stigma and stereotypes about mental illness interfere with attempts at advocacy.

QUESTION 2: *What role does stigma play in behavioral health's receiving so little attention in the public health arena? Discuss the role of professional training in perpetuating or dispelling stigma.*

ANSWER:

a. There is a centuries-long history of stigma associated with mental illnesses. This stigma is reinforced in the press, media, some religious communities, and popular culture.

b. There is broad cultural suspicion that behavioral health disorders are volitional conditions rather than real illnesses. The lack of standardized diagnostic tests to identify and differentiate among mental illnesses amplifies this suspicion.

c. The fact that mental illness is such a common condition is not well understood. The cost to individuals and families is often not recognized.

d. Public health professionals live in the same cultural milieu as the general public and share cultural biases about mental illnesses.

e. Education about behavioral health conditions is limited and often outdated in many professional training programs.

QUESTION 3: *What are potential ways to organize health care delivery to maximize outcomes in behavioral health disorders?*

ANSWER:

a. Increase behavioral health training of medical care staff.

b. Provide easy access to behavioral health consultations in medical settings.

c. Create health homes in specialized behavioral health settings for people with high-risk or complex conditions that integrate medical and behavioral health care.

d. Develop electronic health records with more robust behavioral health content and stronger decision-support tools.

e. Leverage telecommunications and computer supports in a way that highlights the need to assess behavioral health status and support the needs of patients with behavioral health conditions.

QUESTION 4: *Will current efforts at health care reform (ACA for example) result in access for all to appropriate and effective behavioral health services? If not, what else can we do?*

ANSWER:

a. The ACA will broadly improve access to behavioral health services because it will provide insurance coverage for tens of millions of currently uninsured individuals.

b. There is a reasonable set of behavioral health services that the ACA requires of all insurance plans. This stipulation will help assure access to appropriate services and will be an improvement for most Americans.

c. The ACA does not provide adequate support for expanding the size and expertise of the medical workforce, particularly in the area of behavioral health.

d. The ACA provides limited guidance on strategies for the integration of behavioral health and medical services.

e. Meaningful Use regulations have excluded behavioral health providers from receiving HITECH funding, further limiting their ability to leverage technology for use in clinical practice.

QUESTION 5: *Behavioral health services have historically not been addressed in the public health arena. Given the effect of comorbid behavioral health conditions on outcomes in illness, does the continuation of this exclusion make sense? If not, what behavioral health conditions would you identify as priorities for public health?*

ANSWER:

a. Public health professionals historically addressed communicable disease but have expanded their concerns to include chronic disease "epidemics" as these emerged as significant challenges to societal health. Mental disorders are an emerging public health epidemic.

b. Behavioral health issues are pervasive and affect many public health outcomes, making these a significant consideration for public health professionals.

c. Many conditions that are now a focus of public health interventions (such as obesity and smoking) should include robust behavioral health components. One can make an argument for prioritizing many of the serious mental illnesses. Mood disorders are a priority because of their prevalence and the adverse effects of depression on outcomes of comorbid medical illnesses. Substance abuse is a priority because of its associations with injury, violence, and substance-associated medical comorbidities. Schizophrenia is a priority because of its high association with disability and unemployment. Childhood disorders can be prioritized because of the likelihood that effective intervention will improve quality of adult life. Such specific behavioral health issues as suicide, domestic violence, bullying, and a host of others affect the quality of life for individuals and the community. While it is clear that public health can't assume responsibility for all these issues in their entirety, it is clearly appropriate to include consideration of relevant behavioral health issues when developing programs and policy.

CHAPTER 9

QUESTION 1: *Describe why it is important to take into account the unique physical, mental, and psychosocial characteristics of older persons when designing population health approaches.*

ANSWER:

The physical, mental, and psychosocial limitations of the elderly have significant implications for population health management initiatives as social engagement and physical functioning can be important parts of the long-term support services needed to identify health problems early to avoid costly medical care. In addition, the important goal of population health to improve the quality of care and quality of life cannot be achieved without recognizing the unique abilities and disabilities of the population being served and tailoring population health approaches to account for these factors. Without taking these factors into account, it is difficult to appropriately target treatment and care management for this unique patient population.

QUESTION 2: *Describe the goals of population health interventions for older persons in general, including interventions for those with chronic diseases.*

ANSWER:

The focus of health care has shifted from volume to value of services; therefore population health interventions must link their programs, efforts, and products to measurable outcomes. In general, the goals of population health interventions for the elderly are to improve quality of care and quality of life; and to reduce overall costs by tying payment to quality of services to encourage the use of services that can be shown to provide the greatest benefit to both individual patients and to the population at large. More specifically, population health initiatives designed to improve health and reduce costs for the elderly with multiple chronic diseases must be prioritized and tailored. Researchers emphasize that effective population health approaches must identify patients with multiple chronic diseases and apply interventions designed to address the unique needs of this population. Whereas traditional population health approaches emphasize *preventing* the onset of disease (including chronic diseases), for an elderly population in which a large percentage of individuals will inevitably experience chronic disease, an important goal of population health may include *delaying* the onset of chronic disease.

QUESTION 3: *Describe at least two innovations from the private sector that you think are key enablers of effective care management, and why.*

ANSWER:

Digital and online patient tracking tools enable physicians and healthcare systems to improve clinical care for older persons with chronic diseases like diabetes and heart failure. Data management tools (e.g., Phytel) also allow physicians and health systems to support a medical home model and prepare for participation in accountable care organizations.

QUESTION 4: *What are some limitations in population health approaches for an older population identified by researchers?*

ANSWER:

Researchers have documented four fundamental shortcomings with current population health approaches for an elderly population: 1) primary care and other practitioners have not been trained to work in teams to provide complex chronic care; 2) there is a lack of widespread adoption of enabling health technologies and electronic health records; 3) existing fee-for-service payment policies do not encourage or support population health interventions; and 4) payments for medical/health care services and social services are separate and not integrated.

QUESTION 5: *Discuss some of the policy implications of population health for an elderly population.*

ANSWER:

Policy makers should modify current payment policies to remove disincentives that discourage care coordination and adopt payment policies that promote value over the volume of services. In addition, policy makers should adopt quality metrics that transcend sites of care and aggregate these metrics to enable population health approaches to care for the elderly. Policy makers should support such key components of effective population health as electronic health records and other information system solutions. At the same time, policy makers should support development of a well-trained and well-paid workforce through training of primary care physicians and other health care practitioners to meet the unique needs of an elderly population. Finally, policy makers should ensure that elderly individuals, their families, and their social support systems are engaged and empowered to participate in population health approaches.

CHAPTER 10

QUESTION 1: *The methodology used in this chapter is "a case study with an 'n' of one." What do you see as the strengths and shortcomings of this approach?*

ANSWER:

Strengths: this approach calls for reflection and sense-making; and requires attention to process, which may be similar to a future circumstance. Shortcomings: this approach is not generalizable, and because it is not data-driven, some observers may consider it unscientific.

QUESTION 2: *State-sponsored health information exchanges (HIEs) were described as having been given "cult value" status in practice. Explain this concept; and do you agree with the authors that HIEs are an idealized organization "taken as good" by the governmental and research elements of the health care sector?*

ANSWER:

Cult value relates to the treatment of social objects and a special form of social object. Mead held that

> . . . people not only generalise habitual patterns of interaction to imaginatively construct some kind of unity of experience, usually understood as some kind of 'whole', they also inevitably idealise these imaginatively constructed 'wholes.'[11]

The authors asserted that a health information exchange (from the perspective that the HITE-CT was an organization) had a problem with specifying who runs it and what providers are expected to pay for engaging in the use of the system produced by that organization. So in considering whether one agrees that HIEs are an idealized organization "taken as good" in this case as an essential need for population management, one needs to take into account the conflicts between what different people value and need.

QUESTION 3: *Accountability was a theme considered by the authors. Discuss what accountability meant to the authors in regards to the HITE-CT governing board means to you and what is necessary to have someone feel accountable.*

ANSWER:

In the section on "Lack of Diversity and the Domination of Certain Ideologies Lack of Accountability," the authors asserted that the HITE-CT board appointment process allowed for each board member to be chosen by a different political office holder. This being the case, there was no one person accountable for decisions or appointments. Consider how your own organization makes appointments or selections to committees or boards. There should ultimately be a single official or governing body that is accountable for the selections. In the section "Disciplinary Power and Accountability," the authors asserted that accountability is the setting of expectations and the monitoring of performance where there are consequences to meeting or not meeting expectations. They go on to note that in the private setting, accountability is tied to achieving results; and failure to do so can have different consequences in the private sector than in government bureaucracies.

QUESTION 4: *From your own experience, choose a situation in which the result of an interactive process of people was not what was planned or intended; and reflecting on the process, how do you make sense of what happened?*

ANSWER:

Each answer to this question may be based on a unique scenario, but the reader should consider his or her scenario in applying such concepts discussed in the chapter as leadership, policy, power, ideology, and trust.

QUESTION 1: *Select terms in the "terminology terminology" section of this chapter that seem important to you. Arrange them in a graph or table in a way that helps you remember and think about them. Add any terms you think are important that do not appear there. See whether your colleagues agree or disagree, and whether you can reach a kind of consensus on how the terms should be clustered and related to one another.*

ANSWER:

This question is about three things: first, your selection of relevant terms; second, your two-dimensional arrangement of them; and third, the response of others to this arrangement.

Relevant terms: The "terminology terminology" section of this chapter is deliberately historical. We believe that this approach helps explain why things in this context are the way they are. For one thing, we believe this view can help eliminate complaints about the current state of healthcare terminology and focus efforts on going forward. Thus this exercise is an opportunity for you to extract the ideas that you believe will matter.

A two-dimensional arrangement: Chapter 11 is linear by design; but evolution has given us a brain that can detect and remember patterns. So experiment with multidimensional arrangements of your terms and then try to name the relationships between them. Start by collecting the terms that are similar, and then try to name the clusters. For example, some of your terms may be abstract, like "concept," while others are concrete, like "ICD-10-CM." Does "information model" belong by itself, or is it related to "narrative definition"? If you like tables, it's easy to come up with some columns of terms, but harder to decide what a row means. Always try to relate your arrangement to the metabolic syndrome scenario, or a scenario of your choosing.

Your colleagues' response: Spatial organizations can be personal; your brain may work differently from those of others, but it's almost always helpful to see your creation through the eyes of others and then to see theirs. Moreover, are there terms on which there seems to be an arrangement that represents a consensus, and terms on which there is none?

QUESTION 2: *Using metabolic syndrome as the "center," work with your colleagues to explain the details of standard terminologies to one another using one entry from each terminology: one disease, one lab test, one drug, and one procedure. Explore the connections—or lack of connections—among these entries.*

ANSWER:

This question is designed to elicit some important and largely unanswered questions about terminology. Thus the answer to this question is more questions. For example, some believe that "insulin resistance (IR)" is a necessary attribute of "metabolic syndrome." Before trying to assess this hypothesis empirically from EHR data, examine what, if anything, terminologies have to say about it. You will find that IR, and such other diseases as hypercholesterolemia (HC), is represented in disease terminologies, but terminologic connections to metabolic syndrome are weak or nonexistent. You will find a similar state of affairs with laboratory tests. The LOINC test with code 62255-5 seems to test for IR, but only as a predictor of diabetes. And RxNORM lists metformin, used to treat IR, and atorvastatin used to treat HC, but recent evidence indicates that atorvastatin may cause IR. In this context existing inter-term connections may seem impoverished, but to what degree should terminologies represent medical knowledge? Thus, a subtext of this question is another question: "What should be represented in a terminology model?" There is at yet no consensus on the answer to this, so you can contribute. Examine your micro-model of terminology related to metabolic syndrome in this context. What is appropriate, necessary, and helpful in a terminology? And what should be in a disease model and not a terminology model? And therefore, what is the difference? Which relationships could you validate empirically?

QUESTION 3: *Your CMO gives you a journal submission he has been assigned to review. The submission describes a population in which 90 percent of patients get metabolic syndrome and a statistical model that predicts which patients in this population will get it that is 85 percent accurate. Who if anyone is confused?*

ANSWER:

Reflect upon this scenario from a statistics perspective. A casino or an insurance company would go with the background rate—90 percent. In this context the statistical model would seem to be worse than guessing, since we would always guess that an individual in the population has metabolic syndrome, and we would expect to be right 90 percent of the time. But the statistical model may be asymmetric. Maybe it never makes a false positive choice. Think about this possibility until you can express yourself clearly, in a way that you are understood unambiguously. You are likely to face this challenge with any predictive model you develop.

QUESTION 4: *Why does a thesaurus have both a table of contents and an index, and a dictionary has neither?*

ANSWER:

A (real) thesaurus is organized by categories, such as animal-vegetable-mineral. *Roget's Thesaurus* begins with a Class of Abstract Relations, and then moves to a Class of Words about Space, and then Matter, and so on. This organization is analogous to a table of contents: one uses it to find a term by its meaning. One "navigates" to the term through related meanings. Alternatively, if one has a term and wants to find related terms, one can look for the term in the (orthographically organized) index. The latter will link to the location using a physical datum (such as a page number) where the term will be found in its category.

QUESTION 5: *In a dictionary, meaning is defined in a narrative definition. Where and how is meaning defined in a thesaurus?*

ANSWER:

The meaning of a term in a thesaurus is defined through relationships to other terms. This manner of definition is close to what a computer can "understand" about meaning.

QUESTION 6: *Recent work* asserted that a predictor of a terminology quality problem—inconsistency—is the length, in number of words, of a term. Speculate on why this might be so.*

Agrawal A., et al. "Inconsistencies in SNOMED CT ...", AMIA 2013.

ANSWER:

A simple hypothesis is that the longer a term, the more ambiguous it is, and ambiguity can lead to inconsistency. *Longer* could also imply *newer*; and *newer* could predict inconsistency. We won't know for a while whether this observation, namely that inconsistency tends to follow from length, will be sustained. Further reflection reveals a cognitive dimension to this issue. Sturge-Weber syndrome was defined nearly 100 years ago. A more descriptive name is "encephalotrigeminal angiomatosis," but most references to the disease still call it by its syndromic name in spite of increased "molecular genomic" understanding. All this is yet more evidence that naming, especially the naming of diseases, is difficult.

QUESTION 7: *Find CPT "procedures" that might suggest a diagnosis of metabolic syndrome.*

ANSWER:

This is the kind of task that's easier empirically, given some metabolic syndrome electronic health records, than it is normatively from terminologies. Nevertheless, one can reflect about possible associations and browse CPT procedures to find such phrases as "nutritional counseling," "weight loss interventions," and "hypercholesterolemia evaluations."

QUESTION 8: *Given what you know about health care and health status, divide observations with which you are familiar into those that use a reference model and those that use inspection. What can you conclude?*

ANSWER:

Much of traditional history taking involves inspection, including listening to the patient. Increasingly, laboratory tests—using reference models, obviously—are part of physical exams. As longitudinal databases of patient records grow in size to support managing the health of a population; more nuanced tradeoffs between these two approaches will emerge. The skill set required to capture a patient history by inspection and that required to order and interpret laboratory tests using reference models appear to be different.

CHAPTER 12

QUESTION 1: *Since HII is beneficial to both individuals and healthcare stakeholders, why has it been so difficult to implement?*

ANSWER:

1) Existing stakeholders are comfortable in the current paradigm of "health information exchange" that now occurs largely via fax transmissions between providers, and it is difficult for them to envision a new system that solves the problem in an unfamiliar way.

2) The challenges of privacy, information completeness, sustainability, standards, and architecture are highly interrelated and thus resistant to independent analysis. Solving the problem requires simultaneous consideration of all its aspects, which is extremely challenging.

3) The solution to an effective HII represents disruptive innovation, which cannot be easily supported by the incumbent stakeholders. Therefore a new outside organization must be created and funded, and this is very difficult to accomplish.

4) Many of the problems created by the lack of HII are not readily visible; there are no dramatic "plane crashes" even though many lives are being lost unnecessarily and there are numerous avoidable injuries. This relative invisibility results in a lack of public demand for change.

QUESTION 2: *How can an effective HII address concerns about biodefense, the detection and response to intentional attacks with biological agents?*

ANSWER:

An effective HII could provide the real-time data needed for early detection of outbreaks from intentional biological attacks and also help greatly to manage and monitor an effective response. These capabilities are analogous to those needed by public health for naturally occurring diseases and conditions.

QUESTION 3: *Are public health agencies prepared to take advantage of the capabilities of an effective HII? Why or why not?*

ANSWER:

Public health agencies are not prepared because of:

1) Chronic underfunding (e.g., HITECH Meaningful Use requires transmission of data to public health, but provides no funds to public health agencies to build the systems to receive this data).

2) Lack of informatics expertise. There are insufficient personnel specifically trained in public health informatics.

3) Lack of appreciation of the key contributions that informatics can provide. Public health managers and leaders do not have sufficient informatics knowledge to recognize when it is needed and then organize and utilize the capabilities it can provide.

4) The siloed natutre of funding, which often precludes the creation of comprehensive information systems (and forces the development of unnecessarily expensive duplicative systems).

5) The lack of coordination of public health informatics efforts. There is no overall public health informatics plan for the nation to ensure that systems interact appropriately with each other and are not duplicative. There are few mechanisms for developing systems that meet common public health requirements and can thus be used by multiple public health agencies (to reduce development and maintenance costs through sharing).

QUESTION 4: *What public policies need to be adopted to facilitate the more rapid achievement of an effective HII?*

ANSWER:

1) Real protection of personal health information, thus eliminating the HIPAA TPO exceptions and making all health information use subject to individual consent; making the patient the owner of his or her health information while providers are entitled to copies (these changes would need to be gradual).

2) Regulation of health information organizations (HIOs), which includes: (a) making the appropriation or use of health information by an HIO without

consent a crime with substantial fines; (b) requiring HIOs to undergo periodic privacy and security audits with the results publicly available; and (c) requiring criminal background checks for all HIO personnel.

3) Funding large-scale HRB demonstration projects.

4) Requiring assessment of HII efforts using realistic metrics that truly reflect progress toward the goals of comprehensive information for each person (e.g., as described in Labkoff SE and Yasnoff WA. [2007] A framework for systematic evaluation of health information infrastructure progress in communities. *J Biomed Informatics* 40(2):100-105).

QUESTION 5: *Describe a feasible and workable HII architecture consisting of a national network of health record banks (HRBs) as an alternative to current HIE approaches using institution-centric architecture. How would patient records be available and get updated for patients needing care outside the region where their HRB operates? How would searches across multiple HRBs for population health purposes be accomplished?*

ANSWER:

Health record banks in communities across the nation with each person having an account in just one bank are a feasible HII architecture. All banks would use the same deposit and access protocols. Deposits to one bank of information for an account holder in another bank would automatically be forwarded. Records would be available for any patient anywhere via Internet connection directly to their HRB. Deposits could be made to any bank and would be forwarded to the account holder's institution. Searches could be distributed across banks and the query results combined by an umbrella organization (e.g., the Health Record Banking Alliance) because all the banks would satisfy the "independence" criterion for distributed searching (since each patient's complete information would be in one and only one bank). For more details, see the Architecture White Paper of Health Record Banking Alliance:

http://www.healthbanking.org/docs/HRBA%20Architecture%20White%20Pa per%20Jan%202013.pdf (Accessed 26 July 2013)

CHAPTER 13

QUESTION 1: *The explosion of data use has come to be known as Big Data. What differentiates Big Data from traditional data analysis?*

ANSWER:

Traditional analytics involve analyses of relatively small samples of data, certainly less than a million "rows" or cases, and a small number of columns, or "variables." Big Data involves a very large number of cases and variables. The general definition of Big Data includes the property that the data sets are so large (cases and variables) and complex (entity relationship diagrams, numbers of tables, etc.) that traditional data processing tools do not function well, or simply reach their limitations.

QUESTION 2: *What digital storage capacity could store all data available in 2013?*

ANSWER:

One zettabyte (1 sextillion bytes) is the digital storage capacity of the world.

QUESTION 3: *Name the three major categories of data mining, and describe each in a phrase.*

ANSWER:

a. Discovery: non-hypothesis-driven data analysis that includes graphics (i.e., visual data mining); conditional logic (i.e., Boolean algebra expressions); affinities and associations (variable and case correlations); and trends and variation (regression analyses).

b. Predictive modeling: outcome prediction (regression analyses) and forecasting (extrapolation of regression findings).

c. Forensic analysis: deviation detection (outliers) and link analysis (linking anomalous entities).

QUESTION 4: *How does one attack a problem in Big Data that is too huge for CPU-based computing?*

ANSWER:

Divide the problem into pieces, sub-tasks, or "chunks" that can be processed in parallel. Solve the problem in the reduced space of multiple parallel processes, and then bring the solutions together after all parallel tasks have completed for the Big Data solution.

QUESTION 5: *Are there possibilities for data mining and Big Data in medicine and population health, or have all problems been solved? Elaborate and discuss why. Which areas need further research with data mining/Big Data?*

ANSWER:

Medicine and population health are behind the curve in adopting data mining and Big Data technologies. Many opportunities exist in health care (medicine and population health) because the EHR/EMR is itself in the process of being developed. The reason these areas have not fully adopted the Big Data paradigm is because of the secure nature of the data (it contains PII), and acceptable rules of governance are still being formulated. The EHR/EMR is still being developed, and there is at this point no "single version of the truth." As the EHR/EMR matures, it will evolve into a system of standards and practices that will streamline the conduct of research in medicine and population health.

QUESTION 6: *What is the relationship between patient clinical health information and information used in population health studies?*

ANSWER:

Clinical information for each patient is available in the EHR/EMR. Population health data are ideally the subgroup aggregations of EHR/EMR. In the world of practice, however, it is not the usual case for population health researchers to use the same datasets that clinical researchers use, but that is the case in current practice. The barriers include database architecture, disparate data sources, and availability of some clinical data for population health research.

CHAPTER 14

QUESTION 1: *What was the difference discussed in the chapter between traditional public health practice and the concept of population health promotion?*

ANSWER:

One must draw a distinction between the theoretical concepts of traditional public health and the kind of public health activities conventionally practiced in communities. By the book, traditional public health would not be that different from population health as articulated in this book. Unfortunately, conventional public health work is usually practiced in problem-focused silos, not only disconnected from even related problem areas but also disconnected from the healthcare system as a whole. In addition, typical public health is funding-driven rather than driven by careful assessments of needs and assets. Finally, typical public health is microscopic in practice, considering a rather narrow range of interventions and partners. A major disconnect occurs when subject matter experts make efforts to improve conditions without fully engaging those people living in the neighborhoods.

On the other hand, the novel concept of population health promotion initiatives invokes a broader approach to multisectoral and comprehensive community stakeholder engagement. This concept pays attention to population impact, cost/benefit analysis, and linking the usual medical costs with prevention strategy. One of the critical and foundational tenets of this concept is the importance of collaboration and active engagement by multisectoral stakeholders as essential to project success.

QUESTION 2: *What is meant by quality of life, and how does understanding it at the population level aid in health policy development?*

ANSWER:

Quality of life in the population health evaluation encompasses understanding the essential elements of any given segment of the population's state of living. These elements include and are not limited to their lifestyle habits, behavioral health status, epidemiological health conditions, education level, work life, and social support structures. While quality of life can be evaluated at the individual level, understanding it at the population level requires quantitative and qualitative data collection to inventory the nature and extent of quality of life deficits to determine which health problems contribute to them. Obtaining community-level quality of life data is not easy, as the data are scattered across different resources. Moreover, society still needs user-friendly technologies for such qualitative data collection and analysis as what would come from focus groups. As referenced in the chapter and in Chapter 5, Green and Kreuter's PRECEDE-PROCEED model provides a framework for such assessments to support health policy development.

QUESTION 3: *What is asset assessment and how is it different from needs assessment?*

ANSWER:

Needs assessment is a very typical public health activity, in which public health agencies take stock of all the most common and pressing health problems in a community. The assessment will rely on existing and original data, both quantitative and qualitative. Public health agencies are used to using needs assessment data as a guide to or justification for program goals and objectives. Asset assessment, sometimes also called asset mapping, takes a more positive approach: rather than just looking at problems and gaps, asset assessment discovers community resources and strengths that can be tapped for population health promotion efforts. Resources and strengths may include particular agencies or organizations as well as unique advantageous circumstances in the community.

QUESTION 4: *What are asset maps and how do they help communities evaluate and improve population health?*

ANSWER:

Asset maps provide information about the deficits, resources, and strengths in each community and can be used to help prioritize community interventions. They include:

- community-based institutions and agencies;
- community leadership;
- health care and mental health service providers;

- healthy food and active lifestyles;

- large employers;

- educational opportunities; and

- advantages afforded by the community's location.

One of the major benefits of asset mapping to support population health is in its value to health program planning. Understanding available (or absent) resources can better enable policy makers, researchers, and public health practitioners to create and implement targeted health programs that effectively meet the needs of their community's population.

QUESTION 5: *What are the sources of quantitative data and qualitative data, and how can they be merged into a community analysis?*

ANSWER:

Fortunately, public and population health can draw on such abundant sources of quantitative data as the National Health Interview Survey, the Behavioral Risk Factor Surveillance System, County Health Rankings, and many more. The process can move forward if the right organizational and technical linkages can be achieved. The population health enterprise should also have immediate access to mountains of clinical data that will also be instructive for population health, not just for clinical care diagnosis. For the most part, qualitative data are original data. This fact means that full understanding of health needs and assets in communities also has to be grounded in people's views, attitudes, beliefs, perceptions, and values. These are usually quite time- and situation-specific, and therefore, population health practitioners will conduct significant informant interviews, focus groups, community observations (so-called "dashboard diagnosis"), photo voice, town hall meetings, and media content analysis. Qualitative methods may be contextualized with quantitative data findings as a starting point. The rationale is to ask community representatives and stakeholders to reflect on numerical data in light of their values and perceptions. The merging of qualitative and quantitative data is obviously not a mathematical computation but rather a process of thoughtful analysis and reflection. It is one part science, one part art.

QUESTION 6: *In the asthma case study, who were the different stakeholders and what was the importance of their roles in the project?*

ANSWER:

Because public health problems are usually complex, solutions rely on many factors being addressed. These factors often represent the turf of different stakeholders, any one of which cannot solve the problem but must be brought together to obtain a synergistic response. The Louisville asthma case study was focused through the Louisville Asthma Innovation Project. There were several stakeholders who included:

- Schoolchildren dealing with asthmatic conditions in West Louisville and their families;

- The Louisville Metro Department of Public Health and Wellness, which spearheaded the project;

- The University of Louisville School of Public Health and Information Sciences, which brought epidemiological expertise and data analysis resources;

- The IBM Smarter Cities grant program, which supported the innovation demonstration project;

- The Jefferson County public school system, which participated with the children and parents in providing a common setting for health screenings of children;

- Passport Health Plan, the administrator of the Kentucky Children's Health Insurance Program (CHIP), which held Medicaid health data records; and

- Propeller Health, a technology innovation firm that brought a novel technology to the project to be pilot-tested for aiding in the needed health data collection on the use of inhalers.

The combination of all these stakeholders led to a novel population health community level demonstration project on a chronic condition that recurs across many communities in America and abroad.

QUESTION 7: *How is the solution to ED super-utilizers in both the Camden, New Jersey, and Louisville, Kentucky, case studies derived from population health concepts rather than clinical medicine?*

ANSWER:

There are two generic reasons why the ED super-utilizer solution is different from the typical clinical medicine approach. First, we look for resources that lie outside the usual clinical toolbox of surgery, rehabilitation and physical medicine, medications, and so forth, but instead, we think about referrals and access to a wide variety of services and supports needed by individuals in this profile. The solutions discussed in both cases involve partnering of multidisciplinary professionals to address the challenges that patients experience, which are often related to social determinants. Engaging social workers, behavioral health providers, and others along with primary care and acute care resources demonstrated financial cost savings to each community's health system and opportunities to address some of the challenges faced by ED super-utilizers. The second generic difference is that in looking for ways to solve the ED super-utilizer problem with population health approaches means that we don't just find a unique solution tailored for each individual. But in addition, we try to build a system that is broader and with more efficient capabilities to prevent and diagnose individuals early who are at risk of becoming super-utilizers.

QUESTION 8: *What is a novel policy potential that can emerge with implementation of HAPPI?*

ANSWER:

The Health and Prevention Promotion Initiative (HAPPI) suggests the potential for a new community health value alliance combined with HRBs to support new PHOs. Two important policy implications are:

a) Health information about each individual should be controlled by that individual; and

b) Establishing sensible state and/or federal regulations governing the operation of HRBs would help promote the necessary trust in these new organizational custodians of sensitive health information.

QUESTION 9: *What is the role of health promotion programs?*

ANSWER:

Health promotion programs are intended to educate consumers and other stakeholders within communities of the impact of various health behaviors that can be changed over time through increased information or incentives and penalties enacted by local, state, and federal policy—especially through Health in All Policy approaches. Targeted health communication campaigns can be effective in curbing behaviors that have a negative effect on the health of a population. Health promotion interventions in the chapter included: a) entertainment education; b) advocacy efforts; c) Internet-based education; d) policy changes; and e) provider training.

QUESTION 10: *What are the five categories in the recommendations for future leaders, and what is their significance to improving the nation's population health?*

ANSWER:

The five categories of recommendations included: a) partnerships, b) alliances, c) complexity, d) the impact of social determinants, and e) innovation. Many reasons could be stated for the significance of these categories but perhaps most important is their common link to caring for any community's population and the concept of Health in All Policies (HiAP). At the heart of every community are the people who live, work, and play there—people from across all generations. They are the reason for continuous improvement and the search for new interventions to eradicate chronic conditions and health inequities. Health in All Policies is a critical overarching approach to establish the policies needed to help communities grow and help citizens obtain the essential resources that can improve their quality of life.

Appendix D: Selected Sources for Evidence-based Population Health Guidance

Cancer Control P.L.A.N.E.T.

http://cancercontrolplanet.cancer.gov/

Cancer control researchers and practitioners need access to the latest research, data, and resources in order to reduce cancer risk, cancer cases, and deaths from cancer; and to enhance the quality of life for cancer survivors,. Cancer Control Plan, Link, Act, Network with Evidence-Based Tools (P.L.A.N.E.T) is an online directory linking to comprehensive cancer control resources for public health practitioners. Cancer Control P.L.A.N.E.T provides access to online resources that can assist in assessing the cancer and/or risk factor burden; identifying potential partners who may be working with high-risk populations; understanding current research findings and recommendations; accessing and downloading evidence-based programs and products; and finding guidelines for planning and evaluation.

ChangeLab Solutions

http://changelabsolutions.org/

ChangeLab Solutions is an interdisciplinary research and planning organization based in Oakland, California. The following description of its work is from its website: "Throughout the nation, ChangeLab Solutions works with neighborhoods, cities, and states to transform communities with laws and policies that create lasting change. Our unique approach, backed by decades of solid research and proven results, helps the public and private sectors make communities more livable, especially for those who are at highest risk because they have the fewest resources. . . . Our website is packed with model policies, how-to guides, fact sheets, and other policy tools. Be sure to check out the TOOLS tab to search our full library of resources. You can also select a topic area from the four at the top of the page—Healthy Planning, Tobacco Control,

Childhood Obesity, Healthy Housing—and explore the TOOLS tab in that section for resources organized by more specific categories."

The Guide to Community Preventive Services

http://www.thecommunityguide.org/index.html

The Community Guide is an online resource for evidence-based recommendations and findings about effective policies to improve public health and prevent disease in your community. All recommended programs and policies undergo a systematic review by a panel of experts. The Community Guide can be used to assist public health practitioners on a variety of topics including adolescent health, tobacco use, health equity, health communication, obesity, or physical activity. The general public may use the Community Guide to assist decision making in programs and services, policies, education, funding, research, or action.

Healthy People 2020 Topics & Objectives / Interventions & Resources

http://www.healthypeople.gov/2020/topicsobjectives2020/default.aspx

Public health and clinical practitioners can navigate to their chosen health concern in any of the topical areas of *Healthy People 2020* (e.g., heart disease and stroke), and then click on the tab labeled Interventions and Resources. In that folder is found a review of intervention evidence and best-practice recommendations. This website is a dynamic resource updated over time.

High-Impact HIV Prevention: CDC's Approach to Reducing HIV Infections in the United States

http://www.cdc.gov/hiv/policies/hip.html

In the United States, prevention efforts have averted nearly 350,000 HIV infections. However, approximately 1.2 million Americans are currently living with HIV. While new infection rates are currently low, continued growth in the population living with HIV will lead to new infections if prevention and treatment efforts are not intensified. In order to advance prevention efforts, the CDC is supporting high-impact HIV prevention methods, which are scientifically proven, cost-effective, scalable, and targeted to specific populations. High-impact HIV prevention strategies are intended to maximize the impact of prevention efforts for all populations at risk and support the goals of the National HIV/AIDS Strategy (NHAS).

NCI Research-tested Intervention Programs

http://rtips.cancer.gov/rtips/index.do

The National Cancer Institute's Research-tested Intervention Program (RTIP) is an online directory of cancer control interventions and program materials. The purpose of RTIP is to provide program planners and public health practitioners with access to research-tested materials. This online database provides a review of programs available for use in a community or clinical setting. Key features of RTIP include full program summaries; interventions reviewed by an expert panel; links to Using What Works; and links to the Guide to Community Preventive Services.

Public Health Law Center

http://publichealthlawcenter.org

The Center describes itself on its website as follows: "The Public Health Law Center is a national non-profit organization of law and policy specialists that help health leaders, officials, and advocates use the law to advance public health. Founded in 2000, our organization today is a preeminent authority in U.S. public health policy and a respected legal resource for dozens of local, state, national and international health organizations. The center is located at William Mitchell College of Law, the largest law school in Minnesota and one of the top U.S. law schools in public interest law. "

SAMHSA's National Registry of Evidence-based Programs and Practices

http://www.nrepp.samhsa.gov/

The Substance Abuse and Mental Health Service Administration's (SAMHSA) National Registry of Evidence-Based Programs and Practices (NREPP) is an online registry of reviewed, rated, and supported promotions, interventions, and treatments related to mental health and substance abuse issues. The purpose of NREPP is to identify and provide access to quality information on tested interventions for informed decision making. By assisting the public in identifying evidence-based approaches, SAMHSA is helping to reduce the gap between scientific knowledge and practical applications in the field.

Teen Pregnancy Prevention Evidence-based Programs

http://www.hhs.gov/ash/oah/oah-initiatives/teen_pregnancy/db/

HHS's Office of Adolescent Health describes this resource on its website as follows: "To help identify programs effective in reducing these risks, since 2009, the U.S. Department of Health and Human Services has contracted with Mathematica Policy Research and its partner, Child Trends, to conduct an independent systematic review of the evidence base on programs to reduce teen pregnancy, STIs, and associated sexual risk behaviors. The review identifies, assesses, and rates the rigor of program impact studies and describes the strength of evidence supporting different program models. Findings are used to identify program models meeting the criteria for the HHS List of Evidence-Based Teen Pregnancy Prevention Programs."

U.S. Preventive Services Task Force Guidelines

http://www.uspreventiveservicestaskforce.org/

Research in the medical and preventive field is continuously growing. The need for an established set of clinical prevention standards in primary health care is important. The U.S. Preventive Service Task Force (USPSTF) strives to provide the latest recommendations for screening tests, counseling, and preventive medications to primary care practitioners. All recommendations undergo a rigorous review and assessment of existing peer-reviewed evidence. The guidelines include an evaluation of benefits and harms of each service based on demographics (age, sex, etc.). Created by an independent group of experts in prevention and evidence-based medicine, the USPSTF Guidelines highlight the importance of including prevention in primary care and highlight the opportunities for improving delivery of effective services.

What Works for Health

http://www.countyhealthrankings.org/roadmaps/what-works-for-health

Evidence-based strategies implemented at the local, state, and federal levels can have a large impact on population health. What Works for Health is an interactive tool used to search a variety of strategies to improve health within your community. Organized according to health factors of interest, this online resource provides suggested strategies based on current research practices. Strategies are listed based on evidence rating (strength of support/research) and can be filtered by specific decision makers (those who are implementing the program/policy). To help you take action, What Works for Health also provides implementation examples, resources, citations, and the measure's likely impact on health disparities.

Index

CPSIA information can be obtained at www.ICGtesting.com
Printed in the USA
BVOW09s0859230814

363951BV00002B/5/P

9 780983 482499